VASCULAR PROBLEMS

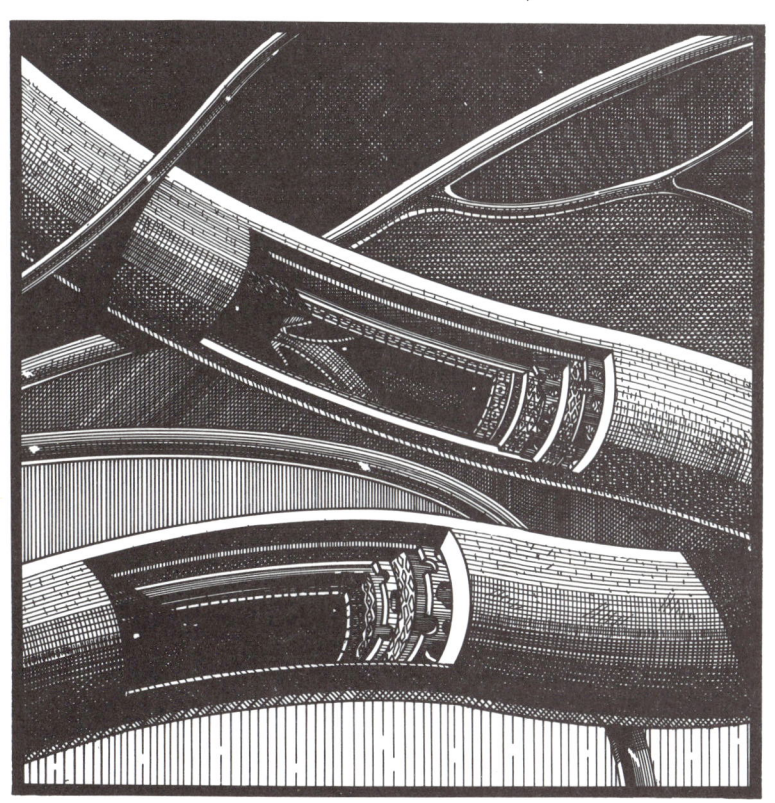

NurseReview

Springhouse Corporation Book Division

Chairman
Eugene W. Jackson

Vice-Chairman
Daniel L. Cheney

President
Warren R. Erhardt

Vice-President and Director
William L. Gibson

Vice-President, Production and Purchasing
Bacil Guiley

Program Director
Jean Robinson

Art Director
John Hubbard

Staff for this section

Book Editor
Kathy Goldberg

Clinical Editor
Diane Schweisguth, RN, BSN, CCRN, CEN

Drug Information Manager
Larry Neil Gever, RPh, PharmD

Designer
Lynn Foulk Purvis

Illustrators
Julia DeVito
Dan Fione
Robert Jackson
Robert Neumann

Project Coordinator
Aline S. Miller

Production Coordinator
Maureen B. Carmichael

Editorial Services Manager
David R. Moreau

Copy Editors
Traci A. Deraco
Diane M. Labus
Doris Weinstock

Art Production Manager
Robert Perry

Artists
Julie Carleton
Mary Stangl

Typography Manager
David C. Kosten

Typography Assistants
Alicia Dempsey
Elizabeth A. DiCicco
Ethel Halle
Diane Paluba
Nancy Wirs

Senior Production Manager
Deborah C. Meiris

Assistant Production Managers
Pat Dorshaw
T.A. Landis

Clinical Consultants for this section

Patricia L. Baum, RN, BSN
Peripheral Vascular Nurse Consultant

Henry D. Berkowitz, MD
Associate Professor of Surgery/Director, Peripheral Vascular Laboratory, Hospital of the University of Pennsylvania, Philadelphia

Irving Huber, MD
Assistant Professor of Medicine, Hahnemann University Hospital, Philadelphia; Attending Physician, Hahnemann University Hospital, Frankford Hospital, and Roxborough Memorial Hospital, Philadelphia; Medical Director, Foster Medical Corp., Conshohocken, Pa.

The clinical procedures described and recommended in this publication are based on research and consultation with medical and nursing authorities. To the best of our knowledge, these procedures reflect currently accepted clinical practice; nevertheless, they can't be considered absolute and universal recommendations. For individual application, treatment recommendations must be considered in light of the patient's clinical condition and, before administration of new or infrequently used drugs, in light of the latest package-insert information. The authors and the publisher disclaim responsibility for any adverse effects resulting directly or indirectly from the suggested procedures, from any undetected errors, or from the reader's misunderstanding of the text.

© 1988 by Springhouse Corporation, 1111 Bethlehem Pike, Springhouse, Pa. 19477

All rights reserved. Reproduction in whole or part by any means whatsoever without written permission of the publisher is prohibited by law. Authorization to photocopy items for internal or personal use, or the internal or personal use of specific clients, is granted by Springhouse Corporation for users registered with the Copyright Clearance Center (CCC) Transactional Reporting Service, provided that the base fee of $00.00 per copy plus $.75 per page is paid directly to CCC, 27 Congress St., Salem, MA 01970. For those organizations that have been granted a photocopy license by CCC, a separate system of payment has been arranged. The fee code for users of the Transactional Reporting Service is: 0874341825/88 $00.00 + $.75. Printed in the United States of America.

NR5-010788

Library of Congress Cataloging-in-Publication Data
Vascular problems.
  (NurseReview)
  Includes bibliographies and index.
  1. Cardiovascular disease nursing.
2. Blood vessels—Diseases.
I. Springhouse Corporation. II. Series.
[DNLM: 1. Vascular Diseases—nurses' instruction. WG 500 V3327]
RC674.V38   1986   616.1
86-15474
ISBN 0-87434-182-5 (sc)

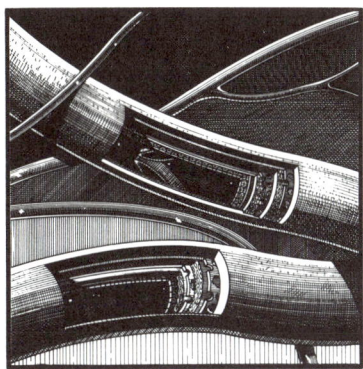

Contents

Shock

1. Patient Evaluation: Assessment Techniques — 3
2. Hypovolemic Shock: Internal or External Fluid Loss — 22
3. Cardiogenic Shock: Impaired Heart Pumping — 43
4. Distributive Shock: Vascular Bed Dilation — 55

Hypertension

5. Hypertension: Disturbed Blood Pressure Regulation — 73

Peripheral Vascular Disease

6. Patient Evaluation: Assessment Techniques — 98
7. Aortic Disorders: Aneurysm, Dissection, and Other Problems — 113
8. Peripheral Arterial Disorders: Chronic Occlusion and Other Problems — 125
9. Peripheral Venous Disorders: Deep-Vein Thrombosis and Other Problems — 140

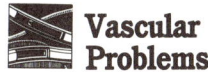 **Vascular Problems** 1

Introduction

The circulatory system is critical to every cell in the body. That's why vascular problems can present such immediate and all-encompassing challenges to your nursing skills.

In just minutes, acute vascular problems can escalate to life-threatening proportions, requiring immediate intervention. Chronic vascular problems, in contrast, require long-term patient management and support. To manage both, you need keen clinical skills and comprehensive information to provide accurate and timely patient care.

Vascular Problems provides a review that can make all the difference in your nursing care. From shock to hypertension to peripheral vascular disease, the text serves as an up-to-date clinical reference written by recognized experts. Throughout the book, you'll find information presented according to the nursing process, outlining your role every step of the way. Sample nursing care plans help you put nursing diagnoses into action by presenting patient goals, detailing nursing interventions, and specifying outcome criteria.

The first section of **Vascular Problems** deals with shock and its critical ramifications, emphasizing your role in its prevention. Techniques for assessing patients at risk and for successfully stabilizing their condition are reviewed in detail. Special inserts diagram and describe shock's effect on cell function. Concise charts help you to understand the stages of shock and what laboratory tests indicate about a patient's condition.

The next three chapters discuss the major types of shock. In "Hypovolemic Shock," you'll brush up on emergency-management skills. Although the cause of hypovolemic shock often is obvious, it may be difficult to detect in some patients. Even as you assess the patient, you must be prepared to intervene quickly.

In "Cardiogenic Shock," you'll review the danger of shock to cardiac patients. Most commonly occurring after acute myocardial infarction (MI), cardiogenic shock kills four out of five affected MI patients. The chapter outlines shock's downward spiral and measures that can halt it before it's too late. The text explains drug therapies and mechanical assist devices.

"Distributive Shock" describes the causes of vascular bed dilation and its effects, including hypotension, venous pooling, and decreased tissue oxygenation. Without intervention, distributive shock leads to anoxia, cell destruction, and death. Anaphylaxis, a sometimes fatal immune reponse, represents an acute form of this type of shock. The text also explains neurogenic shock, commonly caused by spinal cord injury, and assists you in caring for patients with septic shock.

The next section addresses hypertension. It begins by reviewing the mechanisms that regulate blood pressure and the disorder's pathophysiology. Because hypertension can be controlled, thereby limiting its damaging effects, you play a crucial role in educating patients about the need for life-long monitoring and treatment and in offering your emotional support. The chapter outlines barriers you may face—informational, emotional, and behavioral—and techniques for overcoming them.

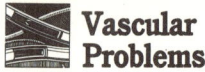

Vascular Problems

Introduction

For some patients, antihypertensive therapy may be nonpharmacologic, involving dietary changes, an exercise program, and other behavior modifications. The text describes these along with drug therapies. A special sidebar provides a quick and easy review of the stepped-care approach to antihypertensive drug therapy, and a detailed chart reviews the most commonly used drugs.

The final section deals with peripheral vascular diseases (PVD). More common now as people live longer, PVD can be acute or chronic and can threaten life or limb. Because your evaluation of PVD is critical to successful management, a chapter is devoted to assessment techniques. A simple guide helps you differentiate between venous and arterial forms of the disease. The text describes diagnostic studies and what they indicate about the patient's condition.

The chapter devoted to aortic disorders describes aneurysms, dissection, and other problems. Because the aorta is the body's largest artery, aortic disorders can affect the entire arterial system. The text reviews aortic function and structure and the effects of aortic disorders.

In the next chapter, you'll review chronic occlusion of the peripheral arteries. The text offers you the tools to identify arterial occlusion through the patient history, physical examination, and diagnostic studies. The chapter outlines drug therapies and various surgeries. You'll gather tips on educating patients about their role in disease management.

The final chapter addresses peripheral venous disorders, such as deep vein thrombosis. You'll review the entire venous system and then focus on the legs, which are involved most frequently. Physical examination, diagnostic studies, and drug intervention all are described to improve your ability to care for these patients.

Concluding with references and an index, **Vascular Problems** promises to be an important and practical addition to your nursing library. Like all the other volumes in the NurseReview series, it provides a professional boost in today's challenging health care environment.

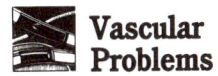

Vascular Problems

3 Shock

Patient Evaluation: Assessment Techniques

Kimberly A. Ramsey, who wrote this chapter, is Education Coordinator at St. John's Hospital and Health Center, Santa Monica, Calif. She received her RN from Akron City Hospital and her BS from the University of Akron, Ohio.

In this chapter, we'll review shock's pathophysiology and describe general assessment techniques for shock: history taking, physical examination, laboratory studies, and hemodynamic monitoring. (For details on how to assess for a specific shock type—hypovolemic, cardiogenic, or distributive—read Chapters 2 through 4.)

Because any patient can develop shock, *preventing* shock should remain the keystone of your nursing care. Remember—once the patient develops signs and symptoms, the shock response has already begun to affect cellular function.

Shock indicates a state of acute circulatory failure causing inadequate tissue perfusion and reduced oxygen delivery to body cells. Shock may stem from any of these conditions:
• reduced circulating blood volume (hypovolemic shock)
• impaired heart pumping (cardiogenic shock)
• widespread arteriolar and venous dilation (distributive shock, also known as vasogenic shock).

These conditions usually produce the signs and symptoms you'll readily associate with clinical shock: hypotension, rapid pulse, and reduced level of consciousness. Such signs and symptoms stem from various physiologic responses to altered circulation and tissue oxygenation. With poor tissue perfusion, cells don't get enough oxygen, glucose, and other essential nutrients and thus can't produce sufficient energy (adenosine triphosphate [ATP]) to power normal cellular functions. Cells then generate excess acids that further inhibit cellular activity. As cellular pH decreases, cells release strong enzymes that destroy the cell membrane and digest cellular contents. Loss of cell membrane integrity causes irreversible cellular changes. Let's examine these changes in detail.

Pathophysiologic dynamics. Shock's cellular effects include the following:
• Cellular metabolism changes from aerobic to anaerobic. Consequently, cells produce less ATP just when the body needs extra energy. This results in lactic acid production.
• As blood flow slows, acid waste accumulation that results from poor blood flow dilates capillaries and decreases resistance. Also, elevated circulating serum acid levels stimulate the medulla to trigger respiratory removal of carbon dioxide. The patient then hyperventilates.
• Vasodilation (from accumulated waste products) reduces venous return, thereby decreasing cardiac output. The body tries to compensate by stimulating the sympathetic nervous system (SNS) to constrict the arteries and thus refill the intravascular compartment. While preserving systemic flow, this reaction also diverts blood away from the tissues, intensifying cellular hypoxia and acidosis.
• Hypoxia and acidosis weaken the cell wall, allowing destructive enzymes to extrude. Increased cellular permeability alters sodium, potassium, and water movement, leading to cellular dehydration and, ultimately, cellular death.

Acute circulatory disruption most severely affects tissues that receive greater amounts of cardiac output (such as the brain, kidneys, liver, and skin). Areas with preexisting circulatory compromise (such as the myocardium of a patient with coronary artery disease) also suffer severely.

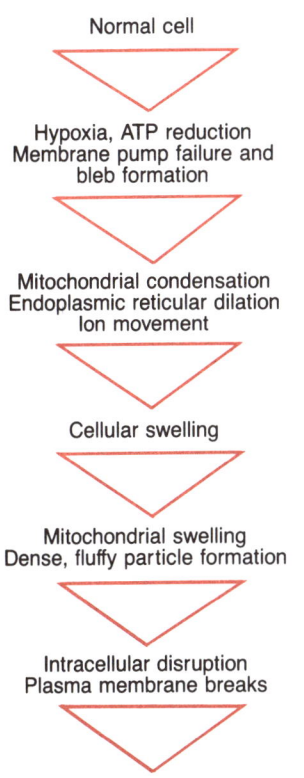

The cell in shock: Tracing injury stages

Normal cell
↓
Hypoxia, ATP reduction Membrane pump failure and bleb formation
↓
Mitochondrial condensation Endoplasmic reticular dilation Ion movement
↓
Cellular swelling
↓
Mitochondrial swelling Dense, fluffy particle formation
↓
Intracellular disruption Plasma membrane breaks
↓
Cell degradation

Note: Mitochondrial swelling and particle formation signal *the point of no return*, after which no therapy can prevent cell death.

Continued on page 4

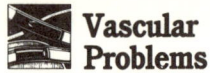

Vascular Problems

4 Shock

Patient Evaluation

Continued

Clinical evidence of the body's response to shock commonly takes place in three stages:
- *early shock* (also called the compensatory, or first, stage)
- *middle shock* (also called the progressive, or second, stage)
- *late shock* (also called the refractory, or third, stage). Multiple organ failure (also known as shock's fourth stage) represents late shock's end result.

No two patients respond to shock in exactly the same way. Shock's severity and duration, specific tissue needs, and the patient's general health, age, and underlying condition determine the individual response. However, each shock stage typically produces the effects described on the next few pages. No matter what you call each stage, keep in mind that shock's cellular effects precede signs and

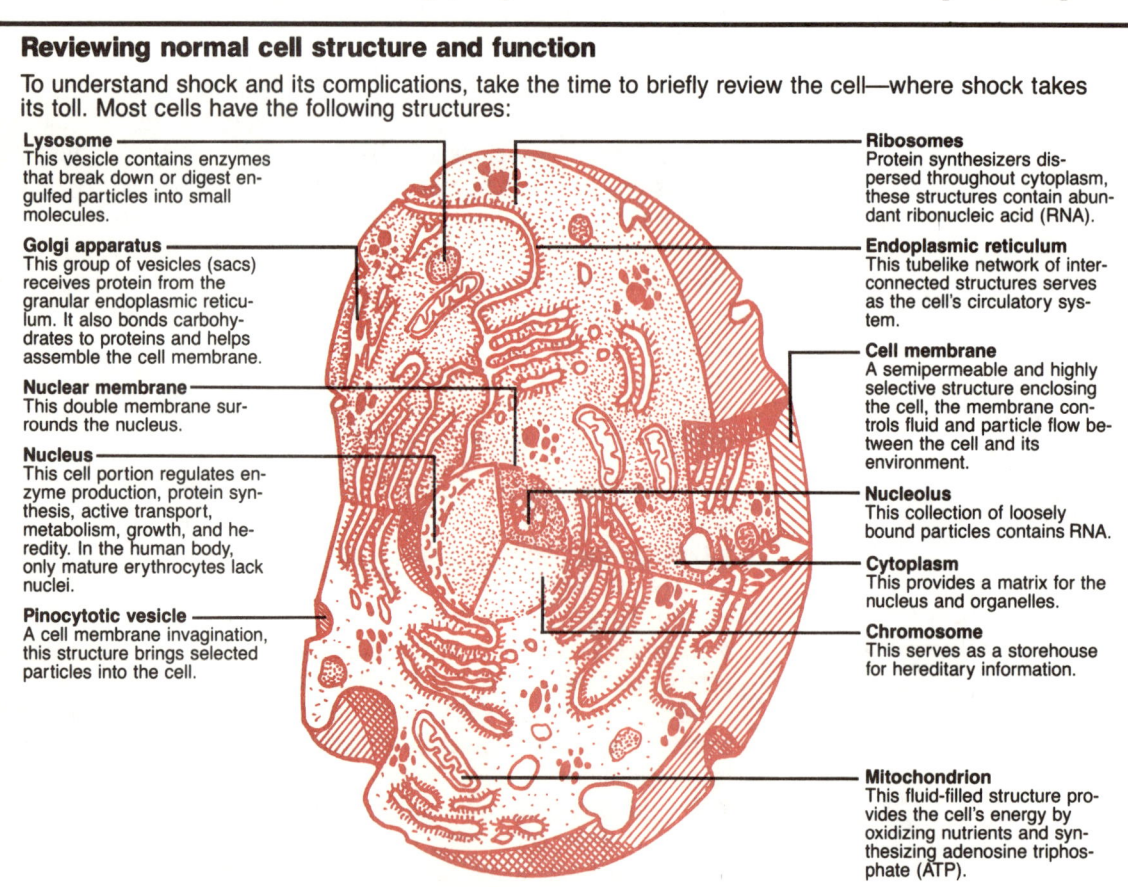

Reviewing normal cell structure and function

To understand shock and its complications, take the time to briefly review the cell—where shock takes its toll. Most cells have the following structures:

Lysosome
This vesicle contains enzymes that break down or digest engulfed particles into small molecules.

Golgi apparatus
This group of vesicles (sacs) receives protein from the granular endoplasmic reticulum. It also bonds carbohydrates to proteins and helps assemble the cell membrane.

Nuclear membrane
This double membrane surrounds the nucleus.

Nucleus
This cell portion regulates enzyme production, protein synthesis, active transport, metabolism, growth, and heredity. In the human body, only mature erythrocytes lack nuclei.

Pinocytotic vesicle
A cell membrane invagination, this structure brings selected particles into the cell.

Ribosomes
Protein synthesizers dispersed throughout cytoplasm, these structures contain abundant ribonucleic acid (RNA).

Endoplasmic reticulum
This tubelike network of interconnected structures serves as the cell's circulatory system.

Cell membrane
A semipermeable and highly selective structure enclosing the cell, the membrane controls fluid and particle flow between the cell and its environment.

Nucleolus
This collection of loosely bound particles contains RNA.

Cytoplasm
This provides a matrix for the nucleus and organelles.

Chromosome
This serves as a storehouse for hereditary information.

Mitochondrion
This fluid-filled structure provides the cell's energy by oxidizing nutrients and synthesizing adenosine triphosphate (ATP).

Cellular metabolism and tissue perfusion. A cell functions most efficiently with the oxygen molecule's help. For example, a cell supplied with one oxygen molecule, another nutrient (for example, glucose, fatty acids, or amino acids), and adequate enzymes produces 36 ATP molecules. A cell with *no* oxygen molecules (which uses anaerobic metabolism) produces 2 ATP molecules. Anaerobic metabolism lacks efficiency because it doesn't break down nutrients completely. Acidic waste products then accumulate, most notably hydrogen ions, carbon dioxide, and lactic acid. Such waste triggers local destructive patterns, such as vasodilation and sluggish blood flow.

A cell's nutritional needs depend on tissue perfusion. Tissue perfusion usually increases when nutritional needs increase, and decreases when needs have been met.

Perfusion depends on the blood's forward flow opposed by vascular resistance. Changes in vessel diameter, circulatory volume, and blood flow rate may alter perfusion.

Autoregulation—vasomotor control of local tissue blood flow over a wide range of systemic blood pressures—aims to normalize tissue perfusion. As resistance pressure approaches forward pressure, perfusion drops to zero and autoregulation fails. Tissue blood flow then falls under both local metabolic and systemic influences. Loss of this important physiologic mediator contributes to organ destruction and death in late shock.

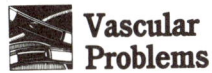
Vascular Problems

5 Shock

Patient Evaluation

How shock causes cellular death

Shock affects an individual cell just as it affects the whole body. Precapillary arterioles normally regulate capillary blood flow by constricting or dilating in response to blood pressure changes, neural regulation, oxygen needs, or vasoactive substances. But when shock develops, the precapillary system in the kidneys, mesentery, and skeletal muscles undergoes vasoconstriction (via direct sympathetic stimulation and catecholamine release). This reduces capillary oxygen and nutrient supply, resulting in selective cellular ischemia.

Tiny cell membrane pores normally permit entry of water, ions, and small molecules. The cell's mitochondria produce adenosine triphosphate (ATP). In early shock, when anoxia impairs ATP output, ions leak from the mitochondria. Eventually, this causes mitochondria dysfunction, which halts ATP production. Sodium-potassium exchange through the cell membrane then diminishes. Electrolyte imbalances within the cell cause swelling that leads to the cell's death.

Now a sequence of broader cellular destruction begins, starting with release of vasoactive and vasotoxic substances. These substances cause intracellular fluid to shift into the interstitial space, further compromising total circulating volume. This sets the stage for vasoconstriction and platelet aggregation and, consequently, sluggish blood flow and worsening ischemia. The destructive process proceeds until it damages body organs and ultimately the entire body.

symptoms. (For more information on signs and symptoms of each shock stage, see *Shock's three stages: Comparing clinical findings,* page 11.)

Early shock. In this stage, the body undergoes a generalized SNS response. Seconds or minutes after cardiac output drops, pressoreceptors in the aorta and carotid arteries sense a blood pressure decrease and send signals to the medulla's vasomotor center. This stimulates the SNS, causing the heart to beat faster and more powerfully to increase cardiac output and blood pressure. To supply more oxygen to the myocardium, coronary arteries dilate. Vessels serving the GI tract, kidneys, and skin constrict to shunt blood to the heart and brain, improving perfusion.

SNS stimulation also causes hormonal or endocrine reactions. In response to vasoconstriction that shunts blood away from the kidneys, the juxtaglomerular apparatus (JGA) releases renin. This substance becomes chemically altered in the blood to create angiotensin I. As angiotensin I circulates through the lungs, it's chemically transformed into angiotensin II, a powerful vasoconstrictor. While increasing blood pressure and expediting venous return to the heart's right side, vasoconstriction also stimulates the adrenal cortex to release aldosterone, which circulates to the kidneys and causes renal tubules to increase sodium reabsorption. This, in turn, causes water reabsorption (controlled by antidiuretic hormone [ADH]). Thus, JGA activation ultimately leads to sodium and water retention, reduced urine output, and increased fluid volume.

SNS stimulation also triggers the anterior pituitary gland to release adrenocorticotropic hormone (ACTH). This substance signals the adrenal cortex to release more glucocorticoids, leading to serum glucose elevation. The adrenal medulla reacts to SNS stimulation by producing more epinephrine and norepinephrine, which help prolong sympathetic effects and elevate the serum glucose level by stimulating glycogenolysis.

Chemical compensation also occurs in early shock. When cardiac output drops, blood flow to the lungs slows, which enlarges physiologic dead space and creates ventilation/perfusion imbalances. As a result, blood oxygenation decreases. Sensing this decrease, chemoreceptors in the aorta and carotid arteries signal the brain to increase ventilatory depth and rate, which reduces the blood's carbon dioxide level. Respiratory alkalosis then develops. (In septic shock, endotoxins may directly stimulate the brain's respiratory centers, contributing to hyperventilation.)

Cerebral blood vessels react to reduced carbon dioxide levels and alkalosis by constricting. This causes cerebral ischemia or hypoxia. Cerebral function also suffers from reduced oxygen levels stemming from decreased cardiac output and ventilation/perfusion imbalances. Chemoreceptor stimulation also activates the medulla's vasomotor center, contributing to SNS responses.

Middle shock. In this stage, decreased tissue perfusion becomes apparent, as compensatory mechanisms can't maintain sufficient cardiac output. This causes reduced tissue perfusion. When prolonged, compensatory vasoconstriction impairs cellular function.

Continued on page 6

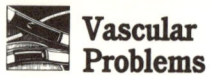

VASCULAR Problems

6 Shock

Patient Evaluation

Continued

Arteriolar vasoconstriction reduces capillary blood flow, which diminishes oxygen delivery to cells. Cellular oxygen deficit, in turn, reduces ATP production and promotes anaerobic metabolism, resulting in local acidosis. Impaired cellular function also causes cells to release toxic substances.

Because capillary flow decreases, these substances build up in the tissues, altering local tissue environment. Precapillary sphincters relax, permitting blood flow into the capillary bed. However, while blood flows freely *into* the bed, it can't flow freely *out* of the bed. Capillary hydrostatic pressure builds, pushing capillary fluid into the tissues. Capillary pores then enlarge, causing protein leakage from the vessels into the interstitial fluid. Protein loss depresses serum colloid osmotic pressure and expedites fluid movement from capillaries into the tissues or interstitial space. This fluid shift decreases intravascular blood volume and increases interstitial fluid volume, causing edema. Fluid also shifts from the interstitial space into the cell, promoting cellular edema and dysfunction. Reduced intravascular volume makes blood more viscous, which increases flow resistance. Capillary sludging then follows, further impairing blood flow.

By compromising venous return and cardiac output, reduced circulating blood volume and capillary flow intensify SNS-induced vasoconstriction. Blood then shunts to priority organs, diminishing peripheral and cutaneous blood flow.

Late shock. As compensatory responses fail, shock's pathophysiologic mechanisms become irreversible. Several vicious cycles lead to death, including these:
• *cardiac failure*, stemming from impaired myocardial contractility—the result of inadequate coronary perfusion, acidosis, and reduced cardiac output
• *acidosis*, which hinders tissue perfusion and impairs renal and respiratory function
• *altered blood clotting*, caused by acidosis, reduced vascular blood volume, and sluggish capillary flow. These alterations lead to platelet and red blood cell aggregation—which may cause disseminated intravascular coagulation (DIC).
• *inadequate cerebral blood flow*, resulting from reduced cardiac output and perfusion pressure (below 50 mm Hg). This triggers a dramatic SNS response. If cerebral ischemia continues, critical brain centers stop functioning. Failure of the medulla's vasomotor center causes sympathetic tone loss, in turn leading to lethal reductions in blood pressure, heart rate, and tissue perfusion. The body's reactions to shock thus culminate in multisystemic failure.

The nursing history

Depending on the clinical situation, shock's cause and/or type may be obvious. If possible, obtain the patient's history while assessing his signs and symptoms.

Chief complaint

If the patient's conscious, begin the history by determining his chief complaint. Suspect shock if he reports extreme lethargy, accompanied by dizziness even when he's in bed. Other common complaints

Normal cardiac output distribution

Organ	Blood flow (ml/min)	Percentage of total cardiac output
Liver	1,350	27%
Kidneys	1,100	22%
Skeletal muscles	750	15%
Brain	700	14%
Skin	300	6%
Lungs and bronchi	150	3%
Heart	150	3%
Other	500	10%

(*Note*: During exercise, skeletal muscles may receive up to 75% of cardiac output, depriving all other organs except the brain.)

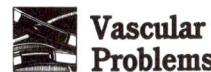 **Vascular Problems**

7 Shock

Patient Evaluation

include blurred vision, thirst, dry mouth, clammy skin, diaphoresis, and numbed extremities (especially the fingertips, toes, nose, earlobes, and lips). He may describe altered body perceptions, such as a vacant feeling. He may also initially seem agitated, then increasingly fearful as circulatory collapse continues. (Generally, agitation briefly accompanies a rapid cardiac output decrease.) Consider such complaints as warning signs that merit immediate attention.

If the patient's unconscious, check for objective signs of shock. Coupled with present illness data, these findings may lead you to suspect shock.

Present illness
Your patient stands a greater risk for shock if his present illness involves any of these conditions:
- *acute or slow blood loss*, as in GI hemorrhage; long-bone fracture; major laceration; extensive kidney, liver, or spleen hematoma; or surgery
- *evidence of fluid shift into interstitial spaces* (third spacing), as in extensive burns, ascites, intestinal obstruction, or pancreatitis
- *volume depletion state*, as in diabetes insipidus, diabetic ketoacidosis, hyperglycemic hyperosmolar nonketotic coma, excessive vomiting and diarrhea, excessive drainage, administration of osmotic cathartics or diagnostic dyes, or therapeutically induced diuresis. *Note*: Monitor your patient carefully for shock if he's receiving a diuretic.
- *mixed volume depletion and third spacing*, as occurs 3 to 4 days after surgery. By this time, the postoperative patient may have gained up to 4 lb (1.8 kg) of water, reflecting a fluid shift from vessels into the tissues. If he's still receiving only dextrose 5% in water instead of food and fluids, he may also be undernourished. This may lead to vascular instability (identified by below-normal serum protein [albumin] and total protein levels).
- *catheter placement in large central veins*, as in I.V. therapy, dialysis, hemodynamic monitoring, or I.V. hyperalimentation
- *infection*
- *blood transfusion reactions*
- *anaphylactic or anaphylactoid reactions*
- *recent multiple or long-bone fractures*
- *acute spinal cord injury*
- *acute myocardial infarction, mitral insufficiency, or cardiac tamponade*
- *aortic aneurysm with vena caval obstruction.*

Other high-risk patients include those with chronic illness or immunosuppression and those undergoing invasive GI or genitourinary procedures. Immune system deficits make pediatric and geriatric patients vulnerable to shock.

Past medical history
Check the patient's past medical history for clues to shock's cause and to organs particularly susceptible to shock's complications (which frequently result from preexisting medical problems). Stay especially alert for shock and its complications when caring for a patient with a history of cerebrovascular disease, end-stage renal disease, liver disease, coronary artery disease, peripheral vascular disease, chronic obstructive pulmonary disease, diabetes mellitus, sickle-cell anemia, or immunosuppression. Preformed antibodies por-

Continued on page 8

Measuring blood pressure

As shock reduces your patient's blood pressure, systolic and diastolic sounds become increasingly difficult to auscultate. When this happens, use one of the following alternative methods to take your patient's blood pressure:
- *systolic blood pressure palpation*
- *Doppler systolic blood pressure measurement*
- *intraarterial catheter placement*
- *noninvasive automatic blood pressure monitoring* (for details, see page 16).

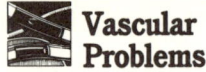

Patient Evaluation

The nursing history—*continued*

tend potential anaphylactic shock and transfusion reactions. The following history findings suggest such antibodies:
• atopy
• multiple blood transfusions (suspect this with a history of blood dyscrasia, cancer, GI hemorrhage, or multiple surgeries)
• multiple births or cesarean births.

Other factors that can increase the risk of shock complications include a history of altered coagulation, anticoagulant therapy (especially in an undernourished patient), liver disease, and cardiac problems (including myocardial infarction, mitral insufficiency, left ventricular aneurysm, and congestive heart failure).

With an unconscious patient, look for a Medic-Alert tag or wallet card listing his medical history.

Family history
Researchers have linked certain familial traits and known genetic relationships with some causes of shock. A history of any of these conditions makes shock more likely: heart disease (such as coronary artery disease or cardiomyopathy), diabetes mellitus, bleeding disorders, or allergies.

Social history
Although the clinical situation may prevent you from obtaining the patient's psychosocial history initially, be sure to gather such information after he's stabilized. Find out how your patient's adapted to past crises. Healthy adaptive behaviors include fear and anxiety in response to real threats and the ability to recognize and request help for specific limitations. Maladaptive responses to crises include persistent feelings of overwhelming powerlessness, anger, and fear when faced with little or no risk; addiction to or dependence on drugs or alcohol; and noncompliance with therapy.

Note: If your patient's psychosocial history suggests maladaptive responses to crises, be aware that he may become extremely agitated if he develops shock. Such a response can increase his energy needs and expenditure. This, in turn, can make complications more likely or exacerbate any complications that develop.

The physical examination

Key signs and symptoms of shock first appear in body systems most sensitive to lowered tissue perfusion. Findings vary with the shock type and with the stage and degree of compensation.

During *early shock* (as SNS compensation begins), expect normal blood pressure (not decreased, as you might expect), accompanied by rapid pulse and respiratory rates. The patient shows heightened mental alertness and apprehension; his pupils may dilate. As circulating blood volume drops, he may complain of thirst; his skin may become clammy and develop goose bumps. *Important*: Although such subtle findings may not suggest critical illness, never overlook them. By recognizing shock's early warning signs and taking appropriate measures, you can boost the patient's survival odds and help reduce the risk of complications.

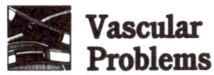

Vascular Problems

9 Shock

Patient Evaluation

Early shock's signs and symptoms may unfold gradually or relatively rapidly. Sudden circulating volume loss or preexisting heart disease, for example, may accelerate this phase.

As circulatory loss continues, *middle shock* begins. As cellular and microcirculatory alterations take place and reduced organ perfusion becomes apparent, signs and symptoms grow more pronounced. Check for the following:

Decreased systolic blood pressure. Venous return drops markedly. Circulating blood volume diminishes as sympathetic arteriolar vasoconstriction traps fluid in the arterial circulatory system. Venous dilation then occurs. As a result, venous return to the heart lessens, causing reduced forward volume and pressure (reduced preload) into the right heart and out the left ventricle (reduced cardiac output).

Systolic pressure drops as blood volume and pressure in the contracting left ventricle decrease. Contraction becomes less competent with left ventricular muscle fiber understretching (as in low-volume states) or overstretching (as in high-volume states). The patient with previously diseased cardiac muscle particularly risks incompetent contraction.

Increased diastolic blood pressure. As sympathetic compensation refills arterial circulation (through arteriolar vasoconstriction), blood volume and pressure rise with diminished forward blood propulsion to the tissues. Vasoconstriction and static fluid in the arterial circulation increase total peripheral resistance. Compensatory tachycardia contributes by shortening diastole and thus increasing diastolic blood pressure.

As systolic pressure decreases and diastolic pressure rises, pulse pressure narrows. An important sign, narrowing pulse pressure signals that compensatory mechanisms have failed to normalize blood pressure.

Tachycardia and pulse changes. Catecholamines released by the SNS stimulate the heart's sinoatrial node to discharge rapidly to provide adequate systemic circulatory volume. This results in tachycardia, which further compromises the patient by boosting his energy needs and, consequently, his oxygen demands. With diminished volume, prolonged tachycardia impairs myocardial contraction—particularly during diastole.

Because tachycardia shortens diastolic filling time, ventricular volume decreases, leading to reduced myocardial fiber prestretching. A minimally stretched fiber won't contract efficiently, resulting in left ventricular incompetence. This further reduces cardiac output.

Remember, coronary arteries undergo perfusion during diastole. As tachycardia shortens diastole, myocardial perfusion diminishes, creating myocardial ischemia. Accompanying signs and symptoms may also appear.

Assess the patient's major arterial pulses for rate, rhythm, amplitude, character, and duration. Suspect shock if you note a rapid, weak, thready, and brief arterial pulse. Rhythm depends on any accompanying dysrhythmias. You can best observe venous pulses

Continued on page 10

Middle shock: Associated signs and symptoms

Cool, moist, pale skin. This indicates that blood's been diverted from the skin to major organs. As blood diversion continues, microcirculation grows sluggish, causing acid accumulation. This leads to mottled skin, particularly in large muscles.

The shock type affects skin color and moistness. In early septic shock, the skin may feel warm and moist and appear flushed. In hypovolemic shock, the skin may seem dry, with poor turgor. Anaphylactic shock causes flushing with macular or papular lesions. In all shock types, the skin generally becomes cool, moist, and pale as shock progresses.

Cyanosis. Peripheral cyanosis (from reduced blood flow or vasoconstriction) suggests blood diversion to major organs. The patient may develop dusky to bluish discoloration of the nail beds, earlobes, and oral mucosa. Central cyanosis (oxygen deficiency) occurs when hemoglobin's oxygen-carrying capacity decreases—usually when the circulatory system contains at least 5 g of unoxygenated hemoglobin. Central cyanosis becomes apparent in the mucous membranes of the mouth and nose, the skin surrounding the lips, and beneath the tongue.

Poor capillary refill. To assess the patient's capillary refill, apply pressure over the nail bed until blanching occurs. Quickly release the pressure and note the rate at which blanching fades (an index of perfusion). In shock, perfusion decreases, which lengthens capillary refill time.

Hypothermia. This usually results from reduced metabolic activity. Although hypothermia lowers metabolic demands, it also causes vasodilation. However, septic shock usually causes an elevated temperature.

Muscle lethargy. Muscle lethargy stems from anaerobic metabolism. Skeletal muscles normally receive approximately 15% of the cardiac output. But during shock, most of this blood gets diverted to other organs, leaving muscles deprived of oxygen and other nutrients. Anaerobic metabolism results, leading to increased lactic acid production. General muscle lethargy sets in, along with increasing soreness and spasm.

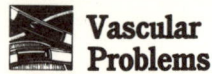
Vascular Problems

10 Shock

Patient Evaluation

The physical examination—*continued*

in the internal and external jugular neck veins. In cardiogenic shock, high right-heart filling pressures may produce full venous pulses and neck vein distention. In hypovolemic shock, filling pressures fall and venous pulses may become too weak to distinguish.

Decreased urine output. Urine output decreases from the following effects:
• Reduced cardiac output. About 22% of cardiac output goes to the kidneys. As circulating blood volume drops, blood and fluid become trapped in the microcirculatory system to enhance blood flow to such organs as the kidneys. Kidney function serves as an especially good index of reduced cardiac output and decreased oxygen delivery; active transport systems responsible for urine formation use 80% of the ATP produced by the kidney's tubular cells. When cellular oxygen supplies diminish—as in shock—urine output reduction becomes an early, reliable sign of reduced cardiac output.
• Direct SNS stimulation of the afferent arteriole. Each kidney nephron has an afferent arteriole leading into the glomerulus and an efferent arteriole leaving the glomerulus and entering the peritubular capillaries. SNS stimulation selectively constricts the afferent arteriole, causing reduced glomerular blood flow and filtration (the first step in urine formation).
• Renin release. In response to glomerular filtration reductions, the JGA within the nephron releases an inactive renin form. A series of enzymatic reactions converts renin to angiotensin II, which acts on the nephron to constrict the efferent arteriole, further reducing glomerular filtration.
• ADH release. As circulating fluid volume drops, solutes become increasingly concentrated. Osmoreceptors then sense the need to conserve water to dilute the solutes. ADH, released by the hypothalamic-hypophyseal (pituitary) axis, acts directly on the nephron's collecting ducts and, to a lesser degree, on the distal tubule, to promote water reabsorption. This produces highly concentrated urine.

ADH also acts (although less effectively) on the intestinal epithelium to conserve water through reabsorption. Tremendous GI tract fluid shifts during SNS stimulation divert conserved water into the third space, preventing it from contributing to circulating volume.

In addition, ADH stimulates adrenal medullary secretion of aldosterone, which aids sodium conservation. This in turn promotes continued serum hyperosmolarity with low circulating fluid volumes. The feedback mechanism that normally stops ADH release now fails because osmoreceptors continue to sense elevated serum osmolarity. Thus, the ADH release cycle continues.

Except in a patient with known renal failure, low urine output signifies developing shock. Urine output below 30 ml/hr indicates a glomerular filtration rate reduction of approximately 60%. At this point, look for signs of reduced glomerular blood flow (indicated by elevated urine osmolarity and urine specific gravity) or reduced

11 Shock

Patient Evaluation

Shock's three stages: Comparing clinical findings

Parameter	Early stage	Middle stage	Late stage
Level of consciousness (LOC)	Alterations caused by hypoxia, hypocapnia, and sympathetic catecholamine release. The patient may initially seem restless, agitated, anxious, or confused and show impaired memory and judgment.	Severe alterations, including bizarre, inappropriate behavior; lethargy; and unresponsiveness. As LOC decreases, the motor response to pain may progress from flexion to extension to no response.	Severe alterations from cerebral ischemia; possibly progressing to unresponsiveness
Blood pressure	Normal or adequate to perfuse vital organs. Systolic pressure rises from increased stroke volume; diastolic pressure, from systemic arteriolar vasoconstriction.	Normal to decreasing. Pulse pressure narrows as systolic pressure drops from decreased stroke volume; diastolic pressure rises from increased vasoconstriction. Hypotension may cause weakness and fatigue. Paradoxical pulse may develop.	Frank hypotension with widened pulse pressure to zero blood pressure, caused by sympathetic tone loss (from dysfunction of the medulla's vasomotor center). Cardiovascular collapse occurs.
Pulse	Possible sinus tachycardia from sympathetic stimulation	Sinus tachycardia continues, but any rate and rhythm disturbances resulting from myocardial ischemia may lead to various dysrhythmias. Peripheral pulses become weak, rapid, and thready as vasoconstriction impairs blood flow to peripheral areas. Lowered stroke volume contributes to pulse degeneration.	Extremely slow, weak to absent pulse from sympathetic tone loss
Respirations	Rapid and deep from respiratory alkalosis and reduced oxygenation	Tachypnea continues. However, breathing becomes shallow from hypoventilation, possibly causing shortness of breath. Expect crackles or wheezes on auscultation. Signs and symptoms of adult respiratory distress syndrome (ARDS, also called shock lung) may develop.	Tachypnea to slow, shallow respirations from ARDS
Urine output	Decreased from reduced blood flow to kidney nephrons	Decrease continues.	Severely decreased to anuria from renal blood flow lack; kidney failure
Skin	Cool, pale, and clammy from peripheral vasoconstriction and enhanced sweat gland activity	Pale or cyanotic and possible cold or clammy from vasoconstriction. Nail beds may show poor capillary refill. You may note edema from fluid shifts. (In septic shock, skin may become warm and flushed, denoting so-called *warm shock*.)	Cold, mottled, ashen, or cyanotic
Other	• Possible thirst • Hypoactive bowel sounds from sympathetic stimulation that diminishes gastric motility (peristalsis) • Possible pupil dilation from sympathetic stimulation; pupils react equally to light.	• Possibly hypoactive or absent bowel sounds from impaired GI motility. Paralytic ileus may develop. GI ulcers may form, with signs of stress ulcer (hematemesis or melena). GI congestion may lead to nausea, vomiting, or anorexia. • Possible body temperature reduction from decreased vasoconstriction, cellular metabolism, and heat production. Muscle aches may develop from lactic acid accumulation.	• Multisystemic failure • Immune system collapse • Coagulation cascade (resulting in disseminated intravascular coagulation)

renal function (assessed by elevated blood urea nitrogen [BUN] and serum creatinine levels, reduced drug clearances, or elevated serum levels of drugs excreted by the kidney, without dosage increase or known competition for excretion with another drug).

However, in *septic shock*, polyuria (a dilute urine output of 100 to 200 ml/hr) may occur, possibly from vasodilation secondary to bacterial toxins—usually in septic shock's warm stage.

Continued on page 12

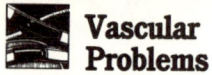

Vascular Problems

12 Shock

Late shock: When body systems fail

In late shock, as compensation falters, the body responds in the following ways:

Brain. As brain perfusion decreases, carbon dioxide levels rise, leading to vasodilation, hyperemia, and cerebral congestion. Oxygen and glucose needs go unmet, leading to progressive ischemia and infarction. Signs of increased intracranial pressure develop as this process continues.

Lungs. Shock promotes capillary endothelial damage, leading to resistance to blood flow. This, in turn, causes systemic hypoxia and interstitial pulmonary edema. Eventually, adult respiratory distress syndrome may develop.

Kidneys. Acute renal failure may reflect a prerenal, an intrarenal, or a postrenal cause. Acute renal failure produces these findings: increasing agitation; oliguria; inability to concentrate urine; rising blood urea nitrogen and serum creatinine, potassium, phosphate, and magnesium levels; and below-normal to normal serum calcium, albumin, and total protein levels. ABG analysis reveals metabolic acidosis.

Liver. Continued hypoperfusion damages the liver's reticuloendothelial cells, which decreases infection resistance. Liver failure also occurs.

Heart. Cardiac failure may occur from myocardial damage and infarction. During shock, coronary artery flow dwindles while myocardial oxygen consumption increases. The combined effects of continued acidosis and myocardial toxic factor release reduce contractility. Hypoxia, acidosis, and reduced coronary artery flow cause myocardial irritability, resulting in dysrhythmias.

GI tract. Ulcers frequently arise, especially in septic shock—probably from blood shunting from the splanchnic area and gastric mucosa and from increased gastric acid production.

Hematologic system. Shock leads to release of procoagulant substances while depleting the body of many clotting factors. This sets the stage for the development of disseminated intravascular coagulation.

Patient Evaluation

The physical examination—*continued*

Increased respiratory rate. As acid levels increase, carbon dioxide stimulates the brain's respiratory center to speed respirations (tachypnea), to facilitate carbon dioxide expulsion and to compensate for acidosis. SNS compensation facilitates this response, as epinephrine dilates bronchioles and relaxes surrounding musculature. Tachypnea requires much energy, thus taxing the brain's respiratory centers, the lungs, and the surrounding musculature.

As shock progresses, toxic metabolic products and insufficient energy production cause generalized muscle weakness, then hypoventilation. The patient develops rapid, shallow breathing that doesn't replenish alveolar air but renews dead-space air. Ventilatory failure follows. As the patient's respiratory function worsens, he'll use the accessory muscles in his neck, shoulders, and abdomen to breathe more easily. You'll also notice nostril flaring and tracheal tugging. Auscultate his breath sounds for crackles and wheezes caused by air movement through fluid, mucus, and narrowed air passages.

Altered level of consciousness. From heightened alertness, the patient deteriorates to mental unresponsiveness as cerebral blood flow slackens. Initially, SNS stimulation causes increased reticular activating system activity and, consequently, increased alertness. This, in turn, may result in such changes as restlessness, agitation, and apprehension. Later, when brain oxygenation drops and acids accumulate, disorientation and lethargy develop. Elevated carbon dioxide levels bring about widespread cerebral vasodilation, which promotes cerebral congestion. As congestion advances to cerebral edema, lethargy intensifies and the patient eventually deteriorates to unresponsiveness. Although reduced consciousness signals worsening of the patient's condition, it also serves as a protective response by conserving the energy expended in a normal conscious state.

For signs and symptoms of late shock, see *Late shock: When body systems fail.*

Laboratory studies

Expect the doctor to order various diagnostic tests to help determine shock's extent and the patient's response to treatment and to help identify any developing complications. Be sure to carefully correlate test results to the patient's clinical condition. (See *Assessing shock from laboratory findings* for test results that suggest shock.)

Arterial blood gas (ABG) analysis

This study helps assess the patient's systemic oxygenation and acid-base response. Initially, the patient develops respiratory alkalosis (high pH, low carbon dioxide [$PaCO_2$] levels) in response to lactic acid production and hyperventilation. Acid accumulation progresses until metabolic acidosis prevails (low pH, low bicarbonate [HCO_3^-] levels). Metabolic acidosis heralds decompensation and organ failure.

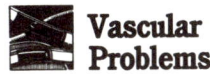

Vascular Problems

13 Shock

Patient Evaluation

When assessing serial ABGs, check inspired oxygen concentration; oxygenation, pH, and $PaCO_2$ changes; and base excess or HCO_3^- findings. Keep in mind that a hemoglobin increase from 10 to 12 mg/dl increases total oxygenation to a far greater degree than does an increased inspired oxygen percentage. Therefore, administering large oxygen amounts won't necessarily improve the patient's condition if his hemoglobin level's inadequate.

Serum lactic acid test

This test also helps evaluate whether oxygen transport's adequate for metabolism. When oxygen supplies drop, anaerobic metabolism predominates, producing lactic acid. The serum lactic acid level rises with continued cellular anaerobic metabolism. Along with

Continued on page 14

Assessing shock from laboratory findings

Test/normal value	Value in shock	Cause
BLOOD CHEMISTRY		
Serum glucose 70 to 100 mg/100 ml	• Above normal in early shock • Below normal in late shock	• Sympathetic stimulation • Glycogen depletion and impaired liver function
Serum proteins *Total:* 6.0 to 7.8 g/100 ml	• Below normal	• Capillary leakage and reduced liver cell synthesis
Albumin: 3.2 to 4.5 g/100 ml	• Below normal	• Capillary leakage and reduced liver cell synthesis
Globulin: 2.3 to 3.5 g/100 ml	• Normal or below normal	• Larger particle size, reduced capillary leakage
Blood urea nitrogen (BUN) 5.0 to 20.0 mg/100 ml	• Above normal	• Decreased renal excretion
Serum creatinine 0.6 to 1.2 mg/100 ml	• Above normal	• Decreased renal excretion
Serum electrolytes *Sodium:* 136 to 142 mEq/liter	• Above normal in early shock • Above or below normal in late shock	• Increased aldosterone secretion leading to renal retention of sodium • Renal function changes
Potassium: 3.8 to 5.0 mEq/liter	• Below normal in early shock • Above normal in late shock	• Increased aldosterone secretion leading to renal excretion of potassium • Acidosis, cell necrosis, and impaired renal function
Chloride: 95 to 103 mEq/liter	• Below normal in early shock • Above normal in late shock	• Alkalosis and bicarbonate excess • Acidosis and bicarbonate deficiency
Carbon dioxide (bicarbonate): 21 to 28 mEq/liter	• Above normal in early shock • Below normal in late shock	• Alkalosis • Severe acidosis
Serum enzymes *Creatine phosphokinase (CPK):* 5 to 35 mu/ml	• Above normal	• Heart and/or muscle cell necrosis
Serum glutamic-oxaloacetic transaminase (SGOT): 15 to 40 units/ml	• Above normal	• Heart and/or liver cell necrosis
Serum glutamic-pyruvic transaminase (SGPT): 15 to 35 units/ml	• Above normal	• Liver cell necrosis
Lactic dehydrogenase (LDH): 150 to 450 Wroblewski units/ml	• Above normal	• Heart and/or liver cell necrosis
Amylase: 60 to 160 Somogyi units/100 ml	• Above normal	• Pancreatic cell necrosis
Lipase: 0 to 1.5 Cherry-Crandall units/ml	• Above normal	• Pancreatic cell necrosis

Continued

Vascular Problems

14 Shock
Patient Evaluation

Assessing shock from laboratory findings—continued

Test/normal value	Value in shock	Cause
HEMATOLOGIC TESTS		
Hemoglobin men: 14.0 to 16.5 g/100 ml women: 12.6 to 14.2 g/100 ml	• Below normal	• Hemorrhage
Hematocrit (packed cell volume) men: 4% to 52% women: 37% to 47%	• Above or below normal	• *Above normal:* capillary fluid leakage • *Below normal:* blood loss (values don't change until approximately 6 hours after blood loss)
Red blood cell count men: 4.6 to 6.2 million/mm³ women: 4.5 to 5.4 million/mm³	• Below normal	• Hemorrhage
White blood cell count 4,500 to 11,000/mm³	• Above normal	• Response to possible infection
Platelet count 150,000 to 400,000/mm³	• Below normal	• Platelet aggregation and microemboli
Coagulation tests Prothrombin time (PT): 12 to 14 sec Partial thromboplastin time (PTT): 45 to 65 sec	• Prolonged • Prolonged	• Possible hypercoagulable state • Possible hypercoagulable state
URINE TESTS		
Creatinine clearance men: 1.0 to 2.0 g/24 hr women: 0.8 to 1.8 g/24 hr	• Below normal	• Impaired renal excretion
Osmolality 500 to 800 mOsm/liter	• Above normal in early shock • Below normal in late shock	• Water retention secondary to ADH secretion • Kidney's failure to concentrate urine
Specific gravity 1.001 to 1.035	• Above normal in early shock • Below normal in late shock	• Water retention secondary to ADH secretion • Kidney's failure to concentrate urine (affected by dextran administration)
Sodium 80 to 180 mEq/24 hr	• Below normal in early shock • Above or below normal in late shock	• Sodium reabsorption secondary to aldosterone secretion • Abnormal renal function
Potassium 40 to 80 mEq/24 hr	• Above normal in early shock • Above or below normal in late shock	• Potassium excretion secondary to aldosterone secretion • Abnormal renal function
ARTERIAL BLOOD GASES		
pH 7.38 to 7.42	• Above normal in early shock • Below normal in late shock	• Hyperventilation and carbon dioxide exhalation • Carbon dioxide retention and lactic acid production
PaCO₂ 35 to 45 mm Hg	• Below normal in early shock • Above normal in late shock	• Hyperventilation • Hypoventilation
PaO₂ 80 to 100 mm Hg	• Below normal	• Hypoventilation and hypoperfusion (ventilation/perfusion mismatch)
Bicarbonate (HCO₃⁻) 22 to 28 mEq/liter	• Below normal in late shock	• Severe acidosis

Laboratory studies—continued

other waste products, lactic acid contributes to metabolic acidosis. Mortality increases as serum lactic acid levels rise above 12 mg/dl.

Other tests. The doctor may also order a chest X-ray and electrocardiogram (EKG) to evaluate the patient's pulmonary and cardiac status.

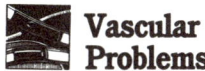 **Vascular Problems**

15 Shock

Patient Evaluation

Invasive hemodynamic monitoring

These techniques yield key information on the patient's cardiovascular and pulmonary function. The doctor may use intraarterial, intracardiac, or central venous pressure monitoring. Regardless of the method used, measurement *trends* prove more crucial than individual values in assessing the patient's status. Some hemodynamic monitoring results may also be used to calculate other hemodynamic parameters (see *Other hemodynamic parameters*, page 20).

Intraarterial pressures

To obtain intraarterial pressures, the doctor will insert an arterial indwelling catheter. An arterial line allows continuous measurement of systolic, diastolic, and mean arterial pressures (MAP). It also provides a source for arterial blood samples, eliminating the need for repeated punctures. In addition, as shock progresses and cuff blood pressure measurements become unreliable, an arterial line permits the most accurate assessment of the patient's status and response to therapy (providing a proper waveform appears on the oscilloscope). *Note:* Expect to obtain a higher systolic pressure

Continued on page 16

Measuring intraarterial pressure

To measure intraarterial pressure, the doctor inserts an arterial indwelling catheter (usually 5 to 6 cm long)—commonly in the radial (preferred), brachial, or femoral artery. (The doctor probably won't suture the catheter if it's inserted into the radial artery.)

Important: Allen's test should be performed before radial artery insertion to assess for collateral circulatory adequacy. To perform this test, simultaneously occlude the radial and ulnar arteries with firm pressure until you see blanching. With sufficient blood flow through the ulnar artery, blanching will disappear quickly after you release the ulnar artery while keeping the radial artery occluded.

The catheter's connected to specialized pressure tubing with a flush system that continuously infuses a heparinized solution (approximately 3 ml/hr). A pressure bag or pump keeps the solution under pressure. The catheter's also connected to a transducer, which senses arterial pressure and converts this measurement to an oscilloscopic waveform. A numerical value also appears on the monitor.

Before reliable pressure readings can be obtained, the system requires calibration and zero balancing (to negate atmospheric pressure effects).

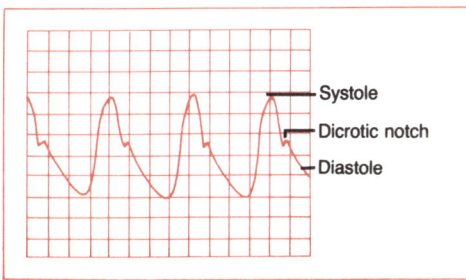

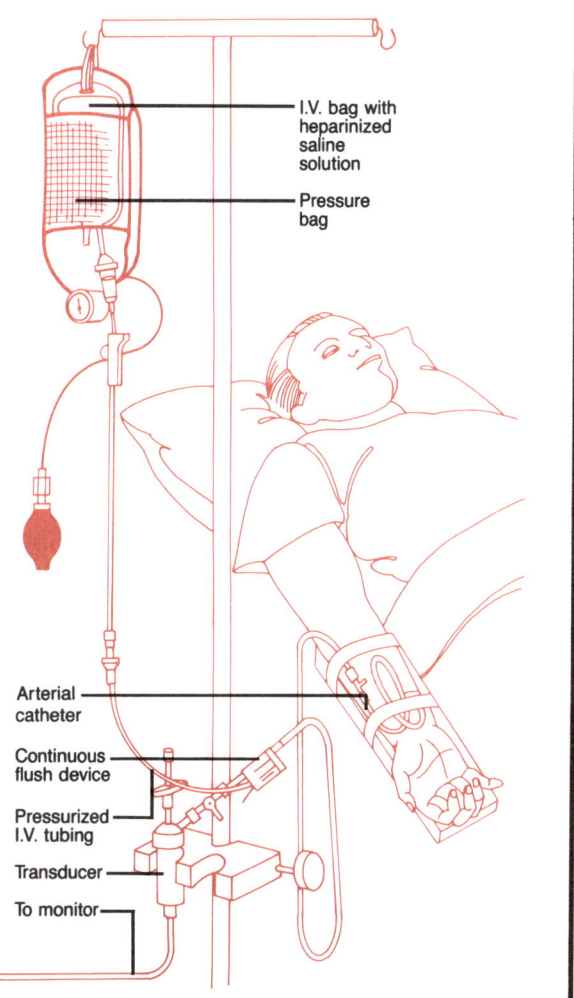

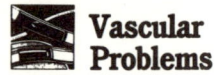 **Vascular Problems**

16 Shock

Patient Evaluation

Noninvasive automatic blood pressure monitoring

The doctor may order this measurement method for a patient who needs frequent blood pressure monitoring but who doesn't need an intraarterial catheter, or for a patient in whom such a catheter can't be placed. The monitor provides highly accurate blood pressure and heart rate measurements at intervals as frequent as every 60 seconds.

The system works by automatically inflating an ordinary pressure cuff around the patient's arm. As the cuff deflates, the monitor's precalibrated transducer detects pressure pulsations. After each inflation, the monitor also displays mean arterial pressure readings.

Invasive hemodynamic monitoring—*continued*

(by about 10 mm Hg) with an arterial line than the systolic pressure obtained by auscultation or palpation.

If an intraarterial catheter can't be placed, the doctor may use a noninvasive automatic blood pressure monitoring device. (See *Noninvasive automatic blood pressure monitoring.*)

Systolic pressure, which normally ranges from 100 to 140 mm Hg, reflects the degree of systemic vascular resistance and arterial compliance. Diastolic pressure, which ranges from 60 to 90 mm Hg, reflects aortic blood velocity, arterial wall elasticity, and the degree of vasoconstriction. MAP, which ranges from 80 to 120 mm Hg, reflects the average pressure pushing blood through the systemic circulation to ensure adequate tissue perfusion. To calculate MAP, use one of these formulas:

$$MAP = \frac{\text{systolic pressure} + 2 \text{ (diastolic pressure)}}{3}$$

or diastolic pressure + ⅓ (systolic pressure − diastolic pressure)

MAP above 80 mm Hg indicates adequate tissue perfusion. If your patient's normally hypertensive, however, his body tissues may have adjusted to higher forward pressures. In this case, MAP above 80 mm Hg may not be adequate.

Compensatory SNS mechanisms elevate MAP more by increasing systemic vascular resistance (SVR) than by increasing cardiac output. With elevated SVR, diastolic pressure increases and pulse pressure narrows. Consequently, pulse pressure becomes a significant index of stroke volume and vasoconstriction.

Although MAP monitoring can determine shock's degree, it doesn't consistently reflect total blood flow. The patient may have insufficient tissue perfusion despite normal blood pressure and cardiac output.

Central venous pressure

Central venous pressure (CVP) measurement helps manage shock by evaluating volume replacement needs and identifying the shock type. To obtain CVP, the doctor will order indwelling catheter placement in the superior vena cava at the right atrium. (See *Measuring central venous pressure* for insertion techniques.) CVP thus indicates superior vena caval pressure at the right atrium, reflecting right ventricular preload or filling response. Total blood volume and venous return influence CVP. (*Note:* CVP reflects conditions in the right heart only.)

Normal mean CVP ranges from 1 to 6 mm Hg (2 to 8 cm H_2O). (To convert mm Hg to cm H_2O, multiply mm Hg by 1.34.) Poor myocardial contractility and subsequently elevated filling pressures may increase CVP above normal in cardiogenic shock. Above-normal CVP may also indicate right ventricular failure, volume overload, tricuspid valve stenosis or regurgitation, constrictive pericarditis, pulmonary hypertension, cardiac tamponade, or right ventricular infarction. Below-normal CVP usually suggests reduced circulating blood volume, as in hypovolemic shock. In septic shock, CVP may fall below normal from reduced venous return resulting from capillary pooling.

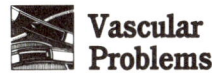 **Vascular Problems**

17 Shock

Patient Evaluation

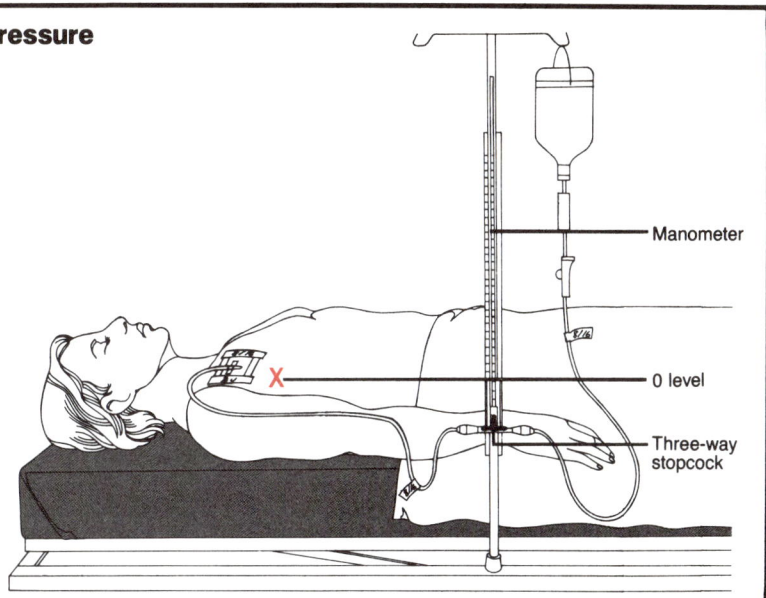

Measuring central venous pressure

To measure central venous pressure, a large-bore indwelling catheter's inserted into a vein (commonly the subclavian, brachial, or jugular vein). The catheter tip lodges in the superior vena cava at the right atrium.

The catheter's connected to a transducer and monitor, which electronically measure the pressure in millimeters of mercury, or to a manometer, which permits manual pressure measurement in centimeters of water (as shown at right). The transducer or manometer should be placed level with the right atrium. No waveform appears with a water manometer. With a transducer, you'll see a right atrial waveform.

However, keep in mind that pulmonary vasoconstriction may increase CVP, regardless of venous return and fluid volume.

Intracardiac pressures

Pulmonary artery (PA) catheter placement allows measurement of right atrial pressure (RAP), right ventricular pressures (RVPs), pulmonary artery pressures (PAPs), pulmonary capillary wedge pressure (PCWP, also known as pulmonary artery wedge pressure [PAWP]), cardiac output, and mixed venous gases. These pressures provide crucial data about the patient's fluid and cardiac status, left ventricular function, and response to therapy. (*Note*: RAP usually reflects CVP.)

Right ventricular pressures

RV systolic pressure normally equals pulmonary artery systolic pressure (PASP); RV end-diastolic pressure, which reflects RV function, equals RAP. Normal RV systolic pressure ranges from 15 to 25 mm Hg; normal RV end-diastolic pressure, from 0 to 8 mm Hg. (Measurement of these pressures usually takes place only during initial PA catheter insertion.)

Pulmonary artery pressures

During systole, when the pulmonic valve opens and the mitral valve closes, the right ventricle and left atrium function as one chamber. PASP reflects right ventricular function and pulmonary circulation pressures—the right heart's peak response during systole.

During diastole, when the pulmonic valve closes and the mitral valve opens, the pulmonary artery and left ventricle function as a single chamber. Pulmonary artery diastolic pressure (PADP) reflects left-heart pressures, specifically, left ventricular end-diastolic pressure (LVEDP), or left ventricular filling pressure (preload) in a patient without significant pulmonary disease. (Because PADP closely correlates with PCWP, it may be used instead of PCWP.)

PASP normally ranges from 15 to 25 mm Hg; PADP, from 8 to 15 mm Hg; mean PA pressure, from 10 to 20 mm Hg. PADP rises

Continued on page 18

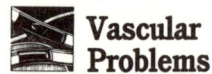

Vascular Problems

18 Shock

Patient Evaluation

Invasive hemodynamic monitoring—*continued*

with left ventricular failure, increased pulmonary blood flow (left or right shunting, as in atrial or ventricular septal defects), and any condition that increases pulmonary arteriolar resistance (for example, pulmonary hypertension, volume overload, mitral stenosis, or hypoxia). Expect above-normal PAPs in cardiogenic shock, normal or below-normal PAPs in septic and hypovolemic shock (unless the patient has a related lung disorder).

Pulmonary capillary wedge pressure
PA catheter balloon inflation permits PCWP measurement (inflation causes the catheter tip to float in the direction of blood flow). When

---

Pulmonary artery pressures: Reviewing measurement methods

To measure a patient's pulmonary artery (PA) pressure, the doctor inserts a flow-directed, balloon-tipped, multilumen PA catheter (for example, a Swan-Ganz catheter) into a large central vein (such as the subclavian, jugular, or brachial vein). After advancing the catheter into the right atrium, he inflates the balloon to help float the catheter through the right ventricle and into the pulmonary artery.

When deflated, the catheter rests in the pulmonary artery, permitting PA diastolic and systolic pressure readings. When inflated, the catheter lodges in a small pulmonary artery branch. An opening in the catheter's tip permits pulmonary capillary wedge pressure (PCWP) readings.

The catheter measures about 110 cm long, with markings in 10-cm increments. It comes with two to five lumens (the number of lumens determines which functions it can perform).

The distal lumen, located at the catheter's tip, measures PA pressures when connected to a transducer and measures PCWP during balloon inflation. This lumen also permits drawing of mixed venous blood samples.

The proximal (central venous pressure) lumen, with its opening in or near the right atrium, measures right atrial pressure. This lumen can be used as a central line for fluid administration (unless it's connected to a transducer). It also serves as the injection site for cardiac output determinations.

The balloon inflation lumen, as its name suggests, inflates the balloon at the catheter's distal tip for PCWP measurement.

The thermistor connector lumen, with its opening in the pulmonary artery, contains temperature-sensitive wires that feed information into a computer for cardiac output calculation.

The pacemaker wire lumen, with its opening in the right atrium, provides a port for pacemaker electrodes or measurement of mixed venous oxygen saturation.

The lumen ports chosen for monitoring will be connected to special tubing with a flush system that continuously infuses a heparinized solution (approximately 3 ml/hr). The solution remains under pressure with a pressure bag or pump.

The lumen ports will also be connected to a transducer—placed level with the heart—that senses pressure and converts it to an oscilloscopic waveform. A numerical value also appears on the monitor.

Like intraarterial pressure monitoring equipment, this system requires calibration and zero balancing (negating the effects of atmospheric pressure) to ensure accuracy.

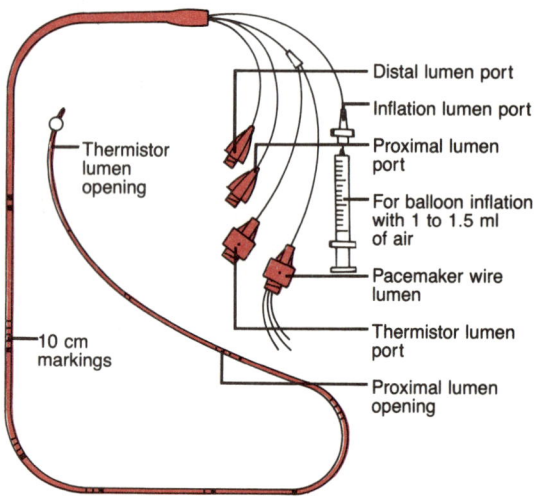

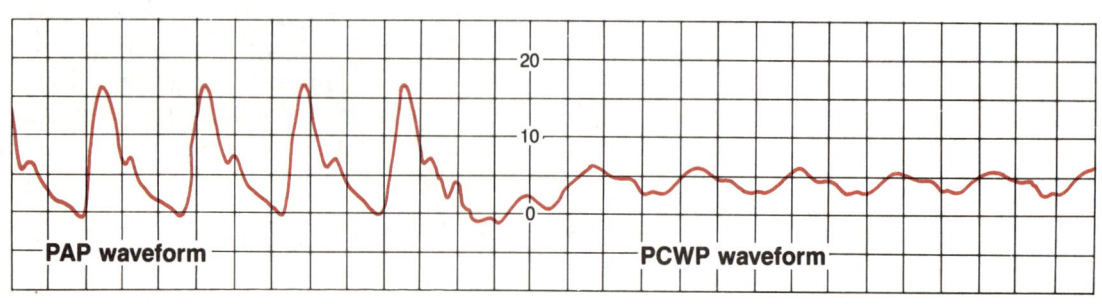

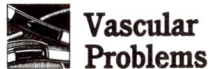 **Vascular Problems** 19 **Shock**

Patient Evaluation

balloon diameter equals or measures slightly less than the capillary's diameter, the catheter wedges in the capillary. Blood then can't flow past the inflated balloon and the catheter tip reflects pressure in the more distal pulmonary capillary system.

Important: Make sure the balloon's totally deflated (except when taking a PCWP reading). Prolonged wedging may cause pulmonary infarction.

During diastole, the heart momentarily relaxes as it fills with pulmonary vein blood. This permits the pulmonary vasculature, left atrium, and left ventricle to act as a single chamber with identical pressures. Thus, PCWP reflects left atrial and ventricular pressures, unless the patient has mitral stenosis. PAPs and PCWP changes reflect changes in LV filling pressure or LVEDP, permitting LV preload assessment. PCWP measurement may also reveal pulmonary congestion. Pressure in the pulmonary capillary reflects fluid movement between the vascular bed and the interstitial spaces and alveoli. Thus, as more fluid escapes into the interstitial tissues, PCWP increases.

Mean PCWP normally ranges from 6 to 12 mm Hg. Hypovolemic shock, which results from reduced circulating volume and venous return, leads to lower filling pressures and, consequently, abnormally low PCWP. In early septic shock, below-normal PCWP indicates relative hypovolemia secondary to diffuse vasodilation and fluid shifts from the vascular space. In neurogenic shock, decreased PCWP stems from peripheral vasodilation and reduced venous return.

Abnormally high PCWP usually accompanies cardiogenic shock, reflecting LV pump failure or inability to accommodate venous return (preload). Pulmonary congestion usually develops when PCWP measures about 18 mm Hg; pressures above 25 mm Hg reflect impending or existing pulmonary edema.

Other hemodynamic parameters
Cardiac output (CO) and mixed venous gases may also be determined via PA catheter placement. CO indicates the amount of blood (in liters) the heart ejects each minute. Calculate CO with this formula:
$$CO = \text{stroke volume} \times \text{heart rate} \ (CO = SV \times HR)$$
In normal adults, CO ranges from 4 to 8 liters.

Transport of blood, oxygen, and other vital nutrients to the tissues depends on CO. Because inadequate perfusion constitutes shock's major physiologic defect, CO measurement helps determine shock's extent, LV function, and the patient's overall cardiac status.

The thermodilution technique helps determine the patient's CO. This involves injection of a solution of known temperature and volume through a PA catheter's proximal lumen. The solution mixes with superior vena caval or right atrial blood (depending on the catheter's location). When this blood flows past a thermistor embedded in the catheter's distal end, the thermistor detects the blood and solution temperatures and relays this data to a computer. After analyzing the information, the computer displays the patient's CO (in liters/min)

Continued on page 20

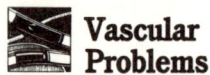

Vascular Problems

20 Shock

Patient Evaluation

Invasive hemodynamic monitoring—*continued*

on a screen. For the most accurate determination, you'll want to average at least three CO measurements.

Adjusting CO to the patient's size yields a measurement called the *cardiac index*, which normally ranges from 2.5 to 4.2 liters/min/m². To calculate cardiac index, first determine the patient's body surface area using a nomogram (such as the DuBois body surface area chart). Then use the following formula:

$$\text{Cardiac index} = \frac{\text{cardiac output (liter/min)}}{\text{body surface area (m}^2\text{)}}$$

In cardiogenic shock, when the left ventricle's pumping capacity declines, expect CO to drop below normal. As the ventricle fails, preload escalates markedly above normal. SVR increases to compensate for shock, causing increased afterload. A cardiac index below 2.2 liters/min/m² usually indicates cardiogenic shock.

In hypovolemic shock, expect abnormally low blood volume, which results in reduced venous return and preload. This leads to abnormally low PCWP and CO. SVR increases to make up for lowered venous return. However, because myocardial function usually remains normal, increased afterload doesn't increase preload, as in cardiogenic shock.

In septic shock, hemodynamic parameters vary depending on the shock stage. In early septic shock, widespread vasodilation and regional pooling produce a relative blood volume reduction. Below-normal PAPs and PCWP reflect lowered venous return. Reduced SVR and various compensatory mechanisms expedite LV ejection. As a result, CO usually rises well above normal.

Despite the vasoconstriction of late septic shock, the patient will have a persistent volume deficit as blood becomes trapped in regional beds and plasma leaks from capillaries into extravascular spaces. Cardiac function worsens and CO drops from depressed myocardial contractility and increased afterload.

Neurogenic shock results from peripheral vasodilation secondary to vasomotor tone loss. Below-normal PCWP and PAPs reflect decreased SVR and venous return. Because lowered SVR helps LV ejection, CO may remain normal or rise abnormally if the patient initially had sufficient blood volume.

Mixed venous gases. Samples drawn from the PA catheter's distal lumen will be analyzed for venous oxygen saturation (SvO_2). Alternatively, SvO_2 may be monitored via a fiberoptic oximeter thermodilution PA catheter. Arterial oxygen saturation (SaO_2) can be determined from ABGs. Calculations using SvO_2 and SaO_2 can then reveal the *arteriovenous oxygen difference (a-vDO₂)*, which helps assess the patient's pulmonary and oxygen transport status. By reflecting the difference between oxygen content in arterial blood and mixed venous blood, a-vDO₂ determines how well blood flow matches metabolic oxygen demands. Normally, a-vDO₂ ranges from 3.0 to 5.5 vol% (ml/100 ml).

Arterial oxygen content derives from SaO_2; venous oxygen content, from SvO_2. Because each hemoglobin (Hb) gram can carry 1.34 ml

---

Other hemodynamic parameters

In addition to the hemodynamic parameters described on the last few pages, other measurements that can help assess a shock patient include those described below.

Stroke volume (SV). You can determine SV—the amount of blood the ventricle pumps with each beat (about 60 to 130 ml)—by dividing cardiac output by heart rate.

$$SV = \frac{CO}{HR}$$

Stroke index (SI). Also known as *stroke volume index (SVI)*, SI adjusts the patient's stroke volume to his body size. Calculate SI by dividing cardiac index (CI; multiplied by 1,000 to convert liters to milliliters) by pulse rate; or by dividing SV by body surface area. SI normally ranges from 35 to 70 ml/beat/m².

Systemic vascular resistance (SVR). This parameter primarily determines venous return—the amount of blood returned to the heart from the peripheral circulation. SVR depends on the degree of cellular vasodilation or vasoconstriction. SVR and venous return increase as vasoconstriction worsens. SVR's a major determinant of afterload.

You can monitor your patient's SVR by calculating it with this formula:

$$SVR = \frac{(MAP - CVP)\ 79.9}{CO}$$

Normally ranging from 900 to 1,600 dyne/sec/cm⁻⁵, SVR usually rises in shock from compensatory sympathetic vasoconstriction. However, when shock causes widespread vasodilation, SVR may decrease.

Left ventricular stroke work (LVSW). This value, which reflects left ventricular work with each beat, helps evaluate ventricular pumping capacity. Normal LVSW ranges from 45 to 85 (g-m/m². Calculate it with this formula:

$$LVSW = \frac{CI\ (MAP - PCWP)\ 13.6}{HR}$$

LVSW usually declines in hypovolemic shock from low circulatory volume; in cardiogenic shock, from impaired pumping ability; in septic shock, from myocardial depressant factor or lowered coronary perfusion.

Patient Evaluation

of oxygen when 100% saturated, the following formula can determine oxygen content:

$$\text{Arterial } O_2 \text{ content (vol\%)} = 1.34 \times \text{Hb value} \times SaO_2$$
$$\text{Venous } O_2 \text{ content (vol\%)} = 1.34 \times \text{Hb value} \times SvO_2$$

Calculate a-vDO$_2$ by subtracting venous O$_2$ content from arterial O$_2$ content.

Normally, oxygen content in arterial and venous circulation should differ by 3% to 5%. In shock, when tissues must extract more oxygen from the blood, the difference widens. This parameter helps determine therapeutic success during all shock phases.

In the normal resting state, body tissues consume only one fourth of the oxygen delivered by cardiac output. As a result of this large oxygen reserve, SaO$_2$ normally measures 96% to 100%; normal SvO$_2$, 75%. Below-normal SvO$_2$ reflects either increased but unmet oxygen demands or reduced oxygen supply. With less oxygen available, tissues must extract more oxygen from the blood. Thus, blood returning to the heart has less oxygen than normal. This reduces SvO$_2$ and elevates a-vDO$_2$ above normal. An a-vDO$_2$ greater than 5.5 vol% reflects reduced cardiac output.

By dividing a-vDO$_2$ by red cell mass (RCM direct measurement), you can evaluate efficiency of tissue oxygen extraction (ETOE). Studies prove this parameter correctly predicts shock survivability in 91% of cases.

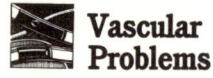

Vascular Problems

22 Shock

Hypovolemic Shock: Internal or External Fluid Loss

Kimberly A. Ramsey, who wrote this chapter, is Education Coordinator at St. John's Hospital and Health Center, Santa Monica, Calif. She received her RN from Akron City Hospital and her BS from the University of Akron, Ohio.

Hypovolemic shock—a complex syndrome that develops when circulating blood volume decreases in relation to intravascular compartment size—reflects a dangerous process. Insufficient blood volume (at least a 15% deficit) initiates a cycle of compensatory and decompensatory responses that can prove fatal without expert assessment and intervention. In this chapter, we'll review the causes of circulating blood volume loss, hypovolemic shock's pathophysiologic stages, and the assessment, planning, intervention, and evaluation techniques to combat this life-threatening condition.

Hypovolemic shock develops when circulating blood volume drops in response to internal or external fluid loss (see *Body fluids: Distinguishing the types*). Read what follows to learn how such loss occurs.

Internal fluid loss. Usually hard to detect initially, internal fluid loss may result from:
• third space shifting. Interstitial, or third space, refers to areas such as those surrounding the viscera, including the peritoneal cavity and the pericardial sac. Capillary permeability and osmotic pressure changes can cause fluid sequestration in these cavities. Peritoneal cavity sequestration (called *ascites* when it accompanies cirrhosis) can reduce circulating blood volume enough to cause hypovolemic shock. Pericardial sac sequestration seldom causes shock from fluid loss because the sac has a small capacity. However, it may lead to shock from impaired left ventricular pumping.
• intestinal capillary fluid leakage into the intestinal lumen. Usually the result of an intestinal obstruction, this decreases intestinal-vein fluid volume and reduces venous return.
• internal hemorrhage. Conditions such as hemorrhagic pancreatitis, hemothorax, and ruptured spleen cause blood pooling in extravascular compartments, thus reducing circulating volume. Long-bone fractures, such as a femur fracture, may lead to internal blood loss of up to 2 pints (950 ml).
• impaired venous return from vena caval obstruction. Conditions such as a tumor or an aortic aneurysm may block blood return to the heart, reducing circulating volume.

External fluid loss. Blood, plasma, or body fluid loss may result from any of the following conditions:
• blood loss. The most common cause of hypovolemic shock, this typically stems from multiple trauma, acute GI bleeding, surgical procedures, or a bleeding disorder.
• plasma loss. Large exposed burns or surface exudative lesions cause plasma loss that may lead to profound hypovolemia.
• body fluid loss. This may arise from the GI tract (from nasogastric suctioning, fistulas, vomiting, or diarrhea) or from the kidneys (from excessive diuretic use, diabetes insipidus or mellitus, or Addison's disease). Such fluid loss can cause severe dehydration or may complicate preexisting dehydration, leading to hypovolemia. Close assessment of fluid, electrolyte, and acid-base balance helps detect hypovolemic shock from body fluid loss—a commonly overlooked cause.

Shock's progression. Left untreated, the patient with hypovolemic shock progresses from compensation to decompensation (see *How hypovolemic shock progresses*). Normally, an adult has approximately

---

Body fluids: Distinguishing the types

Body fluids—water containing electrolytes and other solutes—make up approximately 50% to 60% of an adult's total weight. Body fluid can be intracellular or extracellular. *Intracellular fluid* includes fluid trapped within cells. *Extracellular fluid* includes interstitial fluid (fluid between cells) and intravascular fluid (fluid inside blood vessels).

An adult's total body fluids average 40 liters, distributed as shown below.

Body fluids (40 liters)

Intracellular fluid (25 liters) | Extracellular fluid (15 liters)

Interstitial fluid (10 liters)
Intravascular fluid (5 liters)

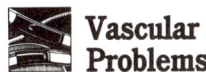 **Vascular Problems**

23 Shock

Hypovolemic Shock

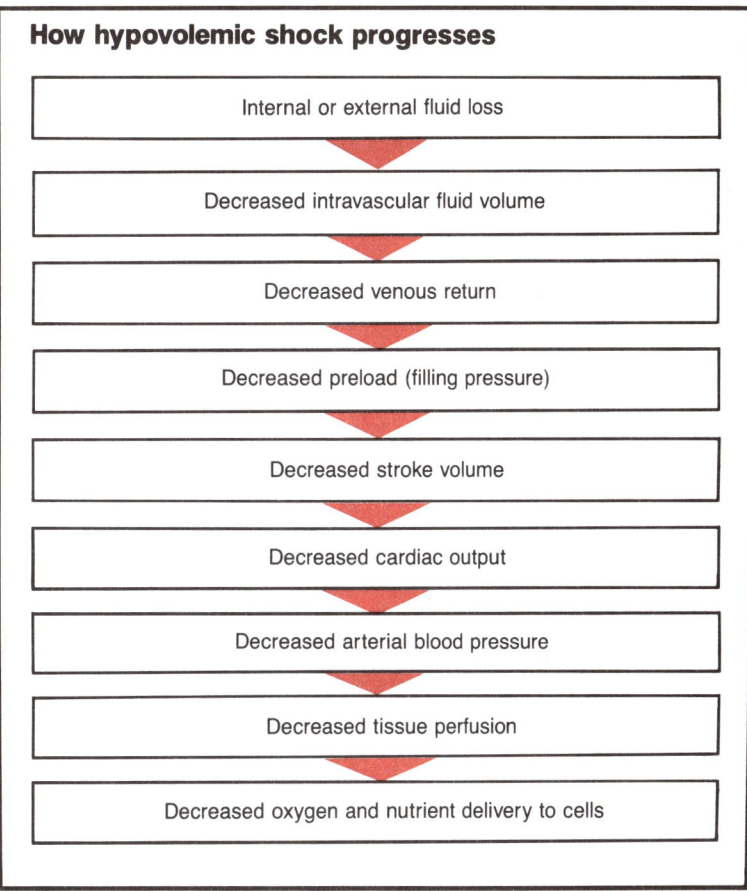

How hypovolemic shock progresses

Internal or external fluid loss
↓
Decreased intravascular fluid volume
↓
Decreased venous return
↓
Decreased preload (filling pressure)
↓
Decreased stroke volume
↓
Decreased cardiac output
↓
Decreased arterial blood pressure
↓
Decreased tissue perfusion
↓
Decreased oxygen and nutrient delivery to cells

Rapid compensatory mechanisms

Rapid compensatory mechanisms take effect 10 to 60 minutes after initial blood or fluid loss. They act primarily to increase mean systemic filling pressures and to improve venous return.

Arteriolar and venous vasoconstriction (resulting from sympathetic compensation) help functionally reduce vascular bed size so that diminished blood volume more completely fills the vascular system. Then the kidneys—selectively sensitive to compensatory vasoconstriction—respond. The afferent arteriole senses reduced pressure and releases renin. Renin undergoes enzymatic conversion to angiotensin (a systemic vasoconstrictor); angiotensin also stimulates aldosterone release, which leads to sodium and water conservation and increases thirst. Rising serum sodium levels (from sodium conservation) stimulate hypothalamic osmoreceptors to release antidiuretic hormone (ADH). This substance acts on kidney tubules, collecting ducts, and (to a lesser degree) the intestinal epithelium, promoting water conservation.

Ultimately, however, these compensatory mechanisms only buy time. Vasoconstriction and hormonal water conservation won't reverse shock without circulating volume replacement. As these mechanisms fail, hypovolemic shock worsens.

5,000 ml of circulating blood volume and can lose up to approximately 10% (500 ml) with little or no blood pressure or cardiac output compromise. However, further loss reduces first cardiac output and then blood pressure. With loss of approximately 40% of total circulating volume, cardiac output and blood pressure fall to zero.

The body strives to maintain homeostasis through compensatory mechanisms. These include:
• sympathetic response. Decreased blood pressure and volume stimulate baroreceptors, which trigger the sympathetic nervous system (SNS) to release epinephrine and norepinephrine. (Keep in mind that some patients, such as the elderly and those under anesthesia, have reduced baroreceptor sensitivity that may inhibit this response.) The SNS attempts to normalize blood pressure by causing *vasoconstriction,* which increases venous return and peripheral resistance, and by *tachycardia,* which boosts cardiac output (see Chapter 1 for details). SNS responses play a protective role; a patient with intact SNS reflexes can lose approximately 35% of his circulating blood volume over a 30-minute period, yet survive with proper treatment. A patient without these reflexes would die after approximately a 20% volume loss. (For this reason, patients receiving sympathetic blocking agents and those with adrenal insufficiency stand a higher risk in hypovolemic shock.) SNS reflexes maintain blood pressure primarily by supporting increased peripheral resistance. However, increased peripheral resistance doesn't improve cardiac output; therefore, as shock worsens, cardiac output falls.

Continued on page 24

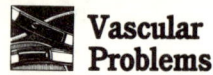

VASCULAR Problems

24 Shock

Hypovolemic Shock

Continued

- central nervous system (CNS) ischemic response. This begins if baroreceptor reflexes fail to maintain mean arterial pressure (MAP) at 50 mm Hg or more. This response attempts to maintain adequate tissue perfusion and blood pressure. However, this response requires considerable metabolic energy just when the body lacks energy sources such as oxygen and glucose. It may also threaten brain cells.
- hormonal response. Stimulation of the renin-angiotensin-aldosterone system and pituitary release of antidiuretic hormone (ADH) cause the kidneys to conserve water and sodium, which leads to increased thirst and salt craving.

In addition to these responses, altered intestinal epithelial permeability promotes water absorption from the intestinal lumen. This helps increase blood volume.

Continued blood or fluid loss or inadequate fluid replacement impairs these compensatory mechanisms, leading to various *decompensatory responses*. Total peripheral resistance (also known as systemic vascular resistance [SVR], or afterload) increases from SNS stimulation, angiotension-promoted vasoconstriction, and increased blood viscosity (from fluid loss without hemorrhage). As total peripheral resistance increases, the heart may fail to push blood forward (fluid flows in the direction of least resistance). Cardiac output and contractility then decrease and myocardial oxygen needs ($M\dot{V}O_2$) increase. The resulting cardiac dysfunction leads to impending cardiac failure. The increased blood viscosity and sluggish blood flow that follow accelerate intravascular clotting, causing disseminated intravascular coagulation (DIC).

Classifying acute hemorrhage

Hemorrhage—escape of intravascular-space blood to an extravascular site—may cause bleeding that's slow or rapid, occult or obvious, chronic or acute. Rapid hemorrhage leading to significant blood loss can trigger hypovolemic shock and diminish blood's oxygen-carrying capacity.

You can seldom judge exactly how much blood a patient may have lost. But assessing his signs and symptoms can help you estimate the loss. Use the table below (based on the American College of Surgeons' classification system) to help correlate your patient's signs and symptoms with blood loss.

	Class I	Class II	Class III	Class IV
Blood loss	up to 750 ml	1,000 to 1,250 ml	1,500 to 1,800 ml	2,000 to 2,500 ml
Blood loss in %[1]	up to 15%	20% to 25%	30% to 35%	40% to 50%
Pulse rate[2]	72 to 84	above 100	above 120	140 or greater
Blood pressure[3]	118/82 mm Hg	110/80 mm Hg	70 to 90/50 to 60 mm Hg	below 50 to 60 mm Hg systolic
Pulse pressure	36 mm Hg	30 mm Hg	20 to 30 mm Hg	10 to 20 mm Hg
Capillary blanch test	Normal	Prolonged	Prolonged	Prolonged
Respiratory rate	14 to 20	20 to 30	30 to 40	above 35
Urine output[4]	30 to 35 ml/hr	25 to 30 ml/hr	5 to 15 ml/hr	Negligible
Central nervous system—mental status	Slightly anxious	Mildly anxious	Anxious and confused	Confused, lethargic
Fluid replacement (use 3:1 rule)	Crystalloid	Crystalloid	Crystalloid + blood	Crystalloid + blood

[1] % of blood in an average 70-kg man
[2] Assume a normal of 72/min
[3] Assume a normal of 120/80
[4] Assume a normal of 40 to 50 ml/hr

Adapted with permission from the *Advanced Trauma Life Support Student Manual*, © 1981 by the American College of Surgeons, Chicago.

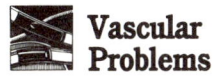
Vascular Problems

25 Shock

Hypovolemic Shock

How hemorrhage causes local responses
If your patient's hypovolemic shock stems from trauma such as a stab wound, expect local as well as systemic compensatory responses. Such local responses, which promote hemostasis and homeostasis, include vessel spasm, platelet aggregation, and clot formation.

Vessel spasm
A broken blood vessel responds by spasmodically contracting to minimize blood loss. Spasm results from stimulation to sympathetic nerves as well as to the involved vessel's smooth-muscle layers. The greater the disruption, the greater the spasm—it can last from a few seconds to 30 minutes.

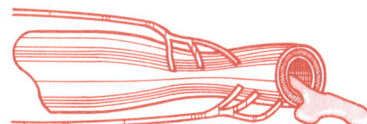

Platelet aggregation
When a blood vessel breaks, circulating platelets flock to the exposed moist, irregular endothelium. They adhere to vessel walls and coalesce, forming a platelet plug. The plug (at least in small vessels) fills the tear but doesn't occlude the vessel.

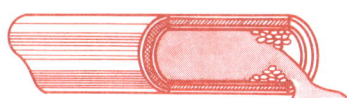

Clot formation
With larger disruptions, bleeding stops only when a clot forms—seconds or minutes after the damaged tissue, altered blood structure, and platelet aggregates together release activator substances. In response, a series of feedback mechanisms lead to fibrin thread formation. These threads, in turn, form a network in which plasma and red blood cells can coalesce into a clot.

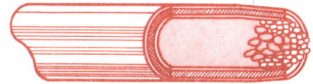

Serum sodium levels rise in response to renin-angiotensin-aldosterone stimulation. Water then moves out of cells toward the bloodstream in an attempt to dilute the solutes. Cells become dehydrated and eventually die, leading to organ failure.

Hypovolemia ultimately causes cellular oxygen deprivation by impairing oxygen delivery, oxygen-carrying capacity, and cellular oxygen utilization.

Assessment
To assess a patient for hypovolemic shock, first try to determine what's caused his condition. Find out whether he's experienced internal or external fluid loss. But remember, hypovolemic shock's an emergency condition, so you'll usually intervene as you perform your assessment. Of course, continue to assess him carefully throughout your care, observing especially for *trends* or changes in his condition. (See Chapter 1 for details on assessing a patient for shock.)

History. Hypovolemic shock and its cause may be obvious. In some cases, however, you'll have to review the patient's history for clues. Check for:
• a history of possible hemorrhage, such as from multiple trauma, GI bleeding, or lacerations (particularly in vascular areas such as the scalp, trachea, perineum, and penis); surgical procedures; or DIC
• conditions associated with external fluid loss, including burns, diabetic ketoacidosis, hyperglycemic hyperosmolar nonketotic coma, diabetes insipidus, and food poisoning
• conditions associated with internal fluid loss, including intestinal obstruction, peritonitis, pancreatitis, cirrhosis, hemothorax, and hemoperitoneum.

Also check for dehydration, which may accompany internal or external fluid loss or reduced fluid intake and may lead to hypovolemia (see *How dehydration can cause shock*, page 26).

You may not have time to obtain a full history, so concentrate on essentials. To quickly gather more information, ask yourself these questions:
• Does the patient have any tissue damage, such as from burns?
• Has he had recent surgery?
• Do you suspect GI bleeding?
• Has he recently experienced prolonged vomiting or diarrhea?
• Has he been taking aspirin or other medications with an anticoagulant effect?
• Has he been taking diuretics? If so, which ones and how often?
• Does he suffer from alcoholism or diabetes?
• Does his job expose him to toxic chemicals or radiation?
• Does he have persistent thirst or complain that his mouth feels dry?
• If you suspect fluid loss, can you determine the source and estimate the volume lost?

Answers to these questions may also provide you with clues to possible complications the patient may develop from hypovolemic shock.

Continued on page 26

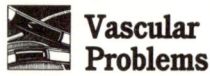

Vascular Problems

26 Shock

Hypovolemic Shock

Hypovolemic shock: Reviewing the causes

External losses
- Whole blood loss from bleeding disorders, surgery, or trauma
- Plasma loss from burns or exudative lesions
- Fluid loss from GI losses, diuresis, or perspiration

Internal losses
- Third-space fluid pooling
- Fluid leakage into intestinal lumen
- Long-bone fracture
- Internal hemorrhage

How dehydration can cause shock

Stay alert for developing hypovolemic shock whenever you assess a dehydrated patient. Suppose, for instance, you're assessing an elderly patient admitted with dehydration. His history includes congestive heart failure controlled with digoxin, furosemide (Lasix), and potassium chloride. He also reports a poor appetite and a 10-lb weight loss over the past 2 weeks. The doctor orders a computed tomography scan with a contrast medium to rule out subdural hematoma (the patient fell several weeks ago). When the patient returns from the radiology department 3 hours later, his condition has worsened and he's developed tachypnea, tachycardia, and hypotension.

Would you suspect hypovolemic shock? You should, given the patient's suggestive history:
- dehydration, a clue to possible intracellular and extracellular fluid loss
- diuretic use, which promotes external fluid loss
- recent weight loss, which may result from poor nutrition. This promotes low colloidal osmotic pressure; fluid tends to move out of the bloodstream and into the interstitial tissue.
- use of diagnostic contrast materials, which have a high osmolarity and promote systemic diuresis.

Continued

Physical examination. Signs and symptoms vary with shock's stage and with the amount and rate of blood or fluid loss. The physical examination can help determine shock's type and cause and can provide baseline information that will help you recognize trends in the patient's condition. While performing the examination, ask yourself questions such as these:
- What's the patient's level of consciousness? Does he appear anxious?
- Does he have rapid, shallow respirations? Do changes in vital signs or behavior accompany such respiratory changes?
- Does his resting pulse exceed 100 beats/minute? Does it feel thready and weak? Does his pulse rate change when he shifts his position?
- What's his blood pressure? Do you note a narrowed (decreased) pulse pressure? Does his blood pressure change when he changes position? (See *Orthostatic vital signs and the tilt test,* page 28.)
- Is his skin cool, clammy, and pale?
- Does he have slow capillary refill?
- Does his urine output measure less than 30 ml/hour (or less than 240 ml/8-hour shift)?

Learn to recognize the signs and symptoms that may occur in hypovolemic shock. These include:
- *hypotension.* Although SNS stimulation may normalize or raise blood pressure initially, hypotension usually develops from reduced cardiac output. (However, keep in mind that a patient with preexisting congestive heart failure [CHF] may not experience effects of SNS stimulation because CHF can diminish the body's responsiveness to catecholamines. Thus, expect this patient to develop hypotension early.)
- *narrowed pulse pressure.* A good blood-flow index, pulse pressure (determined by subtracting diastolic from systolic pressure) narrows, or decreases, in hypovolemic shock. Diastolic pressure rises from vasoconstriction while systolic pressure drops from reduced stroke volume. (Later, as tissue perfusion falls, pulse pressure widens, or increases, as vasoconstrictive compensatory mechanisms fail.)
- *tachycardia.* This takes place in response to SNS stimulation. As heart rate increases, the patient may complain of lightheadedness and palpitations. Peripheral pulses also become weak and thready from widespread vasoconstriction.
- *tachypnea.* Initially, this stems from chemoreceptor stimulation that leads to respiratory alkalosis. Later, it occurs as a compensatory response from direct medullary stimulation caused by metabolic acidosis.
- *irritability and anxiety.* These changes usually occur when hypovolemia develops rapidly. (With rapid hemorrhaging, the patient may become semicomatose.) When hypovolemia develops more slowly, the patient usually experiences heightened awareness or alertness from SNS stimulation. As shock progresses, expect apathy, lethargy, confusion, and coma from metabolic acidosis and decreased cerebral perfusion.
- *cool, pale, clammy, diaphoretic skin.* These changes stem from peripheral vasoconstriction associated with SNS stimulation. They may follow piloerection (gooseflesh), indicating blood shunting away from the skin.

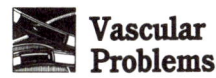

Vascular Problems

27 Shock

Hypovolemic Shock

- *cyanosis.* This usually accompanies significant blood loss.
- *oliguria.* Initially, oliguria stems from reduced renal perfusion; later, from angiotensin, ADH, and aldosterone activity.
- *extreme thirst.* This may accompany decreased extracellular fluid volume; the oral mucosa and tongue become dry. (With extreme blood loss, expect whitened oral mucosa and tongue.)
- *hypothermia.* This develops as inadequate tissue perfusion slows metabolism.
- *angina (chest pain).* Most common in patients with coronary artery disease, angina results from low cardiac output coupled with tachycardia and hypoxemia. These conditions reduce coronary artery perfusion and myocardial oxygenation.

Remember, however, that the patient may not develop signs or symptoms until shock's middle or late stages, when cellular damage has already begun. To help prevent shock from progressing to these stages or to avoid shock's complications, focus early on trends in the patient's condition rather than on individual assessment findings.

Diagnostic studies. Usually, the doctor can't diagnose hypovolemic shock solely from diagnostic findings. For a definitive diagnosis, expect him to correlate test results with the patient's history and physical findings. He'll probably order the following tests if he suspects hypovolemic shock:

Hemoglobin and hematocrit. Values drop abnormally in hypovolemic shock, indicating blood and fluid loss. However, initial values may not reflect such losses. When hypovolemic shock results from volume depletion, hemoglobin and hematocrit levels rise initially from hemoconcentration. Then, as volume's replaced, the hematocrit level drops from hemodilution.

In early hypovolemia, fluids move from the interstitial space into the vascular compartment to maintain homeostasis. In hypovolemic shock caused by hemorrhage, this response leads to an initially normal hematocrit value because the patient has lost proportional amounts of red blood cells (RBCs) and plasma. Then, with transcapillary vascular space refilling, the hematocrit level drops (but usually not for 3 or 4 hours). Although intravascular volume and blood pressure may remain near normal, the patient lacks adequate circulating RBCs to carry oxygen and nutrients.

Hematocrit and hemoglobin levels help the doctor decide which fluids to give: whole blood, packed cells, colloids, or electrolyte solutions. Hemoglobin levels below 9.2 g/dl indicate possible impaired tissue oxygenation and a need for blood. Hematocrit levels below 33% indicate a need for cross-matched blood transfusions; if hematocrit drops below 25%, the doctor may order type-specific blood infusion until cross-matched blood arrives.

Arterial blood gases (ABGs). Initially, these reflect respiratory alkalosis during active SNS compensation to eliminate excess acids (carbon dioxide and lactic acid). A pH above 7.45 and a $PaCO_2$ below 40 mm Hg usually reflect this condition. As hypoxemia progresses to hypoxia, respiratory alkalosis advances to metabolic acidosis. A pH below 7.35, bicarbonate (HCO_3^-) below 25 mm Hg, and oxygen (O_2) saturation below 85% reflect this condition. As shock worsens, $PaCO_2$ rises above 40 mm Hg.

Comparing arterial and venous bleeding

If your patient's bleeding, try to determine the bleeding type—arterial or venous. This may help you identify potential complications.

Arterial bleeding occurs rapidly and produces bright red (oxygenated) blood. Because it's pumped directly from the heart under high pressure, arterial blood spurts with each heartbeat. Rapid exsanguination may result.

Venous bleeding, which occurs more slowly than arterial bleeding, produces dark red (unoxygenated) blood. (However, bleeding esophageal or hemorrhoidal varices produce bright red venous blood.) Moved by gravity flow, venous blood clots more quickly than arterial blood. Therefore, stay alert for disseminated intravascular coagulation.

Continued on page 28

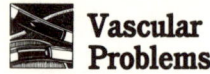

Vascular Problems

28 Shock

Hypovolemic Shock

Continued

Orthostatic vital signs and the tilt test

Orthostatic vital signs and tilt test results may help you assess a patient with possible hypovolemic shock (although you can't rely on them completely).
• *Orthostatic vital signs.* Take your patient's blood pressure and pulse when he's supine, sitting, and standing. (Wait at least 1 minute between each position change.) Consider a systolic blood pressure decrease of 10 mm Hg or more between positions or a pulse rate increase of 10 beats/minute or more a sign of possible volume depletion and impending hypovolemic shock.
• *Tilt test.* With your patient supine, raise his legs above heart level. If his blood pressure rises significantly (indicating autotransfusion from his legs) consider the test positive, indicating volume depletion and possible hypovolemic shock.

Serum lactic acid. Levels rise above normal as cellular metabolism continues with low tissue oxygenation.

Blood urea nitrogen (BUN) and serum creatinine. Levels rise above normal from inadequate renal perfusion.

Serum potassium. Levels rise above normal, possibly from oliguria, inadequate renal perfusion, cellular breakdown associated with GI tract blood loss, and tissue necrosis.

Serum sodium. Levels may rise above normal from dehydration.

Urine specific gravity and urine osmolality. Values rise abnormally with volume depletion.

Urine creatinine clearance. Values drop below normal with reduced renal perfusion.

White blood cell count. Values may initially rise above normal in response to stress; however, persistent elevation suggests developing infection.

EKG (continuous monitoring and 12-lead). Any changes may stem from decreased coronary blood flow.

Chest X-ray. Findings may reveal changes in the patient's pulmonary status.

Invasive hemodynamic monitoring. This technique helps evaluate trends in the patient's condition. *Note:* Assume an increased or decreased value reflects a change from the patient's *baseline* reading—not necessarily a value outside normal range.

Expect any of the following hemodynamic findings for a patient with hypovolemic shock: decreased central venous pressure (CVP) or right atrial pressure, decreased cardiac output, decreased pulmonary artery pressures (PAPs; in a patient with pulmonary disease, PAPs may rise above baseline), decreased pulmonary capillary wedge pressure (PCWP; in a patient with left heart failure, PCWP may rise above baseline), and increased SVR. CVP and PCWP values also help evaluate fluid replacement's effects.

The doctor may also order MAP readings. MAP of 80 mm Hg or more indicates adequate blood flow to maintain tissue perfusion; MAP below 80 mm Hg usually signifies inadequate perfusion.

Tissue perfusion parameters. These serve as the best predictors of hypovolemic shock's progression because they track blood and tissue oxygenation and oxygen-carrying capacity. The most useful parameter—*efficiency of tissue oxygen extraction (ETOE)*—reflects arteriovenous oxygen difference (a-vDO_2) divided by the red cell mass. ETOE predicts survivability in most cases. (For more information on diagnostic tests for hypovolemic shock, see Chapter 1.)

Planning

Nursing care priorities for a patient with hypovolemic shock include providing blood volume expansion (by administering blood, plasma expanders, albumin, or electrolyte solutions, as ordered); providing adequate ventilation and preventing further pulmonary complications; maintaining circulation (by evaluating hemodynamic parameters, cardiac rhythm, and organ function and by implementing

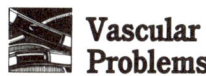

Vascular Problems

29 Shock

Hypovolemic Shock

corrective interventions, as ordered); recognizing acid-base imbalance and correcting it, as ordered; and providing psychological support to the patient and his family.

Nursing diagnoses. Before determining your nursing care plan, develop the nursing diagnosis by identifying your patient's problem or potential problem, then relating it to its cause. Possible nursing diagnoses for a patient with hypovolemic shock include:
• tissue perfusion, alteration in; related to blood's reduced oxygen-carrying capacity, caused by blood loss
• anxiety; related to SNS stimulation and fear of the unknown
• fear; related to feeling of impending doom
• cardiac output, alteration in (decreased); related to reduced circulating blood volume
• fluid volume, alteration in (deficit); related to internal or external blood or fluid loss
• nutrition, alteration in (less than body requirements); related to inadequate nutrient circulation
• sensory perception, alteration in; related to reduced brain oxygenation
• powerlessness; related to life-threatening event
• oral mucous membranes, alteration in; related to hypovolemia and rapid respirations.

The sample nursing care plan below shows expected outcomes, nursing interventions, and discharge planning for one nursing diagnosis listed above. However, you'll want to tailor each care plan to the patient's needs.

Continued on page 30

Sample nursing care plan: Hypovolemic shock

Nursing diagnosis	Expected outcomes
Tissue perfusion, alteration in; related to blood's reduced oxygen-carrying capacity, caused by blood loss	The patient will: • maintain an adequate hemoglobin level. • maintain an adequate PaO_2 level. • maintain an adequate mean arterial pressure (MAP). • maintain a urine output of at least 30 ml/hour.
Nursing interventions • Assess patient's vital signs and level of consciousness every 5 to 15 minutes until he's stable. • Monitor fluid intake and output. Assess urine output every hour. Notify the doctor if output drops below 30 ml/hour. • Assess for effects of fluid, oxygen, and drug administration. • If indicated, warm blood before administration. • Position patient to promote blood return to vital organs. • Monitor hemoglobin and hematocrit levels. Report hemoglobin less than 10 g/dl and hematocrit less than 30%. • If possible, assess hemodynamic parameters every 30 minutes to 1 hour during rapid fluid resuscitation. Assess cardiac output every 2 to 4 hours. • If data's available, calculate cardiac index, a-vDO_2, and SVR. • Monitor and assess ABGs. • If patient's using medical antishock trousers (MAST), assess for effectiveness and complications.	**Discharge planning** Depends on treatment outcome

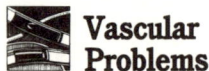
Vascular Problems

30 Shock

Hypovolemic Shock

Continued

Intervention
Treatment goals for the patient with hypovolemic shock include maintaining his airway, breathing, and circulation; providing definitive care by identifying and correcting the cause of his blood or fluid loss; and providing supportive care by maintaining adequate tissue perfusion until treatment takes effect.

To provide definitive care, first identify the blood or fluid loss site. With hemorrhage, intervene as necessary to control bleeding quickly. Also try to identify any internal injuries. The patient may need immediate surgical repair or hemostasis. With severe dehydration, intervene as ordered to correct the underlying cause.

Because hypovolemic shock can stem from various causes, initial treatment will focus on correcting hypovolemia from blood or fluid loss and correcting hypoxemia. Then—because most deaths from hypovolemic shock result from complications—further treatment

---

Using pressure points to control bleeding

If your patient's bleeding from an artery, immediately try to control the bleeding by applying direct pressure to the wound. If this technique doesn't work, apply pressure to the appropriate pressure point, as described below.

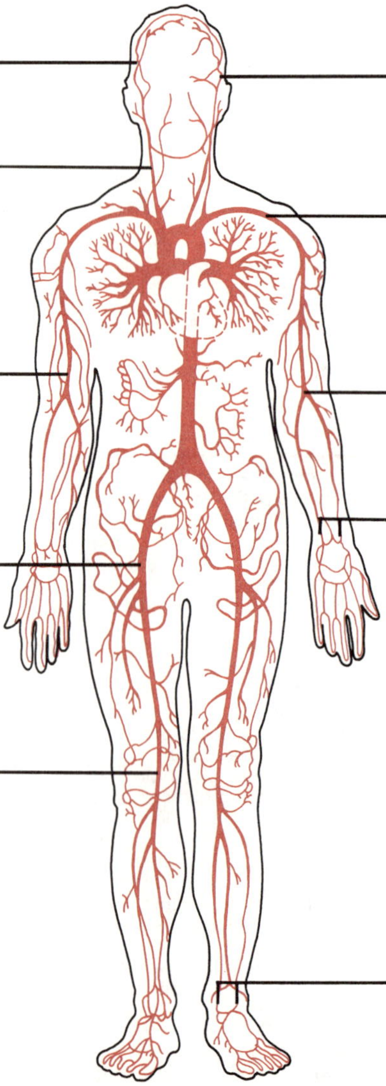

Scalp or temple
Compress the temporal arteries.

Neck
Compress the wound site. But take care not to compress a carotid artery (unless it's the wound site); this may cause cerebral ischemia or cardiac dysrhythmias, possibly resulting in cardiac arrest. Also avoid pressure on the trachea or you'll obstruct the airway.

Elbow or arm just above elbow
Press the brachial artery against the humerus.

Thigh
Press the femoral artery against the femur.

Lower leg
Compress the popliteal artery, located behind the knee.

Face below eyes
Compress the facial artery.

Shoulder or upper arm
Press the subclavian artery against the clavicle.

Lower arm
Compress the ulnar and radial arteries at the antecubital fossa.

Hand
Compress the ulnar and radial arteries at the wrist.

Foot
Apply pressure to all ankle arteries.

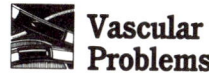

Vascular Problems

31 Shock

Hypovolemic Shock

focuses on correcting the pathophysiologic conditions associated with poor tissue perfusion. Specific interventions include:
• correcting acid-base imbalance
• administering inotropic agents, vasodilators, and other drugs, if needed
• correcting fluid overload associated with initial treatment
• correcting persistent oliguria
• providing nutritional support
• controlling or preventing infection
• providing psychological support.

Correcting hypovolemia from blood loss. Your patient may have hypovolemia from *hemorrhage*—caused by rapid blood loss or slow, uncorrected blood loss. Look for the bleeding site and apply direct pressure over it (see *Using pressure points to control bleeding*). As ordered, initiate I.V. fluid replacement as soon as possible.

Blood pressure and pulse readings can confirm hypotension and tachycardia. However, don't waste precious moments taking vital signs. If the patient's conscious and responsive, assume he has adequate arterial pressure for tissue oxygenation. Position him appropriately (see *Patient positioning: A weapon against shock*, page 33) and insert an I.V. catheter, as ordered, for immediate fluid resuscitation. If the patient's semicomatose, assume he's suffered impaired tissue oxygenation and begin fluid resuscitation immediately. This improves oxygen delivery and tissue oxygen consumption by increasing cardiac output. Use short 14G or 16G I.V. catheters in the patient's forearms or upper arms. Assist with placement of CVP and pulmonary artery (PA) lines.

Until transfusion blood arrives and more specific hemodynamic monitoring can be established, the doctor will probably order crystalloid infusion (lactated Ringer's solution or normal saline solution) at a rate that maintains MAP of at least 80 mm Hg and pulse rate below 120. Stay alert for increased fluid volume (hypervolemia) during this initial fluid replacement stage (before CVP or PA line placement). Use this method to evaluate fluid's effects on the heart's right side: Find a position your patient can tolerate. Then observe his jugular veins for distention. If you note distention, mark across the veins with a pen at this point. As you infuse fluid, quickly compare the distention with the preresuscitation level. A 2″ to 2¾″ (5 to 7 cm) vertical increase indicates either increased circulating blood volume or impaired right-heart pumping ability. Decrease the infusion rate slightly and recheck blood pressure, pulse, and level of consciousness. Auscultate lung bases for crackles and wheezes and the heart for ventricular or atrial (S_3 or S_4) gallops.

Alternatively, the doctor may order infusion of plasma protein fraction, fresh-frozen plasma, or hetastarch (Hespan) until blood's available. Once blood arrives, expect to administer whole blood (in most cases) or packed RBCs (see *Administering blood: Some important guidelines*, pages 40 and 41, and *Guide to blood products*, page 32). The choice depends on the degree of the patient's hypoproteinemia, his preshock condition, and other factors. Packed RBCs may be used for a patient with compromised cardiac function or for one who's received a relatively large volume (0.5 to 1 liter) of plasma protein fraction, fresh-frozen plasma, or Hespan. Blood processing

Continued on page 33

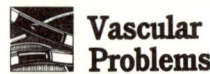

Vascular Problems

32 Shock

Hypovolemic Shock

Guide to blood products

You may be asked to administer whole blood, packed red blood cells (RBCs), plasma, or platelets to a patient with hypovolemic shock. The chart below describes these blood products and reviews benefits and nursing considerations for each. But before studying the chart, refresh your memory of blood groups, Rh typing, and cross-matching.

Blood groups can be differentiated by the antigens (agglutinogens) found on RBC surfaces and the antibodies (agglutinins) found in plasma. Group A blood has A antigens only; group B, B antigens only; group AB, both A and B antigens; and group O, neither A nor B antigens. The person with AB blood lacks plasma antibodies for A and B antigens. Because he can receive any blood type, he's called a *universal recipient*. A person with group O blood has no A or B antigens. His blood won't cause an antibody attack when given to someone with another blood type, so he's called a *universal donor*.

Rh typing determines whether the patient's RBCs contain the Rh factor. *Rh positive* blood contains the Rh factor, *Rh negative* blood lacks it.

Cross-matching assures donor–recipient blood compatibility by mixing specimens together after blood group and Rh factor typing. In an emergency, you may have to administer O-negative blood *before* typing and cross-matching or until proper blood units arrive. However, watch for indications of a transfusion reaction when administering blood that hasn't been properly cross-matched.

Blood product	Benefits	Nursing considerations
Whole blood 500 ml/unit of complete blood (RBCs, leukocytes, plasma, platelets, clotting factors)	• Restores intravascular volume • Improves blood's oxygen-carrying capacity (after several hours)	• Transfuse according to hospital policy and procedure. • Transfuse within 2 to 4 hours after hanging transfusion bag, or as indicated. • Make sure blood's been typed and cross-matched. • Check patient's identification and donor blood unit information before transfusion. • Warm blood before administration. • If possible, give fresh, whole blood rather than stored, banked blood. • Stay alert for transfusion reactions.
Packed red blood cells (PRBCs) *Fresh:* 300 ml/unit of RBCs; about 20% plasma; some leukocytes and platelets *Frozen* (also called leukocyte-poor): 200 to 250 ml/unit of RBCs; no plasma; few leukocytes or platelets	• Helps restore blood volume (especially RBCs) while preventing fluid overload • Improves blood's oxygen-carrying capacity • Reduces risk of metabolic complications	• Transfuse according to hospital policy and procedure. • Transfuse within 2 to 4 hours after hanging transfusion bag, or as indicated. • Make sure blood's been typed and cross-matched. • Check patient's identification and blood unit information before transfusion. • Increased PRBC viscosity causes slow infusion rate. If patient requires rapid infusion, inject normal saline solution into blood bag. • Give 1 unit of fresh-frozen plasma for every 4 units of PRBCs to replenish clotting factors. • Stay alert for transfusion reactions.
Plasma 200 ml/unit of fresh or fresh-frozen plasma (contains all clotting factors except platelets)	• Restores clotting factors (except platelets) • Expands plasma volume	• Transfuse according to hospital policy and procedure. • Transfuse within 2 hours after hanging transfusion bag. • Make sure donor plasma and recipient blood have been typed for ABO and Rh compatibility. • Administer fresh-frozen plasma promptly after thawing to prevent clotting-factor deterioration.
Platelets (platelet concentration) Platelet sediment from platelet-rich plasma, resuspended in 30 to 50 ml of plasma	• Restores platelets • Maintains normal blood coagulability • Helps control bleeding by aiding clot formation	• Transfuse according to hospital policy and procedure. • Transfuse as rapidly as possible. • Make sure donor plasma and recipient blood have been typed for ABO and Rh compatibility. (However, platelets rarely cause hemolytic reactions because platelet concentration contains few RBCs.) • Use a nonwettable filter.

Vascular Problems

33 Shock

Hypovolemic Shock

Continued

techniques increase packed RBC hematocrit from about 30% (whole blood) to about 70% for each unit. As a rule of thumb, hematocrit rises about 4% and hemoglobin rises about 1 g% for each unit of packed RBCs you administer. A patient with a serum albumin level below 2 g% usually requires whole blood.

Follow hospital policy and procedure when administering blood and always give the freshest blood available. Blood cells die as donor blood ages; these cells then liberate harmful acidic substances (potassium and ammonia). Also, coagulation factors (especially platelets and factors V and VIII) decrease in stored whole blood, as does 2,3-diphosphoglycerate (2,3-DPG) content. Decreased 2,3-DPG content inhibits oxygen release by hemoglobin and thus reduces oxygen release to tissues. The patient receiving massive stored blood transfusions may experience metabolic acidosis, hyperkalemia, or coagulation abnormalities that exacerbate shock's long-term effects and lead to complications (reduced tissue perfusion causes anaerobic cellular metabolism).

Other alternatives for the hemorrhaging patient include autotransfusion (see *Autotransfusion: Reviewing benefits and risks,* page 35) and use of medical antishock trousers (MAST) (see *How the MAST suit works,* page 36). The doctor probably won't order colloids for a hemorrhaging patient because they impair coagulation.

Correcting hypovolemia from fluid loss. If your patient's hypovolemic from fluid loss, he'll need both crystalloids and colloids—in most cases, you can expect to administer a mix of 2 liters of crystalloid to 1 liter of colloid. The amount you administer depends on the patient's hemodynamic parameters (such as PaO_2 and $a\text{-}vDO_2$); hemoglobin, hematocrit, and serum albumin values; and clotting factors.

Commonly used crystalloids include lactated Ringer's solution and normal saline solution. Lactated Ringer's solution provides nearly balanced electrolytes. However, doctors disagree about the use of lactated Ringer's solution in hypovolemic shock. Some believe it helps reverse lactic acidosis; others believe it exacerbates lactic acidosis as cellular metabolism becomes anaerobic. (*Note:* Although lactate eventually metabolizes into sodium bicarbonate, it's more stable than sodium bicarbonate, which may precipitate with calcium preparations.)

Normal saline solution helps replace water and salt and may also include selected deficit electrolytes to provide replacement and avoid further dilution. Alternatively, the doctor may order dextrose 5% in normal saline solution (D_5NS), to provide minimal calories (200 calories/liter); or dextrose 5% in half-normal (0.45% NaCl) saline solution ($D_5\frac{1}{2}NS$), most commonly given for patients with known cardiovascular, renal, or liver disease who can't tolerate excess sodium. However, the doctor *won't* order a dextrose solution through the same tubing with a blood transfusion.

Colloids include serum albumin, plasma protein fraction, dextran, and Hespan. To review colloids and crystalloids, read *Guide to commonly used volume expanders,* page 34.

Continued on page 35

Patient positioning: A weapon against shock

When caring for a patient with hypovolemic shock, consider correct patient positioning a priority. The supine position's usually best because it helps direct blood flow to the brain and other vital organs. But you may have to modify this position—in some cases, elevating the legs 20° to 30° may facilitate blood flow to vital organs. However, if you suspect a brain injury, use low Fowler's position to help prevent brain edema and increased intracranial pressure.

Avoid placing your patient in Trendelenburg's position—it encourages vasoconstriction, reduces venous return from the head, inhibits respiration, and hinders blood flow from the lungs to the left atrium.

Vascular Problems

34 Shock

Hypovolemic Shock

Guide to commonly used volume expanders

Volume expanders—crystalloids and colloids—work by refilling the patient's vascular space, increasing his cardiac output, and perfusing his tissues. They don't carry oxygen or replace blood, but they can provide volume expansion, protein, and electrolytes in an emergency. Crystalloids, solutions of low-molecular-weight particles, act quickly to expand plasma volume but last only a short time in the plasma. Colloids, solutions of high-molecular-weight particles, take effect more slowly than crystalloids but have a longer life in the plasma (so you'll give them less frequently). However, colloids increase the risk of fluid shift and overload. The chart below will help you review some commonly used volume expanders.

Solution	Benefits	Nursing considerations
CRYSTALLOIDS		
Normal saline solution 250, 500, or 1,000 ml/unit; 0.9% sodium chloride in water	• Replaces lost body fluids with isotonic solution • Increases plasma volume if patient has adequate red cell mass	• Watch for fluid retention and overload caused by high sodium content. • Use cautiously in patients with congestive heart failure (CHF), renal dysfunction, or hypoproteinemia. • Monitor serum electrolytes and acid-base balance for possible hypernatremia, hypokalemia, and hyperchloremic metabolic acidosis.
Lactated Ringer's solution (Hartmann's solution) 200, 500, or 1,000 ml/unit; 0.9% sodium chloride in water with added electrolytes and buffers (potassium, calcium, and lactate)	• Replaces lost body fluids with isotonic solution • Helps prevent lactic acidosis in aerobic metabolism	• Watch for fluid retention and overload caused by high sodium content. • Use cautiously in patients with CHF, renal dysfunction, pulmonary edema, circulatory insufficiency, or hypoproteinemia. • Monitor for lactic acidosis. During anaerobic metabolism (which may occur in shock), lactate content contributes to acidosis.
COLLOIDS		
Serum albumin (Albuminate) 250 or 500 ml/unit of 5% aqueous fraction of pooled plasma in buffered saline solution; or 25, 50, or 100 ml/unit of 25% aqueous fraction of pooled plasma (salt-poor)	• Increases serum colloid osmotic pressure (draws fluid from interstitial space into intravascular space) • Expands plasma volume rapidly • Helps correct hypoproteinemia • Reduces risk of allergic reactions and hepatitis • Doesn't require typing or cross-matching	• Watch for signs and symptoms of fluid overload. • Use with caution in patients with CHF. • Don't open bottles until you're ready to start the infusion; bottles contain no preservative. • Be sure to give correct concentration—5% albumin osmotically equals plasma; 25% albumin (hyperosmotic) expands plasma volume more quickly.
Plasma protein fraction (PPF) (Plasmanate, Plasma-plex) 250 or 500 ml/unit of 5% human plasma proteins in normal saline solution	• Expands plasma volume • Increases serum colloid osmotic pressure • Helps correct hypoproteinemia • Reduces hepatitis risk • Doesn't require typing or cross-matching	• Watch for signs and symptoms of fluid overload. • Use cautiously in patients with CHF or renal failure. • Infuse no faster than 10 ml/minute. • Check for adverse effects such as hypotension, especially with rapid administration. • Solution contains no clotting factors.
Dextran 500 ml/unit; glucose polysaccharide solution of low molecular weight (Dextran-40, Rheomacrodex, Gentran 40); or higher molecular weight (Dextran-70, Macrodex, Gentran 70-75) in normal saline solution or dextrose 5% in water	• Expands plasma volume rapidly • Reduces risk of allergic reactions	• Watch for signs and symptoms of fluid overload. • Use cautiously in patients with CHF or pulmonary edema. • Avoid using in patients with active hemorrhage or bleeding disorders (at risk for altered platelet adhesiveness). • Dextran may interfere with blood typing and cross-matching if enzyme method's used; draw blood samples for typing and cross-matching *before* starting infusion. • Because dextran may cause renal failure, monitor urine output during infusion. Dextran alters urine osmolarity and specific gravity. • If ordered, give Dextran 1 (Promet) prophylactically to protect against dextran-induced anaphylaxis.
Hetastarch (Hespan, Volex) 500 ml/unit of 6% solution of synthetic polymer of hydroxethyl starch in normal saline solution	• Expands plasma volume for up to 36 hours • Increases serum colloid osmotic pressure • Reduces risk of allergic reactions and hepatitis • Won't interfere with blood typing or cross-matching	• Watch for signs and symptoms of fluid overload. • Use with caution in patients with CHF or compromised renal function. • Monitor clotting times and platelet counts for indications of coagulation disturbance. • Monitor serum albumin levels for decrease below normal.

Vascular Problems
35 Shock

Hypovolemic Shock

Continued

When administering crystalloids or colloids to restore fluids to a patient with nonhemorrhagic shock, place several 16G or 18G I.V. catheters, as ordered, and reserve one line for medications. Infuse solutions as ordered. However, be sure to consider each intervention in light of other treatments your patient's receiving. For instance, if his shock worsens while he's receiving I.V. fluids, you may be tempted to open the I.V. clamp for rapid infusion. But most I.V. solutions contain potassium supplements, so rapid infusion could lead to a dangerously high potassium chloride dose just when hypoperfusion has impaired his renal function. Before administering any drug, ask yourself: Would rapid infusion (if ordered) exacerbate shock? Could the drug's effects negate the value of other interventions?

Correcting hypoxemia. Make sure your patient has an open, patent, unobstructed airway. Airway obstruction may result from:
- a relaxed tongue, caused by a decreased level of consciousness as shock worsens
- pharyngeal secretion accumulation (in a comatose or semicomatose patient)
- blood pooling from nasal, tracheal, or laryngeal fracture
- broken teeth.

Clear the patient's airway as necessary, then begin oxygen therapy as ordered. Provide oxygen sufficient to maintain arterial O_2 (PaO_2) greater than 60 mm Hg. Administer a fraction of inspired oxygen (FIO_2) of 0.35 to 0.40 through a nasopharyngeal catheter, nasal cannula, or mask. Remember, however, that FIO_2 administration above 0.40 for prolonged periods leads to oxygen toxicity and respiratory changes that promote dysfunctional alveoli and reduce lung compliance. Therefore, administer the lowest oxygen amount necessary to achieve a PaO_2 of at least 80 mm Hg. Make sure to provide good oral care—oxygen therapy exacerbates the dry mouth that accompanies hypovolemia. Use lemon-glycerine swabs or ice chips to promote comfort and prevent mouth ulcers.

Keep in mind that the patient needs an adequate hemoglobin level to transport oxygen effectively. Otherwise, raising his FIO_2 may not improve his PaO_2. Also remember that chronic obstructive pulmonary disease (COPD) results in a breathing stimulus triggered by below-normal PaO_2 levels. If your patient has COPD, give him oxygen cautiously and monitor his PaO_2 levels closely.

Throughout your care, keep artificial airways and suctioning equipment at the patient's bedside. If his condition deteriorates, he may need endotracheal intubation and mechanical ventilation.

Correcting acid-base imbalance. Hypovolemia can cause various acid-base imbalances. Initially, your patient will probably have *respiratory alkalosis*. However, as shock progresses, he may develop *metabolic acidosis*. This condition may correct itself as cellular perfusion improves. However, if it persists despite adequate fluid replacement, expect the doctor to order sodium bicarbonate.

Continued on page 36

Autotransfusion: Reviewing benefits and risks

Autotransfusion—now performed in many hospitals—involves collection, filtration, and infusion of a patient's own blood. Used most commonly for patients with chest wounds, it's also an option for patients with hypovolemic shock from hemorrhage, for those with rare blood types, and for those with religious objections to banked blood transfusions. It's fast, safe, and may be used before and after surgery.

Autotransfusion has many advantages. The patient gets compatible blood—his own—and avoids the risk of complications such as transfusion reactions, disease transmission, and isoimmunization. And because the blood's fresh, it has normal levels of potassium, ammonia, hydrogen ions, and 2,3-diphosphoglycerate (2,3-DPG), which helps deliver oxygen to tissues.

An autotransfusion system typically consists of a disposable sterile liner contained in a rigid plastic canister. The liner has two chambers: an upper chamber that collects, filters (through a 170-micron screen), and anticoagulates the blood; and a lower chamber that serves as a reservoir with a 1,900 ml capacity. Special suction tubing mixes an anticoagulant solution (such as citrate phosphate dextrose [CPD]) with blood as it's collected.

After blood's collected (for example, suctioned from the patient's chest via a chest tube), the liner's disconnected from the suction source and compressed to remove the air. Then the blood's infused by gravity or by a pump through a line with a microemboli filter. As soon as the liner's removed, another line primed with CPD can be attached to the system to begin collecting more blood. A broad-spectrum antibiotic may be given to help prevent infection.

Autotransfusion's contraindicated if the patient has a cancerous lesion in the hemorrhage area or if the blood's contaminated with GI secretions such as bile, feces, or other abdominal contents (these could lead to emboli or sepsis).

Vascular Problems

36 Shock

Hypovolemic Shock

How the MAST suit works

The medical antishock trousers (MAST) suit—made of strong, waterproof radiolucent nylon—has three chambers, one for each leg and one for the abdomen. Each chamber can be inflated separately with a foot pump to a pressure of about 104 mm Hg, and each has a pressure-release valve to prevent overinflation (some models have a pressure gauge). Foot and ankle openings allow easy assessment of pedal circulation and permit saphenous vein access. A perineal opening permits bladder catheterization. MAST suits come in adult and child sizes.

Until recently, researchers assumed that a MAST suit produced autotransfusion, squeezing 500 to 2,000 ml of the patient's blood from his legs into his central circulation. However, new research shows that mean arterial pressure rises not from pooled venous blood being forced into the chest cavity and head, but from increased peripheral vascular resistance under the suit.

The MAST suit's generally recommended for such uses as hypovolemia with systolic blood pressure of 90 mm Hg or less; bleeding site compression; and leg and pelvis splinting. The suit may also be used cautiously for pregnant and head-injured patients—contraindicated uses just a few years ago—and during cardiopulmonary resuscitation (CPR). The suit's also been shown to help save victims of cardiopulmonary arrest (although the American Heart Association hasn't firmly recommended this use).

The MAST suit *shouldn't* be used if it would cover a protruding bone fragment or foreign object; if the patient has severe flexion contractures; or if you suspect the patient has cardiogenic shock. Doctors disagree on its use for a patient with severely compromised respiration, as with chronic obstructive pulmonary disease or pneumothorax.

Here's how to inflate and deflate a MAST suit:

Inflation. Position the suit on the patient so that the abdominal chamber's top just touches the lower rib margin. Then, strap on the suit and begin inflating it with the foot pump. Inflate the leg chambers first, then the abdominal chamber. As the suit inflates, check the patient's blood pressure every 15 seconds. Use this as your guide; if blood pressure starts rising after you've inflated one or both leg chambers, you may not need to inflate the abdominal chamber.

If the patient's conscious during inflation, he may complain of respiratory discomfort. As pressure in the suit builds, he may even vomit or defecate. Reassure him that the MAST suit normally causes a feeling of extreme pressure on the legs and abdomen.

After inflation, monitor the patient's vital signs closely and check his blood pressure every minute. Also check his apical pulse, lung sounds, skin color and temperature, and peripheral pulses for signs of fluid overload or constricted peripheral circulation. (*Note:* MAST therapy duration depends on the patient's condition and response to treatment.)

Deflation. *Never* cut a MAST suit off a patient. And don't deflate it until his circulating volume has been restored, he's stabilized, or he's ready to undergo surgery. Suit inflation compresses the patient's lower venous system, inducing lactic acidosis in his legs. This produces carbon dioxide, a potent vasodilator. Rapid deflation will cause carbon dioxide to dilate leg veins and increase the vascular bed enough to cause severe hypotension.

Deflate the MAST suit *gradually* before removing it. Start with the abdominal chamber and continue with the leg chambers one at a time. Monitor the patient's blood pressure after each release of air. If it drops by 5 mm Hg or more, reinflate the chamber and administer I.V. solutions as ordered to increase circulating volume. Continue gradual deflation only when his blood pressure's stable. Deflate a MAST suit rapidly *only* if the patient suffers an abdominal catastrophe and needs immediate surgery.

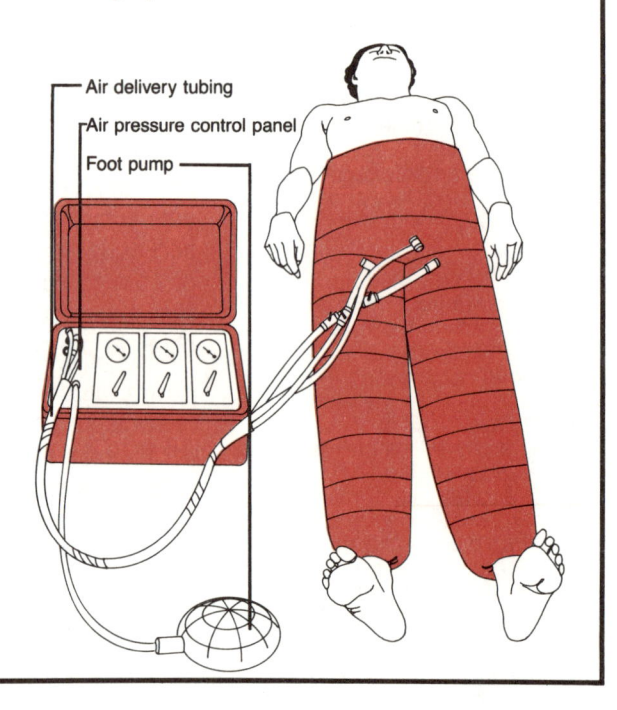

- Air delivery tubing
- Air pressure control panel
- Foot pump

Continued

Calculate your patient's bicarbonate deficit by multiplying his base deficit by his extracellular water volume (5 gal [20 liters] for a man weighing 154 lb [70 kg]). (*Note:* Lactated Ringer's solution contributes only half its base dose toward this deficit.) Give half the sodium bicarbonate dose over 1 to 2 hours, as ordered, then recheck his pH. Administer the remaining dose at 1 mEq/minute and titrate this against pH levels measured every 30 minutes (but use caution to avoid a bicarbonate excess that could trigger metabolic alkalosis).

37 Shock

Hypovolemic Shock

Artificial blood

Researchers continue to investigate the use of artificial blood (blood substitutes) for life-threatening emergencies. Fluosol-DA, the most commonly used substance, contains electrolytes, plasma expanders, and chemicals that carry oxygen; however, it lacks clotting factors. Clinical trials show that Fluosol contributes significantly to oxygen delivery only when given with high fraction-inspired oxygen. Fluosol's oxygen-carrying capacity appears to last about 72 hours. However, it may interfere with normal regulatory microcirculatory mechanisms, making it less useful for treating shock. Currently, it's used only in designated medical centers.

Use a separate I.V. line, if possible, to administer sodium bicarbonate. Given cautiously, sodium bicarbonate improves other drugs' effects by optimizing acid-base level and improving organ performance. However, the high sodium load may cause excess fluid retention and contribute to heart failure. Also, because it's hypertonic, sodium bicarbonate may change serum osmolarity. Therefore, assess your patient continuously for metabolic alkalosis during and after administration.

Metabolic alkalosis may also result from:
- excessive gastric fluid loss from suctioning or vomiting
- massive citrated blood administration (6 to 24 hours after administration)
- impaired sodium bicarbonate removal by the kidney
- massive steroid therapy.

If this occurs, expect to administer lysine hydrochloride; or, if the bicarbonate level rises above 35 mEq/L, ammonium chloride or hydrogen chloride. The doctor may also order treatments for hypokalemia and hypophosphatemia to help correct metabolic alkalosis.

Hypoxia, which accompanies hypovolemia, may result in *respiratory acidosis* with an elevated $PaCO_2$. Respiratory acidosis may also stem from increased alveolar ventilation associated with SNS or hypoxemic compensation. Mechanical ventilation will improve the patient's condition until fluid and sodium bicarbonate resuscitation take effect. If your patient's already on a mechanical ventilator, adding respiratory dead space may correct the problem.

Administering drugs. The doctor may order inotropic agents, vasodilators, or other drugs to help correct your patient's hypovolemic shock. *Inotropic agents* (most commonly low-dose dopamine [Intropin]) improve myocardial contractility and cardiac output. Usually, you'll give these only to a patient with compromised cardiac function. Because inotropic drugs increase myocardial oxygen consumption, the patient's cardiac status may deteriorate from high doses, low preload, tachycardia, or excessively elevated afterload or SVR. These drugs may also exacerbate hypokalemia, partial or complete heart block, and ventricular ectopy. Make sure to start fluid replacement before or during inotropic drug administration. Use an I.V. infusion pump to ensure accurate doses and monitor the patient's response, as ordered, with an EKG and indwelling (Foley) and PA catheters. Titrate the dose according to hemodynamic parameters and urinary output. If you're giving dopamine, keep in mind that this drug has a differential dose-related activity. Titrated doses of 2 to 5 mcg/kg/minute usually cause renal and mesenteric vasodilation, resulting in diuresis. Titrated doses of 5 to 10 mcg/kg/minute usually lead to increased cardiac output and blood pressure without changing SVR. Monitor the patient for increased tachycardia, which may negate cardiac output gains. Doses exceeding 10 mcg/kg/minute produce effects that worsen blood flow to the myocardium and kidney and directly increase tachycardia.

Vasodilators such as nitroglycerin and sodium nitroprusside (Nipride) dilate coronary arteries and increase oxygen delivery. Give titrated nitroglycerin as an I.V. drip at 5 to 10 mcg/minute, increased by 5 to 10 mcg increments every 5 minutes, or as ordered. This helps

Continued on page 38

Vascular Problems

38 Shock

Hypovolemic Shock

Continued

reduce afterload and dilate coronary arteries and may improve cardiac contractility in a patient receiving fluid resuscitation. Titrate the dose to reduce afterload without increasing preload; reduce the dose, as ordered, if the patient develops hypotension, tachycardia, dizziness, and headache. Or, give sodium nitroprusside (Nipride), as ordered, to reduce afterload (however, this drug can cause hypotension). A small, carefully titrated dose (3 to 5 mcg/kg/minute) usually lowers systolic blood pressure by 5 to 10 mm Hg. Additional benefits include coronary artery dilation and increased oxygen delivery. Watch the patient closely for signs and symptoms of thiocyanate toxicity; for example, fatigue, anorexia, weakness, hallucinations, delirium, skin rash, and tinnitus. If you notice these, inform the doctor immediately—the patient may die unless given the antidote (sodium thiosulfate).

Other drugs you may administer include isoproterenol (Isuprel), digitalis, dobutamine (Dobutrex), norepinephrine (Levophed), and epinephrine (Adrenalin). Give these with extreme caution and only in conjunction with fluid therapy. Closely assess the patient's response to the medication. Use of vasoconstrictors (vasopressors) and vasodilators remains controversial—vasopressors given early in shock increase compensatory vasoconstriction and may close arterioles and halt blood flow. Vasodilators increase vascular bed size and may exacerbate hypovolemia.

Occasionally, the doctor may order steroids—corticosteroids and glucocorticoids—to treat hypovolemic shock. *Corticosteroids* help protect cell membranes and reduce inflammation from stress. Steroidal effects on peripheral vasodilation may increase blood flow to poorly perfused organs. And corticosteroids cause sodium and water retention that may help correct hypovolemia. *Glucocorticoids* contribute to the body's compensatory mechanisms by helping epinephrine and norepinephrine constrict blood vessels. However, steroid use remains controversial.

Correcting fluid overload (hypervolemia). During hypovolemic shock, the kidneys function poorly, increasing the risk of intravascular-space fluid overload. I.V. fluids administered during resuscitation may also shift to the interstitial compartment, causing circulating fluid loss and increased tissue edema. Keep in mind that fluid overload accounts for shock's most common serious complications; for instance, acute respiratory distress syndrome (ARDS), sepsis, and renal failure. Stay alert for signs and symptoms of fluid overload: increased preload (indicated by increased CVP and PCWP), muscle weakness, nausea, anxiety, muscle twitching, and indications of CHF.

Expect the doctor to order fluid and salt restriction. As ordered, give 25% albumin along with diuretics such as I.V. furosemide (Lasix) to treat hypervolemia without reducing circulating volume. If the patient develops renal failure, the doctor may order hemodialysis or peritoneal dialysis to reduce fluid overload and remove excess electrolytes and metabolites.

Correcting oliguria. Oliguria usually arises in patients with profound, prolonged hypotension; those who've received large vasopressor dosages; and those with preexisting renal disease. As a first priority for an oliguric patient, try to normalize preload and

---

How pain relief helps fight shock

Prolonged or severe pain can hasten hypovolemic shock's progression by causing vasodilation. This counteracts vasoconstriction—the body's first defense in shock. Thus, pain relief can prove an important weapon against shock.

To reduce your patient's pain, provide emotional support and keep his room quiet. Be prepared to administer analgesics as ordered. Don't be surprised if the doctor orders a small analgesic dose I.V. rather than a larger dose I.M. A small dose in early shock usually combats pain more effectively than a larger dose in late shock; the I.V. route provides almost immediate relief. Also, a small dose reduces the risk of impaired ventilation or cardiovascular function. (During shock, the liver and kidneys don't function normally, so drugs remain in the body longer.) After administering the drug, monitor the patient's blood pressure, pulse rate, and respiratory rate. Note the drug's effectiveness and watch for signs and symptoms of respiratory depression and other possible complications.

Note: Depending on your patient's condition, the doctor may delay giving an analgesic. In this case, use traditional comfort measures and techniques, such as distraction, to minimize pain.

Vascular Problems

39 Shock

Hypovolemic Shock

afterload through fluid replacement. Expect the doctor to order an osmotic agent, such as mannitol or 50% glucose, or a diuretic, such as furosemide (preferred because its rapid metabolization permits more frequent doses). If diuretics alone prove ineffective, the doctor may also order albumin. Monitor levels of BUN, serum creatinine, serum potassium, serum albumin and total protein, urine osmolarity, and electrolytes. Measure urine output hourly to evaluate the patient's response to treatment. If these measures fail, the doctor may institute hemodialysis or peritoneal dialysis to remove excess fluid, electrolytes, and metabolites.

Providing nutritional support. Nutritional support for the hypovolemic patient aims to spare protein resources and promote anabolism (for wound healing and cellular rebuilding). Your patient will require more calories and nutrients than usual to support his increased metabolic requirements. (Remember that shock's anaerobic metabolism—less energy-efficient than aerobic metabolism—increases metabolic demands.) Calories stored as glucose and glycogen become depleted early and decreased blood flow to the GI tract reduces nutrient absorption.

Begin nutritional assessment and support promptly. As ordered, administer simple I.V. substances, such as dextrose 50% solution with amino acids, to help provide efficient energy sources (500 ml of dextrose 50% solution provides 1,000 calories). The doctor may order crystalline insulin (added to the solution or given via I.V. push) at a dose adequate to prevent hyperglycemia. You may also administer an I.V. lipid solution, which provides nearly half the administered calories. This avoids elevated serum CO_2 levels, which result from glucose overutilization as a calorie source (glucose metabolism yields CO_2 as an end product). Consider 3,000 to 4,000 calories for the first 24 hours a reasonable goal (4,000 calories spares protein).

Controlling or preventing infection. Shock-induced stress impairs your patient's immune response, making infection more likely. Observe him closely for signs and symptoms of infection and keep all wounds and incisions clean and dry. Check I.V. insertion sites at least every 2 hours for indications of phlebitis or infection. Follow hospital policy for wound dressing and I.V. care and culture wounds showing gross contamination signs. Administer specific antibiotic therapy depending on culture results.

Providing psychological support. When caring for a patient with hypovolemic shock, you may consider psychological support relatively unimportant. Of course, you can't delay critical interventions just to talk to your patient. But when possible, *do* take time to reassure him as you provide care. Encourage him to draw on his inner resources to survive this crisis and urge family and friends to offer their support (don't forget to reassure *them*, too). Help conserve your patient's energy by keeping his room as quiet as possible. Plan your care to allow for rest periods—uninterrupted sleep provides excellent physical and psychological therapy.

Keep your patient's social needs in mind as well. During treatment for shock, he's the focus of a health care team carrying out life-saving measures that leave little time for social interaction. After he's stable, reorient him to his surroundings and to the staff mem-

Continued on page 40

Vascular Problems

40 Shock

Hypovolemic Shock

Continued

bers involved in his care. Encourage visits by family and friends.

Complications
Your patient may develop complications as a result of therapeutic interventions or from shock's pathophysiologic effects and end-organ deficits. The most common complications include transfusion reactions, ARDS, renal failure, and DIC.

Transfusion reactions. These reactions may occur immediately (during transfusion) or up to 3 weeks later. Their cause may be immunologic or nonimmunologic. To prevent transfusion reactions, always check and double-check your patient's identity, ABO group, and Rh status. Then check your findings against the donor blood label and make sure the blood's not outdated. Even in an emergency, these steps will prove well worth the few seconds they take. If you find any discrepancies or irregularities, *don't* administer the blood. Notify the doctor and blood bank at once.

Immediate, immunologic reactions include:

• *intravascular hemolysis.* This life-threatening condition results from a complete antigen-antibody reaction and usually stems from incorrect identification of the patient, blood sample, or donor blood unit. Signs and symptoms include fever, chills, hypotension, chest and lumbar pain, nausea and vomiting, hemoglobinuria, and hemoglobinemia. At the first sign of these problems, stop the transfusion and send a fresh blood sample and urine specimen to the laboratory, along with blood remaining in the transfusion bag and the I.V. blood tubing (see *Transfusion reaction: What to do,* page 42). Keep the I.V. site open with normal saline solution; hemolysis causes red blood cell rupture, which results in nephrotoxic free hemoglobin that must be flushed through kidney tubules. Expect to administer small dopamine doses to increase cardiac output and improve renal blood flow; you may also give I.V. fluids and diuretics to help maintain urine output near 100 ml/hour.

• *extravascular hemolysis.* In this reaction, an incomplete antigen-antibody reaction causes RBC removal from circulation via the reticuloendothelial system. Like intravascular hemolysis, it usually results from incorrect identification of the patient, blood sample, or donor blood unit. Some patients develop only chills and fever; others develop signs and symptoms that mimic mild intravascular hemolysis. Treatment depends on the patient's condition.

• *febrile nonhemolytic reaction.* This reaction usually occurs in patients with preformed anti-HLA antibodies that react with donor white blood cells. Signs and symptoms may resemble those of a hemolytic reaction, although hemoglobinuria and hemoglobinemia don't occur. Expect the doctor to treat this relatively benign condition symptomatically, through use of comfort measures such as antipyretics.

• *anaphylaxis.* This life-threatening reaction most frequently occurs in an atopic patient (one with chronic allergy) who's received a transfusion in the past 2 weeks. You may note erythema, wheal formation, eyelid edema with visual blurring, laryngeal edema with cough and bronchospasm, and earlobe and hand edema. Fluid shift may cause hypotension, nausea, abdominal pain, and tachycardia. Expect to administer antihistamines. You may also give aminophylline for bronchodilation and sympathomimetics such as epinephrine to support circulation until fluid replacement begins. The

---

Administering blood: Some important guidelines

When you administer blood, always follow hospital policy and procedure. But keep these important guidelines in mind as well:

• Carefully compare patient and donor unit identification. If your patient's hemorrhaging, you may not want to spend time checking identification numbers. However, skipping this step could result in a serious transfusion reaction. Most hemolytic transfusion reactions associated with ABO mismatching stem from identification errors.

• Always administer blood through a filter that removes cellular debris (preferably a microaggregate filter). Cellular debris in donor blood includes leukoagglutinins, which react with the recipient's leukocytes to form a white cell aggregate that becomes trapped in pulmonary microcirculation. This promotes pulmonary congestion with resistance to forward blood flow into the left atrium. The resulting sluggish blood flow may lead to pulmonary edema and poor alveolar gas exchange. Expect such signs and symptoms as respiratory distress, cyanosis, fever, chills, and, eventually, hypotension.

• Always use normal saline solution to prime the tubing. Never mix a drug or another solution with blood. Once you begin the transfusion, monitor the patient for signs and symptoms of immediate transfusion reaction: fever, chills, hypotension, chest and lumbar pain, nausea, vomiting, wheal formation, eyelid edema, bronchospasm, hives, and itching.

• Check the patient's temperature and vital signs before you start the transfusion. Notify the doctor of any temperature elevation and note any increase from baseline during transfusion. Such an increase may indicate transfusion reaction. Document baseline hemodynamic parameters, breath sounds, and urine output and quality.

• Warm banked blood to body temperature (98.6° F. [37° C.]) before administration. Consider this step essential for massive transfusions (replacement of 50% or more of the patient's blood volume at one time or replacement of the patient's total blood volume within 24 hours). Exchange transfusions and potent cold agglutinins also require warming. Banked blood—stored at 33° to 43° F. (1° to 6° C.)—may cause hypothermia if administered without warming. Hypothermia increases the ventricular fibrillation risk, impairs

Continued

41 Shock

Hypovolemic Shock

Administering blood: Some important guidelines
Continued

the patient's ability to withstand further blood loss, and promotes metabolic acidosis. Warm banked blood with an electric blood warmer, if available—this automatically heats blood to body temperature. *Never* warm blood above body temperature or above 107° F. (42° C.) because excessive warming causes hemolysis. (If possible, avoid using a blood-warming coil that you must immerse in warm water. This system takes too long in an emergency and may lead to hemolysis.)

• Provide psychological support. The patient and his family may react to the prospect of a blood transfusion with both relief (because it's a life-saving measure) and fear (because they perceive it as a last-ditch effort). They may also worry about the possibility of disease transmission (especially acquired immunodeficiency syndrome or hepatitis) from donor blood. Some patients may refuse transfusions on religious or cultural grounds. Explain all procedures and reassure the patient and his family.

---

doctor may order I.V. steroids to stabilize cell membranes.

• *urticaria.* This condition, which may follow plasma infusion, results from Ig-A sensitivity. Signs and symptoms include erythema, hives, and itching. Stop the transfusion and administer an antihistamine, as ordered. The doctor may resume the transfusion after the patient's condition improves.

Immediate, nonimmunologic reactions include:

• *bacterial contamination of donor blood.* Expect marked fever and shock with this condition. Also check for hypotension, tachycardia, clammy skin, diarrhea, abdominal cramps, vomiting, muscle pain, and hemoglobinuria. Administer vasopressors, corticosteroids, and antibiotics as ordered.

• *nonsymptomatic hemolysis.* Donor cell destruction may result from freezing, overheating, or nonisotonic supplements. The patient gets no therapeutic benefit when he receives blood containing damaged cells; the cells undergo immediate removal from his circulation. If he's no longer bleeding but his hematocrit remains unchanged and his serum bilirubin level rises after transfusion, consider this hemolysis type a possibility. Retransfuse, as necessary and ordered, and monitor his renal function closely for several days. Prevent nonsymptomatic hemolysis by keeping donor blood in a refrigerator specially designated for blood storage and by using a blood warmer with the designated tubing. Never warm blood above 98.6° F. (37° C.). Prime blood tubing only with an isotonically compatible solution.

• *hypothermia.* This takes place when a patient receives large amounts of cold blood in a short period. Stay alert for chills with shivering and low body temperature.

• *hypocalcemia.* This may stem from citrate overload caused by massive citrated blood transfusions. Excess citrate binds with calcium, reducing serum calcium levels and causing hypocalcemia. Signs and symptoms include tingling fingers, cramps, convulsions, hypotension, prolonged QT interval on EKG, and Chvostek's sign. Administer I.V. calcium gluconate or calcium chloride, as ordered, to replace the deficit. Prevent hypocalcemia by monitoring serum calcium levels after transfusing every fourth unit containing citrate preservative.

Delayed, immunologic reactions include:

• *delayed hemolytic reactions.* Some patients develop antibodies in response to donor blood antigens 2 weeks or more after transfusion. As antibodies multiply, they react with circulating donor cells and accelerate donor cell destruction. Suspect this with an unexplained hemoglobin drop and RBC alloantibody appearance several weeks after transfusion. The patient may require retransfusion.

• *graft-vs-host disease.* This rare reaction occurs when donor (graft) cells react against recipient (host) cells. Check for fever, diarrhea, and signs and symptoms of hepatitis, infection, and bone marrow depression.

• *posttransfusion purpura.* Almost exclusive to women, this reaction stems from development of a platelet-specific antibody. Signs and symptoms include generalized purpura and severe thrombocytopenia. Expect the doctor to order plasmapheresis.

Delayed, nonimmunologic reactions involve the transmission of various diseases, including non-A, non-B hepatitis; malaria; brucellosis; Epstein-Barr virus; cytomegalovirus; toxoplasmosis; trypanoso-

Continued on page 42

Vascular Problems

42 Shock

Hypovolemic Shock

Transfusion reaction: What to do

If you suspect your patient's having a transfusion reaction, take the steps described below (however, be sure to follow hospital policy and procedure).
• Stop the transfusion *immediately* and notify the doctor. But don't remove the I.V. needle.
• As ordered, substitute normal saline solution or another I.V. replacement fluid for the blood transfusion.
• Monitor vital signs at least every 15 minutes, depending on your patient's condition.
• Administer oxygen and other drugs, as ordered.
• Draw blood specimens for laboratory studies and for retyping and cross-matching to help determine the reaction's cause.
• Collect urine specimens to detect any hemoglobin.
• Verify that the patient's name and hospital identification number match those on the blood bank slip and the transfused unit.
• Return the unused blood to the blood bank.
• Document the patient's reaction, noting the time you started and stopped the transfusion, the amount of blood transfused, the patient's signs and symptoms, and all medical and nursing interventions.

Continued

miasis; syphilis (with fresh whole blood transfusions only), and acquired immunodeficiency syndrome.

ARDS. This may develop as capillary stasis and increased vascular resistance lead to interstitial pulmonary edema. Help prevent this by correcting hypovolemia aggressively and promoting adequate oxygenation (however, avoid prolonged high oxygen doses).

Renal failure. This may result from reduced renal perfusion complicated by angiotensin, ADH, and aldosterone activity; or from nephrotoxic agent administration. Renal failure may appear as oliguric or high-urinary-output failure. To help prevent this complication, administer diuretics and albumin, as ordered, after fluid replacement begins to help normalize renal flow. Check urine output hourly.

DIC. This complication results from marked clotting factor consumption during hemorrhagic shock and from blood transfusions low in clotting factors. It probably stems from acidosis, bacterial endotoxins, and thromboplastin (released from damaged cells). Massive injuries cause release of toxic procoagulant factors that promote intravascular clotting. Initially, massive microcoagulation consumes clotting factors, especially platelets, fibrinogen, prothrombin (Factor II), Factor V, and Factor VIII. Then, the fibrinolytic system becomes activated, leading to fibrin clot breakdown that eventually increases fibrin split products (FSP) in the circulation. FSP further decrease clot formation. Diffuse bleeding then develops from clotting factor consumption and active fibrin clot destruction.

You may note petechiae; purpura; blood oozing from orifices, incisions, and I.V. insertion sites; mucosal bleeding; and indications of acute massive bleeding. Expect prolonged prothrombin and partial thromboplastin times. The patient's platelet count will drop below normal and his FSP level will rise markedly above normal. Report signs and symptoms of DIC immediately and prepare to administer blood component therapy—fresh frozen plasma, and/or platelets. Avoid measures that may cause further blood oozing or tissue damage. The doctor will initiate therapy to correct the underlying disorder, compensate for anemia and hypovolemia, and prevent additional bleeding. He may ask you to administer heparin or aminocaproic acid (Amicar), although use of these drugs remains controversial. DIC has a high mortality.

Evaluation

Base your evaluation on the expected outcomes as listed on the sample nursing care plan. To determine if the patient's improved, ask yourself the following questions:
• Does the patient have an adequate hemoglobin level?
• Can he maintain an adequate PaO_2 level?
• Does he show signs or symptoms of decreased tissue perfusion?
• Can he maintain adequate systolic and diastolic blood pressures?
• Can he maintain adequate MAP?
• Does his urine output measure at least 30 ml/hour?

The answers to these questions will help you evaluate your patient's status and the effectiveness of his care. Keep in mind that these questions stem from the sample nursing care plan on page 29. Your questions may differ.

Vascular Problems

43 Shock

Cardiogenic Shock: Impaired Heart Pumping

Suzanne H. Clark, who wrote this chapter, is a Clinical Specialist in the heart transplant program at the University of California, Los Angeles. She received her MSN from the University of California, San Francisco, and her MA in psychology from Pepperdine University, Los Angeles.

Shock, a complex clinical syndrome, describes a state of inadequate tissue perfusion—regardless of the precipitating event. *Cardiogenic shock* results from ineffective heart pumping that leads to reduced cardiac output and subsequent perfusion impairment. This disturbs normal cellular metabolism and triggers systemic responses that exacerbate shock. (See Chapter 1 for more information on shock's pathophysiologic process.)

Acute myocardial infarction (AMI) most commonly causes cardiogenic shock. Up to 15% of patients admitted to coronary care units with AMI develop signs and symptoms of shock; most have sustained damage to at least 40% of the myocardium. Shock after AMI leads to death in about four of every five cases—mainly from extensive ventricular muscle dysfunction.

Cardiogenic shock can also result from end-stage cardiomyopathy; mechanical defects such as acute mitral or aortic regurgitation, ruptured intraventricular septum, and aortic stenosis; severe tachydysrhythmias and bradydysrhythmias; and outflow interference, as in massive pulmonary embolism or cardiac tamponade. Other advanced shock states can also give rise to cardiogenic shock. (See the NURSEREVIEW section on "Cardiac Problems" for details on cardiac function and structure.)

Continued on page 44

Hemodynamics: Reviewing common terms

If you've cared for a patient with a cardiac disorder, you've probably heard many of the terms we'll define here. If you're caring for a patient with—or at risk for—cardiogenic shock, your knowledge of these terms can make a lifesaving difference. Study them carefully. (See Chapter 1 for more on hemodynamics.)

Cardiac output (CO). The blood volume ejected from the heart each minute (expressed in liters/minute). Normal CO ranges from 4 to 8 liters/minute. To calculate CO, multiply stroke volume by heart rate: $CO = SV \times HR$.

Stroke volume (SV). The blood volume ejected from the heart during systole (expressed in milliliters). SV changes can increase or decrease cardiac output. SV depends on *preload, afterload,* and *contractility.*

Preload. Myocardial fiber stretch at the end of diastole. Fiber length depends mainly on ventricular blood volume when diastole ends. As fiber length increases, so does stroke volume. However, if fibers stretch beyond the optimal length, stroke volume decreases—a relationship shown by the left ventricular function curve (see page 46). Factors that can influence preload include the following:
• *atrial filling pressure,* determined by total blood volume and venous return (blood volume distribution) adequacy
• *increased intrathoracic pressure,* for example, from positive end-expiratory pressure (PEEP) ventilation; PEEP can decrease venous return and therefore reduce preload.
• *cardiac dysrhythmias that de-*crease diastolic filling time and preload, such as tachydysrhythmias and frequent premature beats
• *cardiac dysrhythmias that cause atrial component loss,* such as atrial fibrillation and third-degree heart block. Such dysrhythmias, which reduce stroke volume by decreasing preload, may lower cardiac output as much as 30%.

Afterload. The resistance against which the ventricle pumps. The greater the resistance to ventricular systole, the harder the ventricle must work to eject blood. Increased work results in decreased stroke volume. Decreased afterload eases blood ejection, increasing stroke volume.

Contractility. Myocardial fiber shortening force, independent of fiber length (preload). Positive inotropic factors enhance contractility; for example, sympathetic nervous system stimulation and such drugs as digoxin, calcium, and isoproterenol. Negative inotropic factors reduce contractility; for example, anesthesia, acidosis, hypoxemia, and drugs such as propranolol and calcium channel blockers.

Heart rate. The number of heart beats/minute. The body can improve cardiac output by changing the heart rate. A healthy person who can quickly raise his heart rate to 180 beats/minute can double or triple his cardiac output. In a patient with compromised cardiac function, however, an increase to 120 beats/minute may reduce cardiac output by decreasing diastolic filling time and consequently decreasing preload. Also, most coronary artery flow occurs during diastole. Therefore, as heart rate increases, diastolic filling time shortens and coronary blood flow may suffer. Physical activity, fear, pain, fever, hypoxia, and shock can trigger a heart rate increase to meet tissue demands.

Increased preload—a result of greater diastolic filling—can initially compensate for bradydysrhythmias. However, this mechanism may eventually fail if the heart rate drops below 50 beats/minute (particularly in a patient with a damaged heart).

Cardiac index. Cardiac output divided by body surface area. This measurement tells you if the patient's cardiac output can meet his individual needs. (You can obtain the patient's body surface area from a Dubois body surface chart.) Normally, cardiac index ranges from 2.5 to 4 liters/minute/m².

44 Shock

Cardiogenic Shock

Continued

To understand how cardiogenic shock develops and progresses, you'll need to know which conditions occurring in shock can disrupt the myocardial oxygen supply and demand balance and further exacerbate shock. For example, because the resting heart extracts nearly all the blood's oxygen content, increased oxygen extraction won't help meet an increased demand. The major means of boosting myocardial blood supply—enhanced coronary artery blood flow—grows increasingly difficult with blocked coronary arteries (as in most patients with AMI).

In addition, as heart rate increases to compensate for reduced stroke volume, diastolic filling time decreases, compromising coronary filling and consequently oxygen supply. And as mean arterial pressure (MAP) falls, the pressure gradient between the aorta and coronary arteries drops. This may limit blood flow into coronary arteries with preexisting blockage.

The following factors affect myocardial oxygen consumption ($M\dot{V}O_2$):
- As preload, afterload, contractility, and heart rate *increase*, $M\dot{V}O_2$ increases.
- As preload, afterload, contractility, and heart rate *decrease*, $M\dot{V}O_2$ decreases.

Decreased cardiac index (usually below 2 liters/minute/m²) constitutes the major development in cardiogenic shock. This blood supply reduction occurs just when oxygen needs increase. In shock's early stage, the body attempts to adjust to this low flow state by initiating various compensatory mechanisms. For instance, decreased cardiac output stimulates the sympathetic nervous system (SNS) to help boost output through the following responses:

- *vasoconstriction.* This occurs in the skeletal muscles, splanchnic bed, kidneys, and cutaneous vascular beds. Blood then shunts to the heart and brain. Vasoconstriction thus raises systemic vascular resistance (SVR) and maintains arterial blood pressure in response to decreased forward flow.
- *increased heart rate.* The body attempts to compensate for decreased stroke volume by increasing heart rate.
- *increased respiratory rate and depth*
- *increased sweat gland activity*
- *adrenal medulla stimulation.* This results in epinephrine and norepinephrine release. These substances intensify myocardial contractile force and stimulate the anterior pituitary gland to release adrenocorticotrophic hormone (ACTH), which in turn stimulates the adrenal cortex. ACTH causes release of glucocorticoids (primarily cortisol) and mineralocorticoids (primarily aldosterone). Cortisol release increases gluconeogenesis and free fatty acid levels, decreases protein synthesis, and alters the immune system. Aldosterone release improves sodium reabsorption, potassium excretion, and water retention. Hyperosmolarity created by sodium reabsorption stimulates the posterior pituitary gland. Antidiuretic hormone (ADH) release further promotes water retention.

The kidneys also play an important role in shock. Renal arterial vasoconstriction activates the renin-angiotensin cycle, further increasing sodium and water retention, intravascular volume, and venous return.

Tracing cardiogenic shock's progression

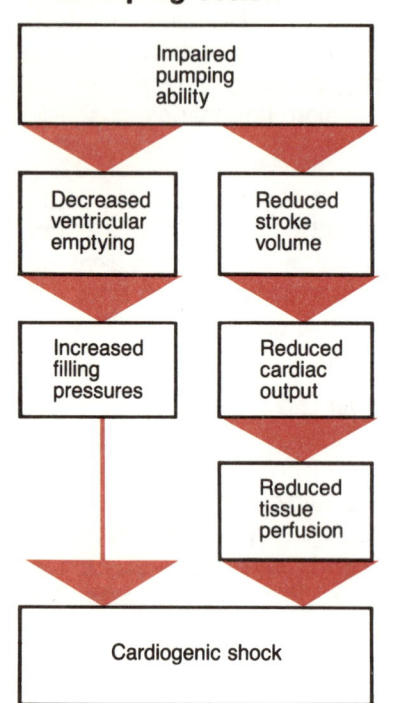

Impaired pumping ability
↓
Decreased ventricular emptying / Reduced stroke volume
↓
Increased filling pressures / Reduced cardiac output
↓
Reduced tissue perfusion
↓
Cardiogenic shock

Vascular Problems

45 Shock

Cardiogenic Shock

Cardiogenic shock from AMI: A downward spiral

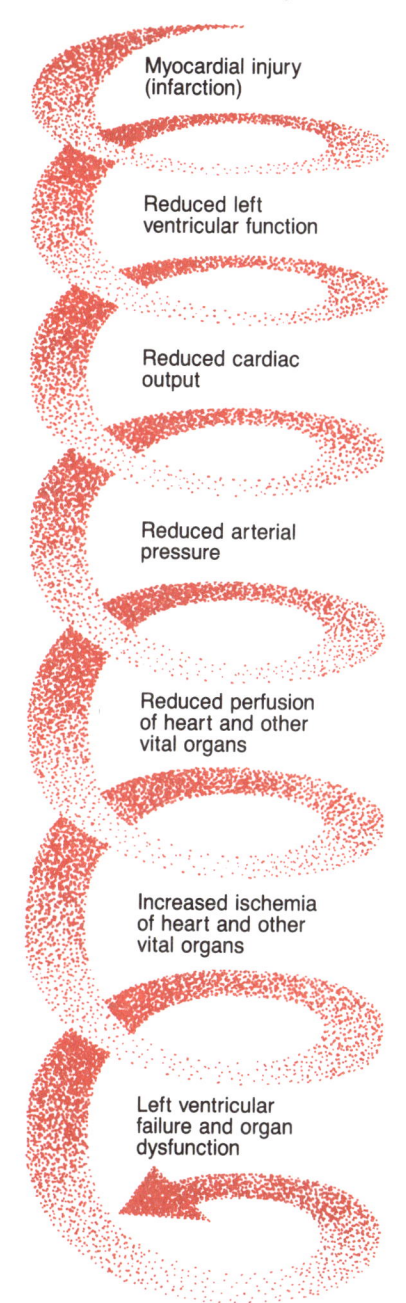

- Myocardial injury (infarction)
- Reduced left ventricular function
- Reduced cardiac output
- Reduced arterial pressure
- Reduced perfusion of heart and other vital organs
- Increased ischemia of heart and other vital organs
- Left ventricular failure and organ dysfunction

These responses occur as part of the body's general response to *any* stressful condition—not just cardiogenic shock (see Chapter 1 for more information on these responses.) Various psychological or physiologic stimuli, including intense fear and anxiety, can activate such responses and compound cardiogenic shock. (Keep in mind that AMI usually causes fear and anxiety.)

All of the mechanisms described above contribute to shock's progression, causing a downward spiral that usually ends in death. (See *Cardiogenic shock from AMI: A downward spiral*.) Let's take a closer look at how these mechanisms can exacerbate the patient's condition:

- *Increased heart rate* increases oxygen consumption and decreases diastolic filling time and coronary artery blood flow.
- *Increased contractility* increases oxygen consumption.
- *Increased vasoconstriction* increases afterload, which increases oxygen consumption and decreases cardiac output.
- *Increased water retention* increases preload, which increases oxygen consumption and may exacerbate pulmonary congestion.

Thus, the body's initial attempts to compensate for diminished cardiac output compound rather than alleviate cardiogenic shock.

Complications. As in all shock types, the major complication—multisystemic failure—results from generalized tissue hypoperfusion. The most vulnerable body systems include:
- respiratory system (causing adult respiratory distress syndrome)
- renal system (causing acute tubular necrosis)
- hematologic system (causing disseminated intravascular coagulation).

The patient also risks infection, especially from these sources:
- invasive lines (such as I.V., intraarterial, and intracardiac lines)
- immune system changes
- decreased blood supply to the GI tract, which can cause mucosal damage and bacteria release into the circulation.

Assessment

The longer cardiogenic shock goes undetected and untreated, the worse the patient's prognosis. If the patient's already in shock, your accurate assessment can help determine his response to treatment, prevent complications, and guide medical and nursing interventions.

To help *prevent* shock, check the patient's history for risk factors. Cardiogenic shock most commonly occurs after AMI. Ask the patient about any chest pain—a sign of reduced myocardial oxygenation that may indicate developing shock. Document the pain's location, radiation pattern, severity, quality, and timing, and note any alleviating or exacerbating factors.

Cardiogenic shock may also occur after open-heart surgery, chest trauma with resulting cardiac tamponade, and end-stage cardiomyopathy.

When assessing a patient for cardiogenic shock, ask yourself: Does he have adequate cardiac output to meet body demands? If it's adequate now, what conditions might jeopardize it in the immediate future?

Continued on page 46

Cardiogenic Shock

Continued

Physical examination. Expect changes in the patient's level of consciousness, blood pressure, pulse, heart sounds, respirations, breath sounds, skin and body temperature, and urine output. The extent of any changes depends on shock's stage (as discussed in Chapter 1). Generally, the patient shows signs and symptoms of decreased peripheral perfusion.

Level of consciousness. In early shock, the patient may respond to cerebral blood flow changes with restlessness, agitation, or confusion. He may also experience personality changes, paranoia, and sleep pattern disturbances. In a patient who risks shock, pay particular attention to behavior changes; don't assume such changes reflect only odd personality traits. As shock progresses, lethargy and coma develop.

Blood pressure. In cardiogenic shock, systolic pressure drops below 90 mm Hg, or at least 30 mm Hg lower than the baseline measurement. Decreased blood pressure may represent prolonged shock, reflecting the body's attempt to compensate for reduced cardiac output. In early shock, systolic blood pressure may rise slightly (if the patient has adequate stroke volume, it may remain normal). Diastolic pressure may rise from vasoconstriction. Narrowing pulse pressure may be an early sign of reduced cardiac output. As shock progresses, arterial blood pressure drops.

Pulse. Expect tachycardia (a weak, thready pulse) from compensatory mechanisms.

Heart sounds. In cardiogenic shock after AMI, you may hear a fourth heart sound (atrial gallop, or S_4), indicating decreased ventricular compliance. In some cases, a third heart sound (ventricular gallop, or S_3) may also develop, meaning increased ventricular filling pressure. A sudden holosystolic murmur may indicate papillary muscle

---

Ventricular function curve

The ventricular function curve (also known as Starling's curve) reflects Starling's law: As preload increases, cardiac output increases—until myocardial fibers stretch beyond their optimal length.

Plotting your patient's curve gives you a visual picture of his overall cardiac function. The curve also allows you to easily monitor therapeutic effectiveness and the patient's clinical trends.

The curve shown at right uses the left ventricular stroke work index (LVSWI—the amount of work the heart performs) and pulmonary capillary wedge pressure (PCWP—preload). *Note:* You may more commonly use cardiac output instead of LVSWI.

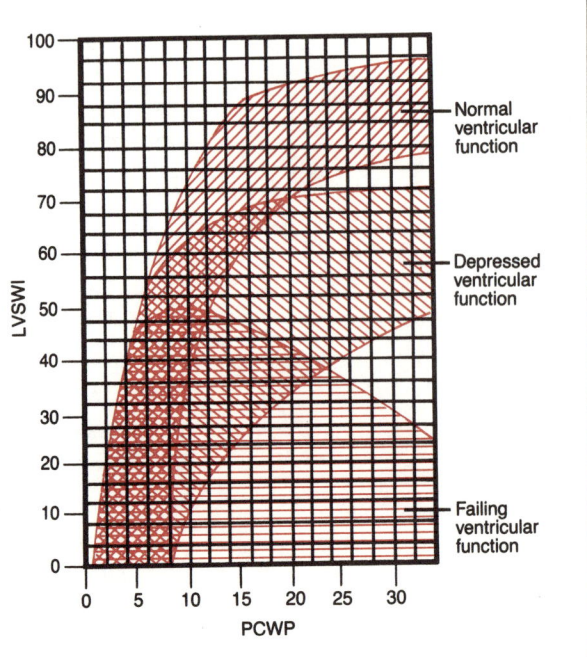

Cardiogenic Shock

dysfunction or rupture or ventricular septal defect—complications that could influence cardiogenic shock's development.

Respirations. In early shock, expect increased respiratory rate and depth. As shock progresses, respirations may grow more rapid and shallow, with signs of respiratory distress. Congestive heart failure and pulmonary edema, which frequently accompany cardiogenic shock, may cause tachypnea and dyspnea.

Breath sounds. Auscultate breath sounds and document any crackles or wheezes, which may arise from narrowed airways and/or increased fluid or mucus.

Skin and body temperature. Decreased peripheral perfusion makes the skin feel cool and clammy and may lead to mottling (especially on the legs). Expect prolonged capillary refill time and possibly cyanosis.

Urine output. Because urine output usually reflects cardiac output, expect *reduced* urine output (below 30 ml/hour) in cardiogenic shock. (However, be sure to assess urinary output *trends,* not just individual measurements.)

Diagnostic studies. As with physical findings, diagnostic test results depend on shock's degree. The doctor will order laboratory studies and hemodynamic monitoring to assess the patient's status.

Laboratory studies. Expect the doctor to order arterial blood gas (ABG) measurements. As shock progresses and tissue perfusion diminishes, cellular metabolism becomes anaerobic. This boosts lactic acid production, reflected in decreased pH—a sign of metabolic acidosis.

ABGs also show worsening hypoxemia. Decreased arterial oxygen (PaO_2) levels may accompany pulmonary edema (common in cardiogenic shock). Such a decrease may also result from inadequate respiratory excursion caused by pain and anxiety. Carbon dioxide ($PaCO_2$) levels may drop below normal (indicating respiratory alkalosis) from alveolar hyperventilation and as compensation for metabolic acidosis. In alveolar hypoventilation, $PaCO_2$ may rise above normal.

Depending on shock's degree, laboratory findings may show the results described in Chapter 1. The doctor may also order cardiac enzyme and isoenzyme tests, an electrocardiogram (EKG), and a chest X-ray to help determine cardiogenic shock's cause.

The patient may also require radionuclide scans, coronary angiography, left ventricular cineangiography, and echocardiography. During shock's acute stage, these tests help assess cardiac status.

Invasive hemodynamic monitoring. Especially important for a patient with cardiogenic shock, hemodynamic monitoring parameters help determine shock's severity, evaluate the patient's response to treatment, and gauge his recovery odds. For the best assessment, correlate measurement *trends* with the patient's clinical condition. (See Chapter 1 for more information on hemodynamic monitoring techniques.)

Continued on page 48

Cardiogenic Shock

Cardiogenic shock: Recognizing warning signs

If your patient's suffered a cardiac injury or myocardial infarction, suspect cardiogenic shock if you note the following assessment findings:
- systolic blood pressure below 90 mm Hg, or at least 30 mm Hg below baseline level
- urine output below 30 ml/hour
- evidence of diminished peripheral perfusion with impaired mental status and peripheral vasoconstriction.

Continued

Assessing preload, which depends mainly on ventricular blood volume at the end of diastole, helps evaluate the patient's volume status. *Right ventricular preload* can be measured from central venous pressure (CVP). With left ventricular compromise (common with AMI), CVP doesn't accurately reflect left ventricular function. However, elevated CVP may help assess cardiogenic shock stemming partly from right ventricular infarction. Patients with elevated CVP also have jugular vein distention.

Pulmonary capillary wedge pressure (PCWP; or pulmonary artery diastolic pressure [PADP] if it correlates with PCWP) proves the most useful parameter for assessing *left ventricular preload*. PCWP helps determine appropriate interventions, assess the patient's response to treatment, and identify any developing complications. Below-normal PCWP or PADP indicates the need for fluids despite pulmonary congestion. Similarities between PADP and PCWP help distinguish cardiogenic shock from massive acute pulmonary embolism. In cardiogenic shock, expect both pressures to rise above normal. In pulmonary embolism, expect above-normal PADP and normal PCWP. The doctor will also order cardiac output and/or cardiac index monitoring.

A ventricular function curve (Starling's curve) also helps evaluate overall heart function and monitor therapeutic effectiveness (see *Ventricular function curve*, page 46).

Afterload reflects the resistance against which the heart must pump (SVR). This parameter helps assess shock's progression and the patient's response to treatment. You can determine *left ventricular afterload* from MAP and CVP using this formula:

$$SVR = \frac{(MAP - CVP)\ 79.9}{CO}$$

SVR normally ranges from 900 to 1,600 dynes/second/cm^{-5}. Cardiogenic shock usually leads to above-normal SVR, which further compromises left ventricular ejection and increases myocardial oxygen consumption. Pulmonary vascular resistance reflects *right ventricular afterload* (not an important index in cardiogenic shock).

Other hemodynamic indexes that help assess shock include mixed venous gases and arteriovenous oxygen difference. Mixed venous blood oxygen saturation measurements help evaluate cardiac output trends. Normally, tissues extract about 25% to 40% of the oxygen from the blood; a 60% to 75% reserve remains in venous blood returning to the heart. If cardiac output falls, tissues extract more oxygen, leaving less remaining in venous blood. A mixed venous blood oxygen saturation below 65% indicates decreased cardiac output. Mixed venous oxygen saturation above 75% indicates blood shunting from the heart's left to right side. This may help diagnose a ventricular septal defect, an AMI complication that could contribute to cardiogenic shock.

An arteriovenous oxygen difference of 6 vol% or more reflects cardiac decompensation—severe heart damage that renders cardiac output inadequate for tissue perfusion.

Vascular Problems

49 Shock

Cardiogenic Shock

Planning
The doctor will order medical interventions designed to increase the heart's oxygen supply while decreasing its oxygen needs. However, in some cases, these interventions could have the opposite effect and worsen the patient's condition. A thorough understanding of shock's pathophysiologic process can help you plan nursing care to enhance rather than compromise the body's adaptive mechanisms. For example, you'll need to keep in mind how preload, afterload, contractility, and heart rate affect cardiac output; how the ventricular function curve can help track the patient's response to therapy; and how certain factors can change the relationship between myocardial oxygen supply and demand.

Nursing diagnoses. Before determining your nursing care plan, develop the nursing diagnosis by identifying the patient's problem or potential problem, then relating it to its cause. Possible nursing diagnoses for a cardiogenic shock patient include the following:
• tissue perfusion, alteration in; related to decreased cardiac output and peripheral vasoconstriction
• skin integrity, impairment of (potential for); related to decreased cardiac output, increased vasoconstriction, and immobility
• gas exchange, impaired; related to decreased pulmonary perfusion and pulmonary edema
• fear; related to acute condition
• activity intolerance; related to decreased cardiac output

Continued on page 50

Sample nursing care plan: Cardiogenic shock

Nursing diagnosis
Tissue perfusion, alteration in; related to decreased cardiac output and peripheral vasoconstriction

Expected outcomes
The patient will:
• maintain stable hemodynamics to support adequate tissue perfusion
 —cardiac index between 2.5 and 4 liters/minute/m^2
 —PCWP and PADP between 15 and 20 mm Hg.
• maintain urine output above 30 ml/hour.
• have warm, dry skin.
• maintain normal mental status (oriented to time, place, and person and appropriate to situation).

Nursing interventions
• Assess vital signs; mental status; skin color, temperature, and moistness; and PCWP and PADP every hour or as indicated.
• Titrate medication doses and/or fluids to patient's condition and hemodynamic parameters.
• Monitor for response to medication.
• Monitor fluid intake and output. Maintain urine output of at least 30 ml/hour.
• Assess cardiac output every 2 to 4 hours or as indicated.
• Calculate cardiac index, SVR, and LVSWI.
• Plot a ventricular function curve to assess trends in patient's condition.
• Provide emotional support to patient and his family.
• If patient's using IABP, monitor for therapeutic response and adverse effects.
• Provide adequate rest periods.

Discharge planning
Depends on treatment outcome

Vascular Problems

50 Shock

Cardiogenic Shock

Continued

- grieving (family); related to patient's acute condition
- injury, potential for (infection); related to invasive procedures and altered immune status.

The sample nursing care plan on page 49 shows expected outcomes, nursing interventions, and discharge planning for one nursing diagnosis listed above. However, you'll want to individualize each care plan to meet your patient's needs.

Intervention
Because most patients can't survive cardiogenic shock, try to *prevent* it whenever possible. Once shock develops, the patient will need prompt, aggressive intervention. Focus on the following goals with a cardiogenic shock patient who's had an AMI:
- improving ventricular function and increasing cardiac output
- increasing myocardial oxygen supply
- decreasing myocardial oxygen demand
- limiting infarction size
- correcting hypoxia
- correcting metabolic acidosis.

The delicate balance between myocardial oxygen supply and demand makes the cardiogenic shock patient a challenge to your nursing skills. You'll need to monitor him carefully for therapeutic effectiveness. However, before initiating any nursing measure, make sure you understand how that measure will affect myocardial oxygen supply and demand. Beneficial actions *increase* supply and *decrease* demand. Use extreme caution when taking any measure that increases demand.

Many interventions with *intended* beneficial effects alter variables that can increase oxygen demand. For example, raising a patient's arterial pressure increases his coronary artery blood flow. However, it also increases oxygen demand. Inotropic agents improve myocardial contractility but also increase demand. In both cases, the intervention's benefits must offset any resultant increased oxygen demand to avoid exacerbating the patient's condition.

Interventions for combating cardiogenic shock include drug therapy, mechanical assist devices, surgery, and independent nursing measures.

Drug therapy. The doctor will tailor drug therapy to the patient's hemodynamic status. The patient with near-normal PCWP will probably need volume replacement. A patient with abnormally high PCWP and SVR frequently benefits from a combination of drugs: one that improves contractility (for example, an inotrope such as dopamine or dobutamine) and another that decreases afterload (for example, nitroprusside). While administering these drugs, closely monitor the patient for signs and symptoms of tissue hypoperfusion in addition to assessing his hemodynamic parameters.

Volume expanders. Approximately 20% of patients with cardiogenic shock have significant hypovolemia from decreased oral fluid intake, emesis, aggressive diuretic therapy, or inappropriate reflex vasodilation. This leads to a decreased cardiac index and signs and symptoms of tissue hypoperfusion. About a third of these patients

---

Classifying cardiogenic shock associated with AMI

Depending on his hemodynamic parameters and clinical condition, a patient who develops cardiogenic shock after AMI falls into one of these four groups:

Group 1: Below-normal PCWP or PADP without pulmonary edema. Expect the doctor to order I.V. fluid replacement.

Group 2: Below-normal PCWP or PADP with pulmonary edema. Expect the doctor to order I.V. fluid replacement.

Group 3: Above-normal PCWP or PADP without pulmonary edema. Expect the doctor to order a vasodilator (such as nitroprusside or phentolamine) and/or digitalis. He may also use a mechanical assist device.

Group 4: Above-normal PCWP or PADP with pulmonary edema. Expect the doctor to order treatment similar to that for a Group 3 patient.

51 Shock

Cardiogenic Shock

How sympathomimetic drugs help reverse shock

If your patient's in cardiogenic shock, the doctor may order a sympathomimetic drug to improve myocardial contractility and organ perfusion. These drugs act on adrenergic nerve fibers—one of two fiber types in the sympathetic nervous system (SNS).

Adrenergic fibers terminate in specific receptor sites, designated as alpha- and beta-receptor sites. Each site stores a neurotransmitter—either epinephrine or norepinephrine.

The eyes, GI tract, sweat glands, skin, kidneys, and blood vessel surfaces contain alpha-receptors. Alpha-adrenergic stimulation causes vasoconstriction.

Beta-receptors come in two types: beta$_1$-receptors, found in cardiac muscle, and beta$_2$-receptors, found in the blood vessels, bronchial tree, and liver. Beta$_1$ stimulation increases myocardial contractile force, heart rate, and impulse conduction through the atrioventricular node. Beta$_2$ stimulation dilates blood vessels—especially coronary and skeletal muscle vessels—and relaxes smooth bronchial muscles (causing bronchial dilation).

Dopaminergic receptor sites, found on the renal and mesenteric vascular beds, respond to small amounts of the neurotransmitter dopamine, causing vasodilation.

Sympathomimetic (or adrenergic) drugs mimic SNS action. Alpha-adrenergic drugs cause vasoconstriction. Drugs that block alpha-receptors (alpha blocking agents) cause vasodilation. Beta-adrenergic drugs increase myocardial contractility and vasodilation. Beta-blocking drugs decrease contractility, slow the heart rate, and, in some patients, cause bronchospasm.

respond well to volume expanders. (Generally, PCWP must increase to 14 to 18 mm Hg [or PADP must increase to 20 to 24 mm Hg] before cardiac output improves.) Because volume expansion affects preload, volume expanders can increase stroke volume and thus improve coronary blood flow and arterial blood pressure.

Expect to administer volume expanders initially in 50- to 100-ml increments given over 5 to 10 minutes (see *Fluid guidelines,* page 52). Recommended solutions include colloids, such as low-molecular-weight dextrans (Dextran 40), albumin, and hetastarch (Hespan). Colloids remain in the vascular bed longer than such crystalloids as dextrose and saline solution, which enter the extracellular space within minutes.

Sympathomimetic (adrenergic) drugs. These agents improve myocardial contractility and blood flow through vital organs by increasing perfusion pressure. Sympathomimetic drugs vary in effect depending on their action on alpha- and beta-receptor sites. Norepinephrine (Levophed), dopamine (Intropin), and dobutamine (Dobutrex) may be used to treat cardiogenic shock.

Norepinephrine stimulates both alpha- and beta$_1$-receptors. At low doses, it increases cardiac output and blood pressure, mainly by improving myocardial contractility and causing moderate vasoconstriction. At higher doses, it leads to marked vasoconstriction, which may reduce cardiac output by increasing afterload (this also increases $M\dot{V}O_2$). Norepinephrine helps patients who have decreased blood pressure that markedly impairs organ perfusion.

Expect to give the drug at an initial I.V. infusion rate between 2 and 8 mcg/minute. Assess the patient for these adverse drug effects: oliguria from severe renal vasoconstriction, ventricular dysrhythmias, increased chest pain from myocardial ischemia, and hypovolemia (with prolonged use) from postcapillary fluid loss related to vasoconstriction. Because necrosis may occur if norepinephrine infiltrates tissues, administer the drug into a large vein. If tissue infiltration develops, discontinue the drug as ordered and inject the site with phentolamine (Regitine). An alpha blocker that causes vasodilation, phentolamine reduces tissue injury. *Note:* Because it increases $M\dot{V}O_2$ and renal perfusion, norepinephrine serves only as a temporary measure.

Dopamine causes varying effects, depending on the dose. Low doses (2 to 5 mcg/kg/minute) cause renal and mesenteric arterial dilation, which improves renal function and reduces preload. In moderate doses (6 to 10 mcg/kg/minute), beta$_1$ stimulation predominates, leading to increased myocardial contractility and blood pressure, with little SVR change. At high doses (above 10 mcg/kg/minute), alpha stimulation causes vasoconstriction. Ventricular ectopy and chest pain may result. The higher the dose, the greater the alpha-receptor effect. (At dosages of about 20 mcg/kg/minute, alpha effects [vasoconstriction] predominate.)

Dobutamine affects mainly beta$_1$-receptors, increasing myocardial contractility. As a result, the ventricles empty more completely and preload decreases. Higher doses create a weak beta$_2$ effect, causing vasodilation. This may decrease afterload and improve cardiac out-

Continued on page 52

Vascular Problems

52 Shock

Cardiogenic Shock

Continued

put. As ordered, administer dobutamine as a continuous I.V. infusion at 2.5 to 20 mcg/kg/minute.

Other sympathomimetic drugs that help treat cardiogenic shock include metaraminol (Aramine), methoxamine (Vasoxyl), phenylephrine (Neo-Synephrine), isoproterenol (Isuprel), and epinephrine (Adrenalin).

Diuretics. These drugs help treat patients with above-normal PCWP and pulmonary venous congestion. The doctor may order furosemide (Lasix), ethacrynic acid (Edecrin), or bumetanide (Bumex) for a patient with decreased urine output. When left ventricular filling pressure exceeds 20 mm Hg and pulmonary edema develops, the patient requires diuresis. However, in acute pulmonary edema, correcting volume deficits and maintaining adequate perfusion pressure most effectively reestablish adequate urine output.

A hypotensive, hypovolemic patient who receives a diuretic may suffer impaired tissue perfusion, which further exacerbates shock. To prevent this, carefully monitor his hemodynamic parameters.

Vasodilators. The body attempts to compensate for decreased cardiac output through vasoconstriction, which normally helps maintain adequate perfusion pressure. However, in cardiogenic shock, this response contributes to the vicious cycle of growing myocardial ischemia. Increased afterload further diminishes cardiac output and blood flow to the coronary arteries. Vasodilators can help break this cycle by decreasing afterload and preload. This permits more complete ventricular emptying, which improves cardiac output and blood pressure.

The most commonly used vasodilators for cardiogenic shock include nitroprusside (Nipride), nitroglycerin, and phentolamine. Nitroprusside acts directly on vascular-bed smooth muscle, causing arteriolar and venous dilation; preload and afterload reductions increase cardiac output. Expect to administer nitroprusside by I.V. infusion, usually beginning at 0.5 mcg/kg/minute. Titrate the dose to achieve the desired effect. The dose averages 3 mcg/kg/minute. Use caution when administering nitroprusside; severe hypotension can develop rapidly. Avoid giving nitroprusside (or any other vasodilator) to a patient with inadequate intravascular volume.

Nitroprusside's normally converted to cyanide by red blood cells, then to thiocyanate in the liver. Excreted by the kidneys, thiocyanate has a half-life of about 1 week. In a patient with impaired renal function, serum thiocyanate levels may rise dangerously and lead to fatigue, anorexia, delerium, and even death. A patient with hepatic congestion may lack the ability to convert cyanide to thiocyanate and thus may develop cyanide poisoning. Make sure to carefully monitor serial thiocyanate and cyanide levels in such a patient.

Nitroglycerin acts primarily as a venodilator, reducing venous return, preload, and $M\dot{V}O_2$. Expect to titrate the dose to achieve the desired effect. Administer this drug in glass bottles (it can adhere to plastic bags) and avoid polyvinyl chloride tubing.

An alpha blocking agent, phentolamine causes vascular-bed dilation. Arterial dilation leads to decreased afterload and increased cardiac

Fluid guidelines

The doctor can determine how much I.V. fluid replacement your patient needs by giving the fluid tolerance tests described below.

If the patient has an initial PCWP/PADP below 15 mm Hg:
• Give 100 ml of fluid over 5 minutes. Then give an additional 200 ml over 10 minutes *if* the patient meets these criteria:
—blood pressure and urine output increase
—clinical signs of shock and pulmonary congestion decrease
—PCWP/PADP remains unchanged or doesn't rise more than 2 mm Hg above initial level.

If the patient's PCWP/PADP remains stable or doesn't rise more than 2 mm Hg or exceed 16 mm Hg; blood pressure remains stable or rises; and signs of pulmonary congestion don't appear:
• Continue I.V. infusion at 500 to 1,000 ml/hour until hypotension and other signs of shock disappear. Check PCWP/PADP, blood pressure, and lung sounds every 15 minutes. (Consider a PCWP/PADP increase to 15 or 18 mm Hg satisfactory.)

If the patient has an initial PCWP/PADP between 15 and 18 mm Hg:
• Give 100 ml of fluid over 10 minutes. Further fluid administration depends on clinical signs and symptoms.

If the patient has an initial PCWP/PADP of 20 mm Hg or higher:
• Don't give fluids. Instead, administer a vasodilator cautiously, as ordered.

If the patient's PCWP/PADP rises to 16 mm Hg or higher after the initial fluid tolerance test:
• Discontinue fluids. The patient's response suggests pump failure—not hypovolemia—as shock's cause. If PCWP/PADP falls to the initial level, use the fluid tolerance test if the patient shows signs or symptoms of shock.

If the patient develops pulmonary edema after receiving I.V. fluids (indicated by PCWP/PADP of 25 to 30 mm Hg):
• Stop the infusion and give a rapid-acting digitalis preparation or vasodilator as ordered.

If the patient has a PCWP/PADP of approximately 5 mm Hg or lower:
• Give fluids according to the patient's response (low PCWP/PADP may stem from excessive diuretic or vasodilator use resulting in hypotension and shock).

Adapted with permission from Emanuel Goldberger, *A Textbook of Clinical Cardiology,* St. Louis: C.V. Mosby Co., 1982.

53 Shock

Cardiogenic Shock

Intraaortic balloon pump

To improve the recovery odds for a patient with cardiogenic shock, the doctor may order an intraaortic balloon pump.

The balloon catheter's connected to a pump console. The doctor usually inserts the catheter into the aorta via the femoral artery. The console determines inflation and deflation cycles according to the patient's EKG or arterial waveform.

Inflated with helium or carbon dioxide during diastole, the balloon increases aortic diastolic pressure, which in turn enhances coronary blood flow and perfusion.

Immediately before systole, the balloon deflates, permitting the left ventricle to eject blood into the aorta at lower pressure.

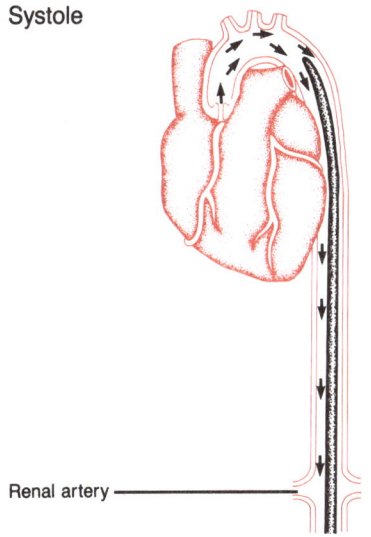

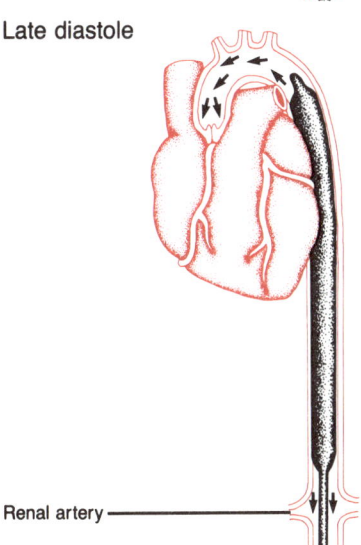

Systole

Renal artery

Late diastole

Renal artery

---

output; venous dilation causes venous pooling and decreased preload. In a patient with rising PCWP, this effect also helps improve cardiac output. However, in a patient with decreasing PCWP, phentolamine can decrease cardiac output and worsen hypotension. Give this drug cautiously to avoid decreasing systolic blood pressure more than 10 mm Hg, or below 80 mm Hg.

The doctor may also order sodium bicarbonate and oxygen to correct any hypoxia and metabolic acidosis; and dextrose in normal saline solution or Dextran 40 to correct hyponatremia (the most common electrolyte disturbance in AMI patients with cardiogenic shock).

Digitalis—usually ineffective in cardiogenic shock—may help treat a patient with uncontrolled or recurrent supraventricular dysrhythmias that don't respond to vagal stimulation. The doctor may order a rapid-acting digitalis preparation for a patient who develops acute pulmonary edema.

Mechanical assist devices. A cardiogenic shock patient with above-normal PCWP and below-normal cardiac index has the poorest recovery odds. Such a patient typically doesn't respond to maximum-dose drug therapy. However, he may benefit from a mechanical assist device that reduces ventricular workload and allows the ischemic myocardium to recover.

The *intraaortic balloon pump (IABP)*, also known as intraaortic balloon counterpulsation, ranks as the most widely used mechanical assist device. The balloon catheter, inserted through the femoral artery into the descending aorta, inflates during diastole (diastolic augmentation) and deflates just before systole. Inflation increases diastolic perfusion and blood flow into the coronary arteries. Deflation decreases afterload. Therefore, the IAPB may improve cardiac output (as afterload decreases, forward flow increases). The balance between myocardial oxygen supply and demand also improves: as more blood flows to the coronary arteries, the heart's oxygen supply grows and decreased afterload reduces oxygen demand.

An *external counterpulsation device* provides noninvasive diastolic augmentation and afterload reduction. Inflated bag units enclose each leg from ankle to thigh. Usually using air, an electronic control console applies alternating positive and negative pressure. Diastolic bag inflation (positive pressure) squeezes the legs, exerting uniform pressure on vessels. This forces arterial and venous blood back to the heart. Diastolic pressure then rises, and coronary artery filling and myocardial perfusion improve. Negative pressure during systole diminishes afterload and pulls arterial blood into the legs.

The *ventricular assist device (VAD)*—a blood pump—temporarily replaces failing ventricular function to allow for a recovery period. Still under investigation, the VAD diverts blood from the left ventricle to the ascending aorta, reducing left ventricular work load and maintaining circulation (see *Ventricular assist device,* page 54).

Surgery. The doctor may consider coronary artery bypass graft (CABG) surgery for a patient with cardiogenic shock. Technical advances have made CABG surgery possible for these severely ill patients. (For details on CABG surgery, see the NURSEREVIEW section on "Cardiac Problems.")

Continued on page 54

Shock

Cardiogenic Shock
Continued

Ventricular assist device
Still investigational, a ventricular assist device (VAD) augments heart action in a patient with inadequate cardiac pump function (such as in cardiogenic shock). A VAD may also serve as a temporary support for a patient awaiting heart transplantation or one who can't be weaned from a heart-lung machine. These devices may eventually provide an alternative to the artificial heart.

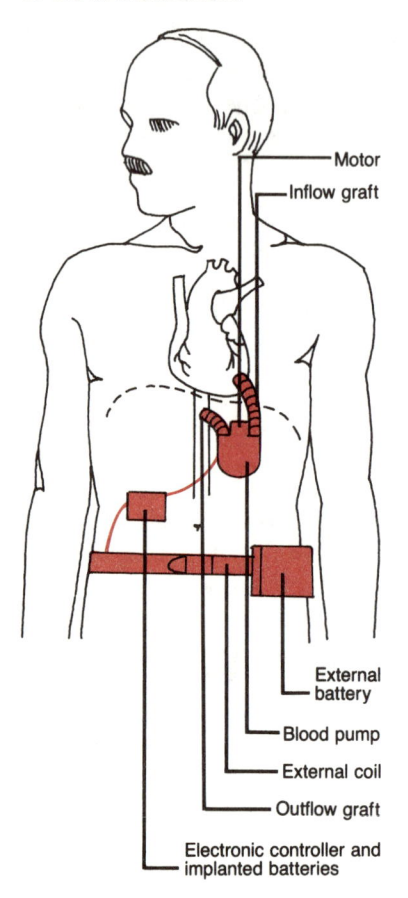

Independent nursing measures. Direct your nursing interventions toward reducing myocardial oxygen demand. To help achieve this goal, take measures to reduce the patient's pain, decrease his anxiety, and provide rest.

Reducing pain. Pain causes catecholamine release, which increases $M\dot{V}O_2$ and exacerbates any dysrhythmias. When carrying out pain-relief measures, first assess the patient's usual response to pain. Does he wait until pain grows severe before asking for relief? If so, encourage him to report even mild pain so that appropriate relief measures can begin early.

Decreasing anxiety. A patient with cardiogenic shock—usually surrounded by sophisticated lifesaving equipment in a tension-filled environment—may become extremely anxious. This may exacerbate the stress response (described earlier in this chapter) and worsen shock. To reduce anxiety, take the following steps whenever possible:
• Organize the patient's environment so that activities take place with minimal confusion.
• Don't talk about the patient where he can hear you—unless you intend to include him in the discussion. Also, avoid talking with other staff workers about nonclinical matters. Otherwise, the patient may feel he's receiving impersonal care.
• If the patient's conscious, explain procedures as you perform them.
• Allow the patient's family to visit—even if you must perform clinical procedures during their stay. He'll need their emotional support.

Providing rest. This may prove the most difficult goal with a critically ill patient because he'll need continuous vital sign assessment. However, try to control noise and traffic flow around him and schedule his activities to allow short, uninterrupted rest periods.

Evaluation
To best evaluate the patient with cardiogenic shock, assess his cardiac output. Consider increased cardiac output a sign of therapeutic effectiveness.

Base your evaluation on the patient's expected outcomes as listed on the nursing care plan. To determine whether his condition's improved, ask yourself the following questions:
• Can the patient maintain adequate tissue perfusion?
• Does his cardiac index fall between 2.5 and 4 liters/minute/m² and his PCWP between 15 and 20 mm Hg?
• Does he show signs of adequate tissue perfusion, such as warm, dry skin; urine output of at least 30 ml/hour; and mental alertness?

The answers to these and other questions will help you evaluate your patient's condition and determine his future needs. Keep in mind that these questions stem from the sample nursing care plan on page 49. Your questions may differ.

Vascular Problems

55 Shock

Distributive Shock: Vascular Bed Dilation

Judith K. Bobb, who wrote this chapter, is Critical Care Nurse Coordinator at the Maryland Institute for Emergency Medical Services Systems in Baltimore. She earned her BSN from the University of Colorado and her MSN from the University of Maryland.

Distributive shock—also called vasogenic shock—results from changes in intravascular volume distribution or location. Unlike other shock types, distributive shock doesn't initially include myocardial performance and blood volume disturbances. Although the vascular bed enlarges, increasing its volume capacity, volume remains unchanged. Because the patient doesn't have enough blood to fill the enlarged vascular bed, his peripheral resistance decreases, reducing his blood pressure. The resulting vasodilation leads to venous pooling, which decreases oxygen and nutrient supplies to tissues and limits cellular waste removal. If the condition persists, anoxia and cell destruction result.

The three main causes of distributive shock include:
- massive antibody-antigen reactions (anaphylactic shock)
- sympathetic tone loss (neurogenic shock)
- widespread infection (septic shock).

Anaphylactic shock

An acute and life-threatening syndrome, anaphylactic shock (also termed anaphylaxis) results from an immune system response to an antigen to which the body's been sensitized. The victim suffers immediate, dramatic vascular and bronchial changes that produce profound hypovolemia and severe respiratory distress. Without prompt identification and immediate intervention, the victim will die.

Almost any foreign material can cause an anaphylactic or anaphylactoid reaction. (An *anaphylactoid* reaction—clinically identical to anaphylaxis—doesn't involve IgE antibodies.) The most common allergens include penicillin and venom from stinging insects of the Hymenoptera order (bees, wasps, and yellow jackets).

Allergens most commonly enter the body through one of two routes:
- injection (drugs, serum, contrast media, and insect or animal venom)
- ingestion (foods and drugs).

An all-or-nothing response, anaphylaxis depends on various factors. A small allergen dose may not produce the typical systemic response. For example, a wasp sting may not inject enough venom to cause anaphylaxis. Delayed absorption of an ingested allergen can also keep allergen levels too low to cause a reaction.

The severity of the victim's response also depends on his predisposition to anaphylaxis. A person with asthma or atopy (hypersensitivity) has an increased anaphylaxis risk and may develop anaphylaxis from even a minute allergen dose. Antibody levels also affect response. After a variable number of years, antibody levels gradually decrease. Eventually, too few antibodies remain to produce anaphylaxis—even in a high-risk individual.

An allergen's chemical makeup also helps determine the response. Soluble antigens produce the most overwhelming reaction—usually within a few minutes. Soluble antigens include I.V. agents such as contrast media, analgesics, and antibiotics. The allergen's entry site can prove crucial, too. For example, insect venom can produce a response within minutes if the sting occurs in a highly vascular area, such as the lips.

A glossary of terms

Anaphylactoid reaction. Clinically identical to anaphylaxis, but without apparent IgE immunoglobulin antibody involvement. It typically involves a reaction to nonprotein substances, such as diagnostic contrast media. An anaphylactoid reaction requires the same treatment as anaphylaxis.

Anaphylaxis. An immediate hypersensitivity reaction resulting from an antigen-antibody reaction in a sensitized person (also called anaphylactic shock). It involves the following:
- an antigen or allergen
- an IgE immunoglobulin antibody
- mast cell and basophil degranulation.

Antibody. An antigen-attacking protein molecule in the circulation or produced in response to an antigen.

Antigen. A foreign substance that stimulates antibody formation.

Basophil. A white blood cell that presumably brings heparin to inflamed tissue and participates in phagocytosis.

Mast cell. A cell in pericapillary connective tissue that releases chemical mediators during antibody-antigen interactions.

Continued on page 56

Vascular Problems

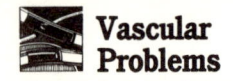

56 Shock

Distributive Shock

Anaphylactic shock—*continued*

The two-phase response. Anaphylaxis starts with a *sensitization phase*, when initial exposure to an antigen occurs. The immune system forms antibodies—usually IgE immunoglobulins—that bind to receptors on mast cells or basophils. At this point, the mast cells or basophils remain inactive. In 3 to 5 days, antibody titer usually rises high enough to produce anaphylaxis with a second exposure to the sensitizing antigen. Although immunologists don't know exactly how long the high antibody level persists, many suspect it may last several years.

The second anaphylaxis phase—the *mediator release phase*—takes place on the next antigen exposure (immunologists first used the term *shock* to describe this second "shocking" antigen dose). Interacting with IgE antibodies on mast cells and basophils, the antigen now triggers degranulation. Anaphylaxis signs and symptoms develop as mast cell and basophil granules release vasoactive substances, including:
- histamine
- slow-reacting substance of anaphylaxis (SRS-A)
- prostaglandins
- eosinophil chemotactic factor of anaphylaxis (ECF-A)
- bradykinin
- serotonin
- platelet activating factor (PAF)
- heparin.

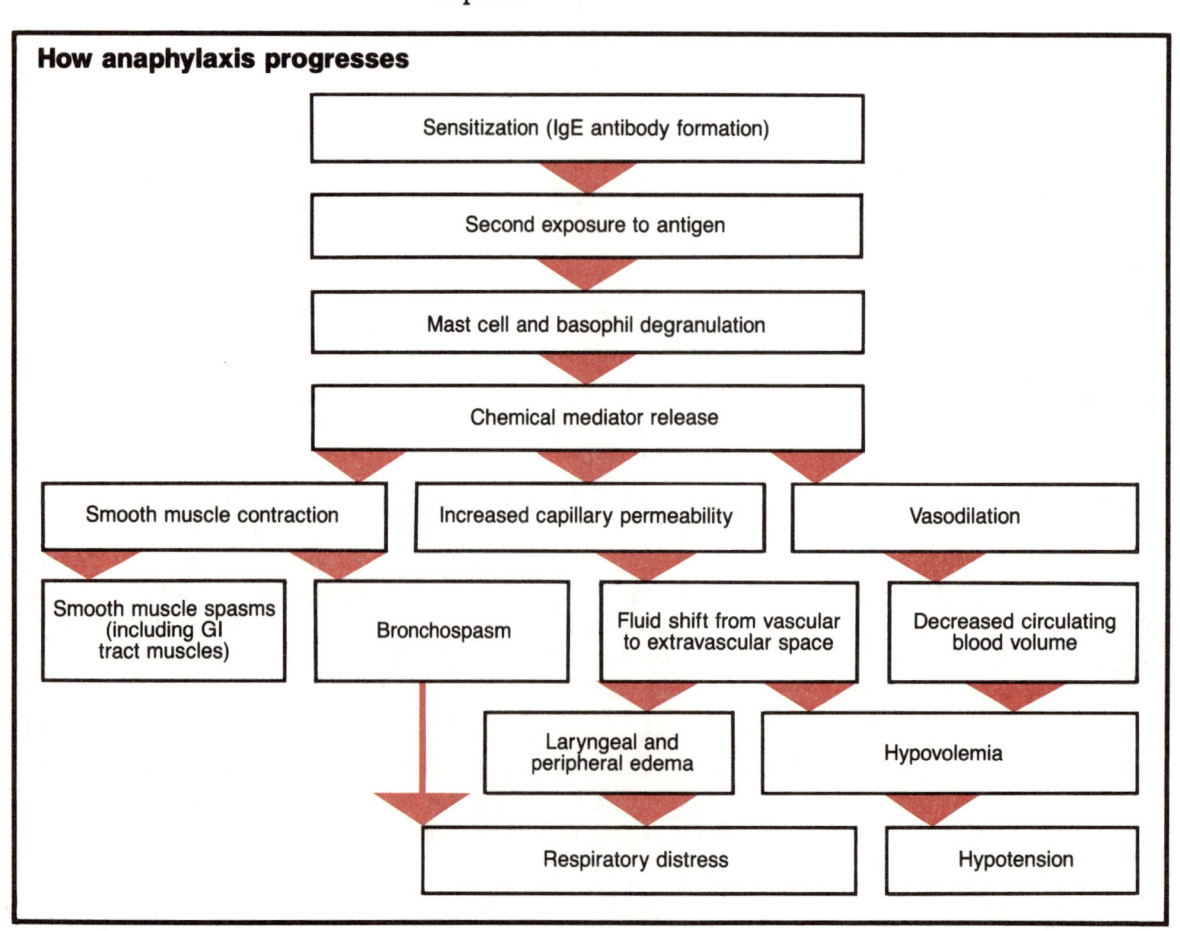

How anaphylaxis progresses

Sensitization (IgE antibody formation)
↓
Second exposure to antigen
↓
Mast cell and basophil degranulation
↓
Chemical mediator release
↓
- Smooth muscle contraction → Smooth muscle spasms (including GI tract muscles)
- Smooth muscle contraction → Bronchospasm → Respiratory distress
- Increased capillary permeability → Fluid shift from vascular to extravascular space → Laryngeal and peripheral edema → Respiratory distress
- Vasodilation → Decreased circulating blood volume → Hypovolemia → Hypotension

Vascular Problems

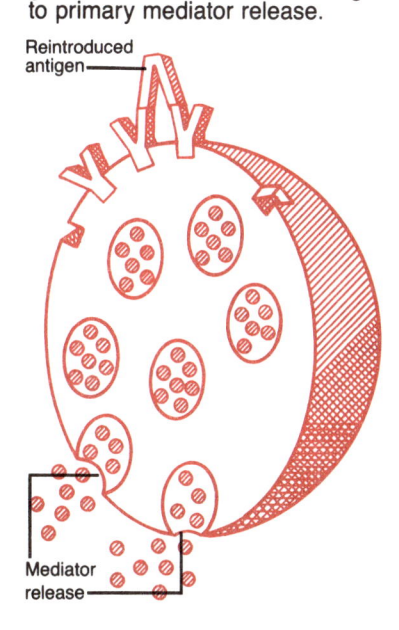

57 Shock

Distributive Shock

The major chemical mediator of anaphylaxis, *histamine* causes smooth muscle contraction, blood capillary dilation, increased capillary permeability, and decreased blood pressure. Experts have described two histamine receptor types—H_1 and H_2. H_1 receptor stimulation dilates blood vessels, increases capillary permeability, and contracts nonvascular smooth muscles. H_2 receptor stimulation increases gastric acid secretion.

While histamine causes some smooth muscles (such as bronchial and intestinal muscles) to contract, it causes others (such as those in smaller blood vessels) to relax. Vasodilation, which can lead to reduced blood pressure, probably results from the combined effects of H_1 and H_2 receptor stimulation.

Capillary dilation, histamine's most characteristic effect, stems from direct action on vessels, regardless of specific innervation. Most obvious in the face and upper body, dilation results from histamine's inhibitory effects on terminal arteriolar smooth muscle. Dilation in postcapillary venules, which lack smooth muscle, occurs mainly passively. Resistance decreases in terminal arterioles and rises in larger veins, which histamine constricts.

Histamine's effects on the microcirculation trigger a chain of events that shifts plasma proteins and fluid from vascular to extravascular compartments. Histamine also increases endothelial cell adhesiveness.

Histamine released from basophils and mast cells causes a typical inflammatory response to tissue injury. However, unlike normal inflammation that develops only at the injury site, anaphylaxis causes an inflammatory response that affects the entire body, producing a potentially lethal crisis.

SRS-A, which contracts bronchial smooth muscle and increases vascular permeability, contains metabolites called leukotrienes. A lipid, SRS-A potentiates histamine's effects.

Prostaglandins have various effects depending on the prostaglandin involved. These substances change vascular permeability, contract smooth muscle, and enhance other mediators' effects.

ECF-A acts on eosinophils to keep them from neutralizing other mediators. ECF-A also stimulates bradykinin and serotonin release.

Bradykinin, an extremely potent kinin (a polypeptide released during inflammation), stimulates smooth muscle contraction, including bronchoconstriction. It also causes vasodilation and increased capillary permeability.

Serotonin, like histamine, increases capillary permeability—especially in pulmonary capillaries.

PAF and *heparin* affect the blood. PAF causes platelet release and aggregation. Heparin may create the clotting abnormalities that frequently accompany anaphylaxis.

Release of these primary chemical mediators may also trigger release of secondary chemical mediators, such as those of the complement system. This results in further physiologic damage that exacerbates anaphylaxis.

Continued on page 58

Tracking an anaphylactic reaction

Sensitization phase
During initial antigen exposure, plasma cells synthesize antigen-specific IgE molecules. Portions of these molecules then bind to receptors on mast cells or basophils.

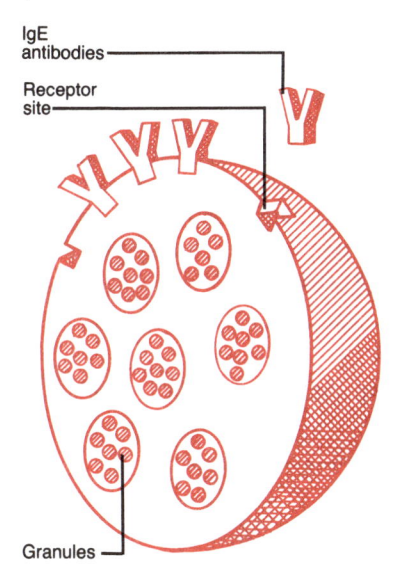

Mediator release phase
On reintroduction, the antigen interacts with IgE molecules. Known as antigen bridging or cross-linking, this interaction triggers biochemical events leading to primary mediator release.

Vascular Problems

Distributive Shock

Anaphylactic shock—*continued*

Assessment

Consider anaphylaxis a possible cause for any unexplained acute respiratory distress. The patient's history can provide crucial information about recent exposure to a potential antigen. Note the time from exposure to symptom onset: although serious, reactions delayed for more than 1 or 2 hours after exposure don't qualify as anaphylaxis. Remember—anaphylaxis means *immediate* hypersensitivity.

If you suspect anaphylaxis, be prepared to intervene as you assess the patient. Make sure he has a patent airway and adequate breathing and circulation. If his condition permits, ask him about any allergies or atopy, such as asthma. Try to find out whether he's had similar reactions before and, if so, to which substance. A patient who's had an anaphylactic reaction to one substance may react the same way to a chemically similar antigen. (If the patient can't

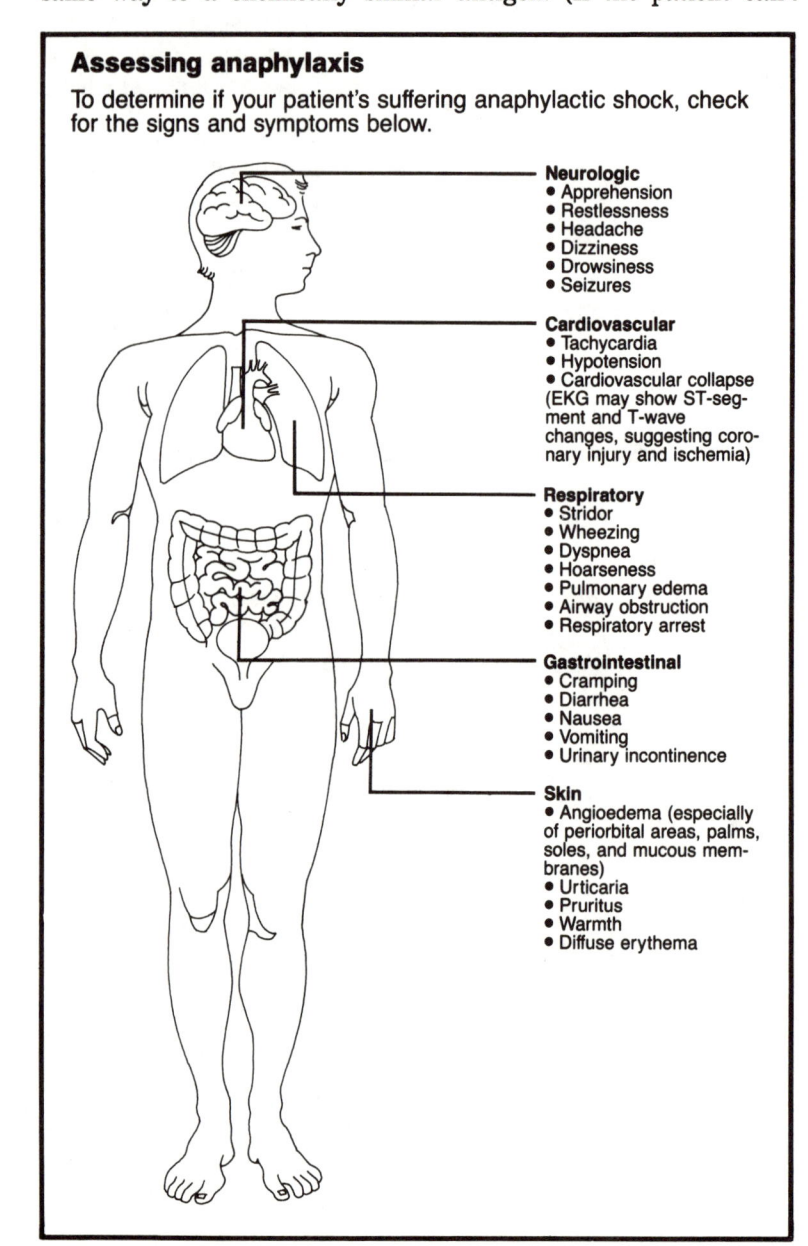

Assessing anaphylaxis

To determine if your patient's suffering anaphylactic shock, check for the signs and symptoms below.

Neurologic
- Apprehension
- Restlessness
- Headache
- Dizziness
- Drowsiness
- Seizures

Cardiovascular
- Tachycardia
- Hypotension
- Cardiovascular collapse (EKG may show ST-segment and T-wave changes, suggesting coronary injury and ischemia)

Respiratory
- Stridor
- Wheezing
- Dyspnea
- Hoarseness
- Pulmonary edema
- Airway obstruction
- Respiratory arrest

Gastrointestinal
- Cramping
- Diarrhea
- Nausea
- Vomiting
- Urinary incontinence

Skin
- Angioedema (especially of periorbital areas, palms, soles, and mucous membranes)
- Urticaria
- Pruritus
- Warmth
- Diffuse erythema

59 Shock

Distributive Shock

Anaphylactic and anaphylactoid reactions: Some common causes

Anesthetics: cocaine, lidocaine, procaine, thiopental

Antibiotics: penicillin and penicillin analogs, cephalosporins, tetracyclines, erythromycin, streptomycin

Blood products and antisera: red and white blood cell and platelet transfusions; gamma globulin; rabies, tetanus, and diphtheria antitoxin; snake and spider antivenom

Diagnostic agents: contrast media containing iodine

Foods and dyes: eggs, milk, nuts, peanuts, soybeans, kidney beans, shellfish, fruits (especially strawberries), tartrazine, yellow dye No. 5

Hormones: insulin, pituitary extract, adrenocorticotropic hormone

Narcotic analgesics: morphine, codeine, meprobamate

Nonsteroidal anti-inflammatory agents: salicylates, aminopyrine, indomethacin

Other drugs: iodides, thiazide diuretics, protamine, chlorpropamide, parenteral iron

Pollens: ragweed, grasses

Venoms: from bees, wasps, hornets, yellow jackets, snakes, spiders, jellyfish

---

respond, ask any bystanders or family members about his history and look for a Medic Alert tag or wallet card.)

Always review any medications the patient took within the hour before signs and symptoms appeared. Also determine whether he's taken any emergency medication (such as that in an anaphylaxis kit) or a beta blocker (for example, propranolol). Beta blockers may inhibit the action of epinephrine—the main anaphylaxis treatment.

Death from anaphylaxis most frequently stems from asphyxiation secondary to bronchoconstriction. To prevent asphyxiation, carefully and continually assess your patient for adequate respiration and ventilation.

Anaphylaxis signs and symptoms depend on the allergen's entry route, the amount of allergen absorbed, the absorption rate, and the degree of patient hypersensitivity (in an immune-mediated reaction). For example, an antigenic food may cause nausea, vomiting, abdominal cramping, and diarrhea before producing severe systemic signs or symptoms. Or a sensitized person may develop localized pruritic urticaria at an insect sting or drug injection site before experiencing more generalized signs and symptoms.

The most lethal reactions typically occur within minutes of exposure to the offending agent. The victim may experience chest tightness or a feeling of impending doom, possibly without preceding symptoms. Generalized skin signs—diffuse erythema, flushing, urticaria, and periorbital and mouth angioedema—may precede severe, rapidly progressing respiratory distress (caused by laryngeal edema and bronchospasm). The posterior pharynx, vocal cords, and uvula commonly become swollen and edematous. Auscultation may reveal diffuse wheezes and prolonged expirations. Hypotension and other signs of shock may follow, although such signs sometimes occur first.

Changes in level of consciousness usually parallel respiratory effects: initial alertness gives way to decreased responsiveness as the patient's arterial oxygen (PaO_2) level and/or brain perfusion decreases. (See *Assessing anaphylaxis* for details on assessment.)

Diagnostic studies. The doctor will rely on history and physical findings rather than on specific tests to diagnose anaphylaxis. After recovery, allergy tests (skin and use tests) may help identify causative agents. (However, these tests may provoke another episode.) The doctor may perform serial skin tests, using intradermal testing, scratch testing, or patch testing.

With *intradermal testing*, the doctor injects allergens into spaced skin intervals on the patient's forearm or intrascapular area. At the same time, he injects a control substance (diluent). After 15 to 30 minutes, he inspects the injection sites for wheals with surrounding erythema—a positive sign. Intradermal testing detects allergies to pollen, feathers, animal dander, and dust.

In a *scratch test*, which reveals sensitivities to the same allergens identified by intradermal testing, the doctor first cleanses the patient's skin with alcohol and allows it to dry. Then he makes a superficial scratch (usually 1 to 4 mm long) and applies extracts

Continued on page 60

Vascular Problems

Shock

Distributive Shock

Cost-cutting tip

If your patient's at risk for a severe anaphylactic reaction, advise him to carry an emergency kit with him at all times. Emergency medication can help prevent a severe reaction, decrease the cost of medical care, and reduce the length of hospitalization.

For a patient allergic to insect stings, for example, you might recommend any of the following:
- Ana-Kit (Hollister-Stier Laboratories), which includes epinephrine 1:1,000 (two 0.3-mg doses) in 1 ml; one disposable sterile syringe; chlorpheniramine maleate, 2 mg (four chewable tablets); sterile alcohol pads (two each); tourniquet (one each)
- EpiPen Auto-Injector (Center Labs), which delivers a 0.3-mg I.M. dose of epinephrine 1:1,000 in 2-ml disposable injectors
- EpiPen Jr. Auto-Injector (Center Labs), which delivers a 0.15-mg I.M. dose of epinephrine from epinephrine injection 1:2,000 in 2-ml disposable injectors.

Also advise the patient to wear a medical identification tag (such as a Medic Alert tag) to inform health care workers of his allergy.

Anaphylactic shock—*continued*

containing the allergen to be tested. Erythema after 30 minutes indicates a positive test.

If the doctor suspects an allergy to clothing, detergents, perfumes, or cosmetics, he may perform a *patch test*. This test uses 1″ gauze squares, soaked with the suspected allergen and taped to the patient's skin. After 48 hours, the doctor removes the patch and inspects the skin. He grades the responses + (erythema only), ++ (erythema and papules), +++ (erythema, papules, and vesicles), or ++++ (erythema, papules, vesicles, and bullae or ulceration).

Use testing helps identify food allergies. The patient keeps a food diary for at least a week. Then he removes potentially allergenic foods (such as wheat, eggs, and milk) from his diet. Once his symptoms subside, he adds these foods back to his diet one at a time. A reaction (immediate or delayed) after reintroduction of a particular food identifies the offending agent.

Planning

Before planning your nursing care, develop the nursing diagnosis by identifying the patient's actual or potential problem, then relating it to its cause. Possible nursing diagnoses for a patient with anaphylactic shock include:
- gas exchange, impaired; related to bronchoconstriction
- breathing patterns, ineffective; related to bronchoconstriction
- fluid volume, alteration in (deficit); related to increased capillary permeability
- cardiac output, alteration in (decreased); related to hypovolemia
- tissue perfusion, alteration in; related to hypovolemia
- injury, potential for (cerebral hypoxia); related to inadequate gas exchange
- anxiety; related to inadequate gas exchange
- fear of dying; related to airway compromise.

The sample nursing care plan below shows expected outcomes, nursing interventions, and discharge planning for one nursing di-

Sample nursing care plan: Anaphylactic shock

Nursing diagnosis	Expected outcomes
Gas exchange, impaired; related to bronchoconstriction	The patient will: • maintain adequate gas exchange. • show reduced respiratory effort. • maintain adequate arterial blood gas (ABG) values. • maintain clear breath sounds.

Nursing interventions	Discharge planning
• Ensure airway patency. • Help the patient find a position that optimizes breathing efficiency and reduces oxygen consumption. • Evaluate oxygen therapy's effectiveness and notify doctor of any changes. • Assess and record vital signs, including breath sounds, as indicated. Notify doctor if you hear crackles or wheezes. • Assess hemoglobin, hematocrit, and ABG values, as indicated. Notify doctor of any abnormalities.	• Discuss the disorder and its process with patient and his family. • Encourage patient to wear a medical identification tag, such as a Medic Alert tag. • Teach patient and his family how to recognize anaphylaxis signs and symptoms. Also teach them how to contact emergency medical services. • Advise patient when to seek medical attention. • Arrange for follow-up care as needed. • If indicated, teach patient how to use anaphylaxis self-medication kit.

Vascular Problems

61 Shock

Distributive Shock

agnosis listed on the previous page. However, you'll want to tailor each care plan to fit your patient's needs.

Intervention
Regardless of how severe anaphylaxis becomes, treatment goals always include:
* providing ventilation
* restoring adequate circulation
* preventing future episodes.

Remember, your patient's condition may change rapidly, so be sure to assess him continuously as you carry out immediate interventions.

Providing ventilation. To maintain airway patency and adequate ventilation, be prepared to intervene with airway control measures or to assist with artificial airway placement—intubation or tracheotomy. As ordered, administer high oxygen concentrations to help protect vital organ function. Be sure to watch for signs and symptoms of laryngeal edema.

Take immediate measures to promote ventilation and reduce oxygen demand. For example, help the patient into a comfortable position and tell him to inhale slowly and exhale through pursed lips, if possible.

While ensuring ventilatory adequacy, try to prevent further exposure to the causative agent; such exposure will exacerbate the patient's condition. For anaphylaxis caused by I.V. drugs or contrast media, stop the drugs or procedure immediately. For venom-induced anaphylaxis, apply a tourniquet to the patient's arm or leg above the sting, if appropriate. Some doctors advocate removing the stinger by scraping the site with a dull object, because grasping and pulling could contract the venom sac and release more toxin.

Besides supporting ventilation, expect to administer drugs to block or counteract histamine's effects. Epinephrine, the preferred drug, prevents further histamine release and counteracts bronchoconstriction, hypotension, and vasodilation (see *How epinephrine reverses anaphylaxis,* page 62). The drug's dosage and administration route depend on the patient's condition. In early anaphylaxis, the doctor may order subcutaneous or I.M. injection of 0.3 to 0.5 ml of a 1:1,000 solution (0.01 ml/kg for a child). If the patient's in acute respiratory distress, expect to give up to 5 ml of epinephrine I.V. of a 1:10,000 solution. If vascular collapse prevents venous access, give epinephrine endotracheally, or inject it into the vascular tissue beneath the tongue, as ordered.

Because epinephrine's action lasts only 3 to 5 minutes, the patient may need repeated doses if he doesn't respond rapidly. To help assess epinephrine's effect on heart rhythm, begin continuous cardiac monitoring, as ordered.

If bronchoconstriction persists despite initial relief from epinephrine, the doctor may order I.V. aminophylline, a bronchodilator with a longer duration of action. Like epinephrine, aminophylline helps block additional mast cell or basophil degranulation.

Continued on page 62

Anaphylaxis care priorities

If your patient develops anaphylaxis, follow these care priorities:

Ensure ventilation by inserting an artificial airway or assisting with intubation or tracheotomy, as ordered and needed. Also, administer epinephrine, bronchodilators (such as aminophylline), and oxygen, as ordered.

Restore adequate circulation by administering epinephrine, I.V. fluids (crystalloids or colloids), vasopressors, antihistamines, or corticosteroids, as ordered. Also, place the patient in Trendelenburg's position to help improve circulation.

Prevent future episodes by taking measures, as ordered, to desensitize the patient to the offending agent. Also, urge him to carry a wallet card or to wear a medical identification tag describing his allergic sensitivities. If he can't avoid potential anaphylactic agents, suggest that he obtain an anaphylaxis self-medication kit.

Distributive Shock

Anaphylactic shock—*continued*

Antihistamines usually don't relieve severe bronchoconstriction, but they can help counteract peripheral signs or symptoms, such as pruritus. The doctor usually orders diphenhydramine (Benadryl).

Corticosteroids may be used as supportive therapy. These drugs stabilize capillary walls, reduce fluid shifts by decreasing capillary permeability, maintain blood pressure, and minimize further systemic reactions by halting degranulation.

Restoring adequate circulation. Once you've ensured the patient's ventilation, expect to begin fluid replacement to correct intravascular fluid loss from third-space shifts and vasodilation. As ordered, insert I.V. lines and administer crystalloid and/or colloid solutions. Titrate fluid doses according to your patient's blood pressure and perfusion status. *Important:* Watch carefully for signs or symptoms of fluid overload, which may cause serious complications.

The doctor may order a vasopressor, such as norepinephrine (Levophed) or dopamine (Intropin), if fluid therapy fails to maintain adequate blood pressure. These drugs improve cardiac contractility and counteract vasodilation. However, because they cause vasoconstriction, they may further compromise tissue perfusion. Monitor your patient carefully if he's receiving either drug.

Placing the patient in a supine or Trendelenburg's position may also help circulation. However, be careful not to compromise ventilation.

A terrifying experience, anaphylaxis can increase your patient's heart rate and oxygen needs. Calm him by providing continuous emotional support. Explain that he's having an allergic reaction, and assure him that you and other health care workers will monitor him closely and treat him appropriately. Explain procedures as you perform them, answer his questions, and don't hesitate to touch him reassuringly.

Preventing future episodes. Once the patient's stable, continue to observe him for several hours, watching for indications of delayed reaction to anaphylaxis or its treatment. Instruct him to avoid any vasodilatory stimulation (such as from vasodilatory drugs, alcohol, and hot showers or baths) for at least 24 hours.

Once the causative agent's been identified, instruct the patient to avoid substances likely to cause future reactions. The doctor may recommend desensitization to alleviate allergic reactions and reduce the risk of future episodes. This method works by introducing small antigen amounts that gradually exhaust antibodies bound to mast cells or basophils. The body then can't release enough chemical anaphylaxis mediators to cause an attack.

Advise the patient to wear medical identification that lists allergens to which he's sensitive. Also urge him to carry a wallet card describing his allergic sensitivities.

If the patient can't avoid potential anaphylactic agents, such as bee venom, he may need a prophylactic antihistamine and/or a sympathomimetic drug to reduce the severity of any future reactions. Suggest that he obtain an anaphylaxis kit so he can give himself epinephrine injections.

How epinephrine reverses anaphylaxis

Epinephrine, an adrenergic drug, mimics the effects of naturally occurring catecholamines on the body's alpha-receptors and beta-receptors. Alpha-receptors (located in veins and arteries) control vasoconstriction. Beta-receptors (located in the heart, bronchioles, and peripheral vessels) control heart rate, myocardial contractility, and bronchiolar and peripheral vessel dilation.

Epinephrine has a potent effect on both receptor types. Consequently, it constricts dilated blood vessels (alpha stimulation) and increases heart rate, improves myocardial contractility, and dilates bronchioles (beta stimulation). These effects counteract anaphylaxis signs and symptoms.

Epinephrine also inhibits histamine release and negates the effects of any circulating histamine. This reverses histamine-related bronchiolar constriction, vasodilation, and edema. Epinephrine also prevents further mast cell or basophil degranulation.

Note: A patient receiving a beta blocker, such as propranolol, may not respond to standard epinephrine doses. If he gets no relief within 1 to 2 minutes after receiving epinephrine, consider asking the doctor to increase the dose and/or frequency of administration.

63 Shock

Distributive Shock

To help prevent anaphylaxis in any patient, ask about known allergies or a history of anaphylactic reactions. Be sure to document the information in the patient's record.

Complications. These vary with shock's severity and with the patient's response to treatment. Cerebral hypoxia can develop from impaired oxygenation and reduced cerebral blood flow.

Evaluation
Base your evaluation on the expected outcomes listed on your nursing care plan. To help determine whether your patient's improved, ask yourself the following questions:
- Has the patient's breathing improved?
- Can he maintain adequate gas exchange?
- Do his arterial blood gas values fall within his normal range?
- Does he have crackles or wheezes?

The answers to these questions will help you evaluate the effectiveness of your patient's care and determine his future needs. Keep in mind that these questions stem from the care plan on page 60. Your questions may differ.

Neurogenic shock

Neurogenic shock can result from any condition that interrupts vasomotor impulses. As vasomotor tone fails, peripheral resistance decreases. Massive vasodilation develops as blood vessels lack sympathetic innervation. In arterioles, vasodilation causes hypotension; in veins, decreased stroke volume and venous return to the heart. Although the patient's blood volume may remain normal, blood pooling in peripheral arterioles and veins disturbs volume distribution. This results in relative hypovolemia. Usually transitory, neurogenic shock causes reduced filling pressure, blood pressure, peripheral resistance, and tissue perfusion.

The term *neurogenic shock* can be misleading. Unlike other shock types, neurogenic shock usually doesn't impair tissue perfusion severely. However, it does cause decreased cardiac output, leading to hypotension.

Neurogenic shock can stem from the following conditions:
- *upper spinal cord injury or disease.* A lesion above the midthoracic region may interrupt sympathetic nervous system (SNS) impulses from the medulla's vasomotor center to peripheral vessels. The most common cause of neurogenic shock, spinal injury may also lead to cord edema, temporarily stopping impulse transmission. (For more on this condition, called spinal shock, see *Spinal shock,* page 64.)
- *high spinal anesthesia.* An anesthetic that travels up the spinal cord may block SNS outflow from the medulla.
- *vasomotor center depression.* Severe pain, hypoglycemia (insulin shock), or use of such drugs as barbiturates can cause this.
- *exposure to noxious stimuli.* Excessive vagal stimulation, such as from fear or pain, can cause syncope. In this condition, the heart rate slows, cardiac output drops, peripheral vessels dilate, and the victim loses consciousness (which removes the stimulus). Compensatory mechanisms then restore normal cardiac output.
- *massive head injury* (rare). This results from vasomotor center damage that causes wildly fluctuating blood pressure. Profound hypotension eventually develops, leading to shock.

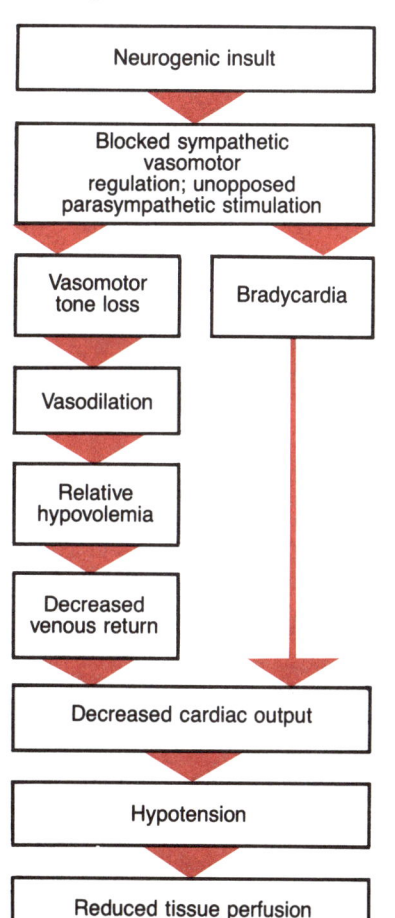

Continued on page 64

What happens in neurogenic shock

Neurogenic insult
↓
Blocked sympathetic vasomotor regulation; unopposed parasympathetic stimulation
↓
Vasomotor tone loss → Bradycardia
↓
Vasodilation
↓
Relative hypovolemia
↓
Decreased venous return
↓
Decreased cardiac output
↓
Hypotension
↓
Reduced tissue perfusion

Vascular Problems

64 Shock

Distributive Shock

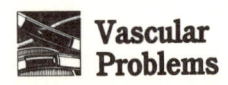

Spinal shock

The most common neurogenic shock type, spinal shock usually occurs within 30 to 60 minutes after spinal cord injury. Researchers don't fully understand the disorder, but they know that spinal cord edema develops in response to the injury, blocking all, or nearly all, reflex activity below injury level.

Spinal shock probably results from sudden impulse loss from the descending pathways, which normally maintain spinal cord neuronal excitability. Disrupted impulse flow causes the spinal cord to undergo an abrupt but transient change that markedly reduces the cord's resting excitability. During this period, the patient experiences spinal shock. Tendon reflexes diminish or disappear, and the patient loses temperature control and vasomotor tone. Hypotension and bradycardia result from vasomotor tone loss. Urinary retention, ileus, and fecal retention result from bladder and bowel paralysis.

Spinal cord damage above the sixth thoracic vertebra severely impairs sympathetic nerve stimulation to peripheral blood vessels. Consequently, the vessels can't constrict, resulting in generalized vasodilation. Venous return to the heart declines and blood pools in veins and capillaries, leading to decreased cardiac output and hypotension.

Spinal shock can last from days to months. However, sympathetic stimulation eventually returns.

If the patient's blood pressure stabilizes at approximately 100/60 mm Hg, he probably won't need corrective measures unless his urine output falls below 30 ml/hour or his mental status deteriorates. If his mean systemic arterial pressure falls below 70 mm Hg, he'll need fluid replacement.

Spinal shock also disturbs cardiac rate and rhythm. Because the disorder blocks sympathetic impulses that normally speed the heart rate, cardioinhibitory impulses predominate. Bradycardia develops, requiring symptomatic treatment.

Spinal shock doesn't inhibit vagal impulses to the heart's sinoatrial node. Therefore, try to minimize vagal stimulation by avoiding Valsalva's maneuver and by giving adequate oxygenation before and after any tracheal suctioning.

Because the patient with spinal shock has neurologic deficits, be
Continued

Neurogenic shock—*continued*

Assessment

When assessing a patient for neurogenic shock, be sure to obtain his history to help determine what's caused his condition. Try to find out why he was admitted or what produced a change in his condition. Check his medication history for any drugs that may affect cardiac output or neurologic function.

Ask yourself the following questions to explore the patient's condition:
• Why was the patient admitted?
• Does he have a history of spinal cord injury? Has his spine been stabilized with a cervical collar or backboard?
• Did he lose consciousness at any time?
• Does he show sensory or motor impairment in his arms or legs? Does he complain of numbness, weakness, or a tingling sensation?
• What's his level of consciousness now? Can he follow simple commands? Does he respond appropriately to questions?
• Did he have recent surgery? What type of anesthesia did he undergo? General? Spinal?
• If he had a general anesthetic, did he experience *deep* anesthesia?
• Does he have a history of hypoglycemia?
• Has he been receiving insulin or an oral antibiotic?

Note: During your assessment, be prepared to take initial interventions, especially to ensure your patient's airway, breathing, and circulation.

Physical examination. Record baseline vital signs (including temperature) and assess the patient's neurologic status. Hypotension associated with bradycardia (neurogenic shock's hallmark) helps rule out other shock types. (Remember—tachycardia usually accompanies other shock types.) However, if your patient's blood pressure remains normal, don't assume he *doesn't* have neurogenic shock. In most cases, neurogenic shock doesn't reduce systolic pressure below 100 mm Hg.

The patient's respiratory rate may increase from anxiety and fear or—if he's suffered spinal cord injury—from damage related to the injury's level and severity. Vasodilation typically makes the patient's skin warm and dry and, in some cases, flushed. Expect adequate renal blood flow to produce normal urine output.

Also document level of consciousness, pupil size and reaction, Glasgow Coma Scale score, and arm and leg strength and movement. Depending on the patient's condition or on the shock's underlying cause, you may need to perform a more detailed neurologic assessment.

Neurogenic shock usually produces neurologic deficits even in its early stage. Specific deficits depend on the brain area suffering reduced perfusion. When recumbent, the patient may not show impaired consciousness unless he has other injuries. (For more information on neurologic assessment, see the NURSEREVIEW section on "Neurologic Problems.")

Assess your patient frequently and document your findings. Keep in mind that signs of SNS disruption may last from hours to weeks if the patient has a spinal injury. To recognize complications early, monitor trends in the patient's condition.

Vascular Problems

65 Shock

Spinal shock
Continued

sure to test his sensory and motor function to document the lesion's level and degree. A severe but incomplete lesion may allow transmission of some impulses, such as those through sacral nerves. Check for sacral sparing, indicated by anal sphincter contraction. Also look for additional evidence of impaired sympathetic function. The patient's temperature may fluctuate with ambient or room temperature (a condition called poikilothermy) because of interrupted feedback pathways to the hypothalamic thermoregulatory center. Take special care to keep the patient's room temperature as moderate and constant as possible. Temperature fluctuations may cause hyperthermia, which increases oxygen demands, or hypothermia, which increases the risk of life-threatening dysrhythmias.

The patient may also show GI or genitourinary disruptions. Peristalsis stops within 24 hours after spinal cord injury and usually doesn't resume for about 3 or 4 days. This can lead to gastric dilation and paralytic ileus. As ordered, insert a nasogastric tube, connected to suction, until bowel sounds return. Carefully monitor serum electrolyte levels to help prevent complications associated with electrolyte and acid-base imbalances.

After spinal cord injury, the urinary bladder can't contract, leading to urine retention. This may persist for weeks or even months. Use an indwelling (Foley) catheter, as ordered, to monitor the patient's fluid balance. Until the acute injury phase passes, the doctor will avoid intermittent catheterization—the preferred treatment.

Distributive Shock

Diagnostic studies. No test definitively diagnoses neurogenic shock. The doctor will base the diagnosis on the patient's history and on physical findings.

Planning
Before determining your nursing care plan, develop the nursing diagnosis by identifying the patient's problem or potential problem, then relating it to its cause. Possible nursing diagnoses for the patient with neurogenic shock include:
- injury, potential for; related to disturbed thermoregulation
- tissue perfusion, alteration in; related to decreased venous return
- mobility, impaired physical (potential for); related to spinal cord injury
- sensory perception, alteration in; related to injury
- airway clearance, ineffective (potential for); related to injury level
- anxiety; related to injury and hospitalization
- coping, ineffective family (potential for); related to injury and prognosis
- self-concept, disturbances in; related to injury.

The sample nursing care plan below shows expected outcomes, nursing interventions, and discharge planning for one nursing diagnosis listed above. However, you'll want to tailor each care plan to fit your patient's needs.

Intervention
Treatment for neurogenic shock centers on maintaining adequate perfusion, oxygenation, and cardiac output and on identifying and correcting shock's cause.

To maintain adequate perfusion, preserve a patent airway and provide ventilatory assistance, as ordered and needed. Minimize any vagal stimulation, such as from suctioning, to avoid further heart rate slowing.

To maintain cardiac output, the doctor will probably order crystalloids or colloids. Titrate all fluids to achieve adequate urinary output and blood pressure. If the patient doesn't respond to fluid administration, he may need vasopressors to increase cardiac output.

Continued on page 66

Sample nursing care plan: Neurogenic shock (spinal shock)

Nursing diagnosis Injury, potential for; related to disturbed thermoregulation	Expected outcome The patient will maintain normal body temperature.
Nursing interventions • Monitor and record patient's body temperature as indicated. • Maintain stable environmental temperature whenever possible. • Prevent patient exposure to drafts and direct sunlight. • Adjust patient's clothing and/or coverings according to body temperature changes. • Keep patient's skin dry. • Sponge patient's skin and increase his fluid intake to counteract slight body temperature elevations. • If fever persists despite cooling measures, assess for possible infection.	**Discharge planning** • Teach patient and/or family members how to take and monitor temperature. • Teach patient to avoid ambient temperature extremes, such as prolonged exposure to direct sunlight. • Teach patient how to control body temperature deviations; for instance, by keeping bath water at moderate temperatures and by avoiding drinking hot or cold fluids. • Teach patient to recognize infection signs and symptoms.

Vascular Problems

66 Shock

Distributive Shock

Neurogenic shock—*continued*

The doctor may order a vagolytic drug, such as atropine, to increase heart rate.

Identifying what's caused neurogenic shock helps determine appropriate treatment. If your patient's suffered spinal cord injury, he'll require spine immobilization with a cervical collar or traction. For neurogenic shock associated with high spinal anesthesia, expect to administer ephedrine or phenylephrine to increase cardiac output and constrict peripheral vessels. For shock from vasomotor depression (for example, insulin shock), expect to administer glucose.

Throughout your nursing care, try to prevent further injury or complications. Once the patient's vascular status stabilizes, try to allay his fears and provide emotional support.

Complications. The result of shock itself or of any spinal cord injury, complications may include the following:
- prolonged tissue perfusion impairment (more than 1 hour). This typically causes organ damage, particularly to the brain, kidneys, lungs, and heart. The spinal cord may also suffer damage from increased ischemia. When prolonged, shock can lead to multiple organ failure and eventually death.
- fluid overload and pulmonary edema from fluid replacement
- complications of spinal cord injury, including additional neurologic impairment. Specific complications depend on the injury's level.
- impaired airway and ventilation from cervical cord damage. With phrenic nerve or intercostal muscle involvement, the patient may have trouble coughing and clearing secretions, thus increasing the risk of aspiration or pulmonary infection.
- aspiration of gastric contents. This complication, which can develop secondary to paralytic ileus and gastric dilation, may require stomach decompression. Avoid nasogastric and nasal endotracheal tubes, which increase the risk of sinus infection.

Evaluation

Base your evaluation on the expected outcomes listed on your nursing care plan. To determine if your patient with spinal shock has improved, ask yourself these questions:
- Does the patient's body temperature fluctuate?
- Does his body temperature shift with room temperature changes?
- Does he sweat or shiver in response to body temperature changes?

The answers to these questions will help you evaluate your patient's care and determine his future needs. Keep in mind that these questions stem from the care plan on page 65. Your questions may differ.

Septic shock

Septic shock, first described in the early 1950s, probably didn't exist before the development of antibiotics. It now affects several thousand patients each year. Involving impaired cellular function and altered hemodynamics, septic shock usually occurs as a complication of another illness or injury involving hospitalization and invasive therapy. It carries an extremely high mortality.

Consider any patient with impaired immunity at risk for septic shock. Such patients include the elderly, those receiving immuno-

---

Autonomic hyperreflexia

About 1% of patients with spinal cord injury experience autonomic hyperreflexia in addition to neurogenic shock. This disorder, which reflects excessive sympathetic stimulation, can develop after injury above the sixth thoracic vertebra. Conditions such as urinary retention, infection, pain, decubitus ulcers, or room temperature changes may provoke autonomic hyperreflexia.

Autonomic hyperreflexia can cause hypertension, potentially lethal fever, flushed skin, and a throbbing headache. The patient's heart rate decreases as baroreceptors attempt to control blood pressure.

Treatment initially focuses on controlling the patient's blood pressure to prevent intracerebral bleeding. Ganglionic blocking agents may also help relieve severe signs and symptoms. To avoid further episodes, try to eliminate or minimize causative stimuli whenever possible.

Shock

Distributive Shock

suppressive drugs, those who've undergone invasive procedures, and trauma victims. (See *Septic shock: Recognizing risk factors* for a more detailed list.)

Any pathogenic organism can cause septic shock. Gram-negative bacteria, such as *Escherichia coli, Klebsiella pneumoniae,* and *Enterobacteriaceae* and *Pseudomonas* organisms, rank as the most common causes. Many such organisms normally inhabit the skin and intestines, where they act beneficially and pose little threat. But when they spread throughout the body via the bloodstream, they can produce overwhelming infection. Unless body defenses destroy them, septic shock develops.

Sepsis-causing organisms can invade the body through any breach in the body's normal defenses or through any artificial device that penetrates protective skin barriers. I.V. and intraarterial catheters

Continued on page 68

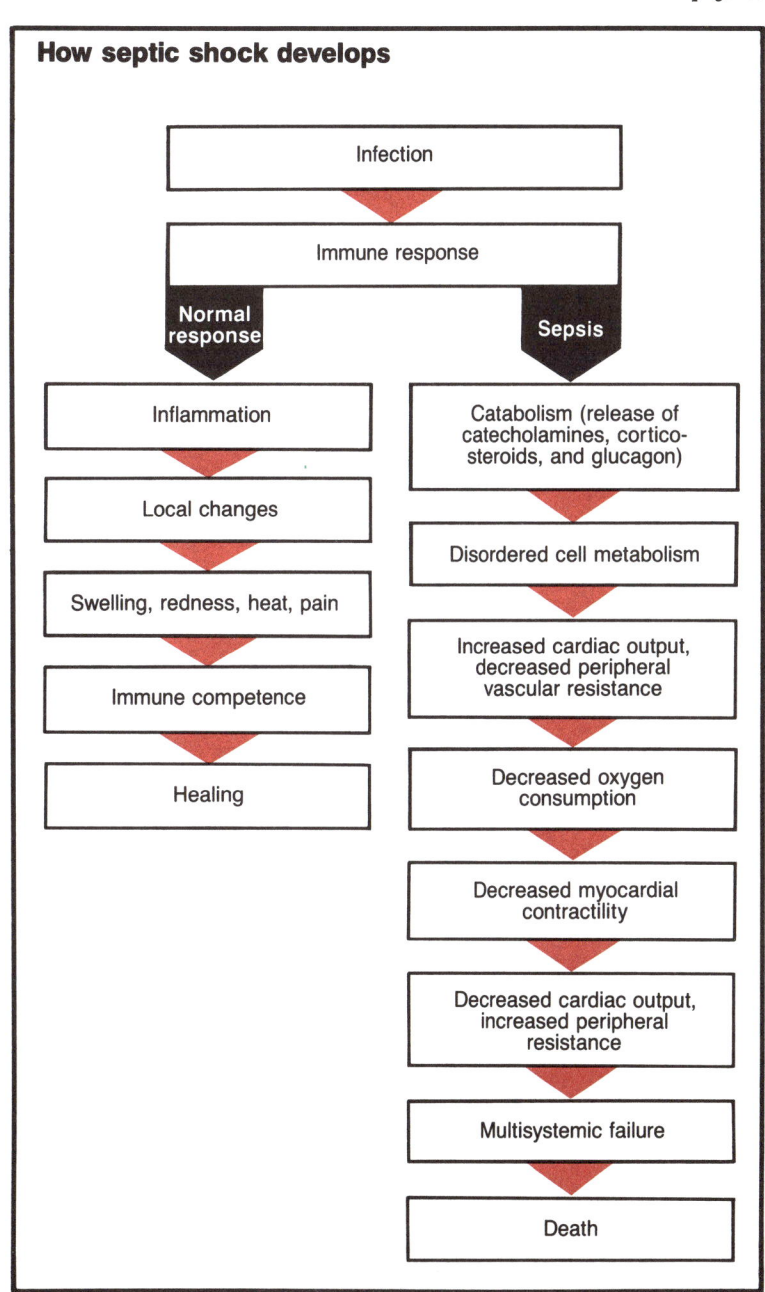

Septic shock: Recognizing risk factors

Consider your patient at risk for septic shock if his medical history includes any of the following:
- burns
- chronic disorders: hepatic dysfunction, cardiac or renal disease, diabetes mellitus, or alcoholism
- immunosuppression from neoplastic disorders, radiation therapy, cytotoxic drug therapy, corticosteroid therapy, or immunosuppressive drug therapy
- invasive diagnostic procedures or devices, such as I.V. lines and catheters
- malnutrition
- stress
- surgical procedures and wounds
- excessive antibiotic use.

Pregnant patients and those over age 65 or under age 1 also have an increased risk.

How septic shock develops

Infection → Immune response

Normal response:
Inflammation → Local changes → Swelling, redness, heat, pain → Immune competence → Healing

Sepsis:
Catabolism (release of catecholamines, corticosteroids, and glucagon) → Disordered cell metabolism → Increased cardiac output, decreased peripheral vascular resistance → Decreased oxygen consumption → Decreased myocardial contractility → Decreased cardiac output, increased peripheral resistance → Multisystemic failure → Death

Vascular Problems

68 Shock

Distributive Shock

Toxic shock syndrome

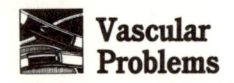

Toxic shock syndrome (TSS), a septic shock type first described in 1978, results from toxins released by gram-positive organisms such as *Staphylococcus aureus*. The condition occurs most commonly in menstruating women using tampons, although it can affect anyone with an *S. aureus* infection. TSS has a mortality between 3% and 15%.

Diagnostic criteria for TSS, established by the Centers for Disease Control, include:
- fever (at least 102° F., or 38.9° C.)
- diffuse macular erythrodermal rash
- desquamation (especially on the palms and soles) 1 to 2 weeks after TSS onset
- systolic blood pressure below 90 mm Hg
- evidence of multisystemic involvement.

The doctor will order initial treatment to correct hypovolemia and hypotension, then take measures to control infection, such as tampon removal, abscess drainage, and specific antibiotic therapy. Because a TSS patient has an increased risk of future episodes, some experts advocate prophylactic antibiotics before and after menstrual periods.

Septic shock—*continued*

offer direct access. Other devices, such as urinary catheters and drains, provide indirect access.

Septic shock has a complex pathophysiologic process. Early researchers believed its effects stemmed from endotoxins released from gram-negative bacteria killed by the body's defenses. However, other studies implicate vasoactive substances released during the immune response.

Although the specific mechanism remains a mystery, researchers now know much more about how the body responds to septic shock. Once infection begins, blood-borne microorganisms invade body organs and produce effects specific to the involved organ. The immune system responds to pathogenic invasion and subsequent infection by producing various defensive changes at the infection site. Initial changes include phagocytosis and complement activation. By-products of this response (such as heat) and biologically active molecules released from dead cells cause formation of vasoactive substances that produce local changes. These changes, including increased capillary permeability and blood flow, produce classic indications of local infection: redness, swelling, pain, and heat. Intravascular infection also causes these changes. However, in septic shock, such changes affect the entire body.

The stress of infection increases catecholamine, corticosteroid, and glucagon release. As a result, the patient's metabolic, heart, and respiratory rates increase and his body temperature rises. At this stage, you may suspect infection, although the patient can still fight it off. But eventually, the normal stress response gives way to septic shock's typically disturbed metabolism.

Glucagon, catecholamine, and corticosteroid elevations in early septic shock increase protein and lipid breakdown. The body then diverts branched-chain amino acids, normally metabolized to provide energy (adenosine triphosphate), into glucose production cycles. Consequently, the serum glucose level rises. However, the body can't use glucose appropriately because of epinephrine-induced insulin resistance. Glucose production also creates heat.

Ureagenetic amino acid breakdown increases blood urea nitrogen levels. Aromatic amino acids may degrade, producing false neurotransmitters (such as octopamine), which increase cardiac output but decrease peripheral vascular resistance.

Triglyceride breakdown increases free fatty acid plasma levels, leading to damaged vascular endothelium, elevated ketoacid and pyruvate-lactate levels, and hyperglycemia. Despite gluconeogenesis, nutrient delivery to tissues slows and energy production begins to fail. (For a summary of septic shock development, see *How septic shock develops*, page 67.)

Initially, these metabolic changes produce a hyperdynamic cardiovascular response—increased cardiac output and decreased peripheral resistance—known as *hyperdynamic* (warm) shock. Uncontrolled sepsis progresses to *hypodynamic* (cold) shock, resulting in shock's more typical clinical changes: cardiac output and blood pressure reductions, leading to vasoconstriction.

69 Shock

Distributive Shock

Assessment

Consider septic shock possible in any high-risk patient, especially one who's undergone many invasive tests or treatments. Throughout your nursing care, keep in mind that *trends* in the patient's condition yield more valuable information than do individual assessment findings.

Ask about any history of genitourinary tract procedures, immunosuppressive drug use, trauma, or major surgery. Note your patient's age; elderly patients run a greater risk of septic shock.

Physical examination. Check for signs and symptoms of septic shock's two phases:
• *hyperdynamic phase:* increased cardiac output and full, bounding pulse
• *hypodynamic phase:* decreased cardiac output and weak pulse. Impaired tissue oxygenation occurs in both phases.

If you suspect septic shock, focus your assessment on organ systems that usually show early signs of impairment. Note the patient's level of consciousness, respiratory function, and urine output; these may decline long before cardiovascular changes or fever appears. To assess for altered mental status, check for increasing agitation, anxiety, or irritability and a shortened attention span. If you note these signs, look for evidence of respiratory impairment.

Monitor urine output for additional evidence of decreased organ function: abruptly decreased output may appear as the first overt sign of shock. (For details on assessment findings in septic shock's two phases, see *Hyperdynamic and hypodynamic septic shock: Comparing signs and symptoms.*)

Diagnostic tests. The doctor will base his diagnosis mainly on the patient's history and physical examination. Laboratory tests, such as blood cultures and white blood cell counts, can help confirm sepsis.

Cardiovascular studies help distinguish septic shock from other shock types. These studies may include measurements of cardiac

Continued on page 70

Hyperdynamic and hypodynamic septic shock: Comparing signs and symptoms

Parameter	Hyperdynamic (warm) septic shock *Signs and symptoms reflect increased cardiac output, peripheral vasodilation, and decreased systemic vascular resistance.*	Hypodynamic (cold) septic shock *Signs and symptoms reflect decreased cardiac output, peripheral vasoconstriction, increased systemic vascular resistance, and inadequate tissue perfusion.*
Blood pressure	Normal or slightly elevated	Hypotension (systolic blood pressure below 90 mm Hg or 50 to 80 mm Hg below patient's previous level)
Pulse	Increased rate; full, bounding peripheral pulses	Increased rate; possible dysrhythmias; weak, thready, or absent peripheral pulses
Respiration	Rapid, shallow	Rapid, shallow; pulmonary congestion may develop
Level of consciousness	Altered	Severely reduced
Urine output	Below normal	Below normal to absent
Temperature	Above normal	Possibly below normal
Skin	Pink, flushed, warm, and dry	Cold, pale, and clammy, with peripheral mottling; cyanosis

Vascular Problems

70 Shock

Distributive Shock

Septic shock—continued

output, peripheral vascular resistance, oxygen consumption, and blood gases. (For more information on assessing shock, see Chapter 1.)

Planning
Before determining your nursing care plan, develop the nursing diagnosis by identifying the patient's problem or potential problem, then relating it to its cause. Possible nursing diagnoses for a septic shock patient include:
• fluid volume, alteration in (deficit); related to increased capillary permeability
• cardiac output, alteration in (decreased); related to hypovolemia
• tissue perfusion, alteration in; related to hypovolemia
• injury, potential for (cerebral hypoxia); related to inadequate gas exchange.

The sample nursing care plan below lists expected outcomes, nursing interventions, and discharge planning for one nursing diagnosis listed above. However, you'll want to individualize each care plan to meet the patient's needs.

Intervention
Initial septic shock therapy aims to maintain adequate perfusion and oxygenation. Your patient may also need fluid replacement and/or drugs to support cardiac output. The doctor may order crystalloids, colloids, or blood products to increase intravascular volume and maintain urine output. In all shock phases, administer fluids cautiously with the guidance of hemodynamic measurements (for example, central venous pressure, pulmonary capillary wedge pressure, and/or cardiac output) to avoid such complications as fluid overload.

Preventing septic shock
You can play a major role in preventing septic shock by identifying patients at risk and reducing their exposure to pathogens. Always maintain strict aseptic technique, and wash your hands frequently and carefully. Check all potential pathogen entry sites regularly, noting any signs of local inflammation or systemic infection. Stay alert for potential pathogen transmission resulting from ventilator tubing connections, contaminated stethoscope chest pieces, or moist soap bars.

Also take steps to promote the patient's immune response by ensuring nutritional adequacy and giving antibiotics properly. Remember—the earlier you recognize septic shock and begin interventions, the better your patient's recovery chances.

Sample nursing care plan: Septic shock

Nursing diagnosis	Expected outcomes
Fluid volume, alteration in (deficit); related to increased capillary permeability	The patient will: • maintain adequate perfusion. • maintain urine output of at least 30 ml/hour. • maintain adequate blood pressure.

Nursing interventions	Discharge planning
• Assess and record vital signs, including level of consciousness, as indicated. • If possible, monitor and record central venous and pulmonary capillary wedge pressures as indicated. • Assess and record fluid intake and output hourly. • Measure urine specific gravity. • Obtain daily weights. • Reduce oxygen demands by minimizing patient's activities. • Monitor for effects of fluid, oxygen, and drug therapy. Notify doctor of any abnormalities. • Assess for and record skin turgor, edema, and mucous membrane color and moistness. • Assess breath sounds for crackles or wheezes. Notify doctor if you hear these sounds. • Assess hemoglobin, hematocrit, and arterial blood gas values.	Depends on treatment outcome

Vascular Problems

71 Shock

Distributive Shock

To ensure adequate perfusion and oxygenation, protect the patient's airway and assist ventilation, if necessary. Because septic shock causes pulmonary dysfunction, the patient may need mechanical ventilation (such as high oxygen concentrations and positive end-expiratory pressure) to maintain adequate arterial oxygenation.

The doctor may also order vasopressors and positive inotropic drugs in the hyperdynamic phase. Vasopressors, such as metaraminol (Aramine), norepinephrine (Levophed), and dopamine (Intropin), help reverse vasodilation. Positive inotropic drugs, which increase myocardial contractility, include dopamine, dobutamine (Dobutrex), isoproterenol (Isuprel), norepinephrine, and digitalis. As ordered, always administer these drugs in conjunction with fluid therapy. (*Note:* Always use a central line when administering norepinephrine.)

Other drugs used during the hyperdynamic phase may include sodium bicarbonate (to correct acidosis) and steroids (although their role in septic shock remains controversial).

Medications ordered during the hypodynamic phase may include vasodilators to reverse vasoconstriction and positive inotropic drugs to improve blood ejection from the heart into the pulmonary and general circulation. Vasodilators used for hypodynamic shock include nitroglycerin (Tridil) and sodium nitroprusside (Nipride). You may also need to administer chlorpromazine (Thorazine) and phentolamine (Regitine). Positive inotropic drugs useful in hypodynamic shock include dopamine and dobutamine.

Once measures to support perfusion begin, treatment focuses on identifying, localizing, and controlling the causative organism. Until tests identify it, expect the doctor to order antibiotic therapy with agents effective against both gram-negative and gram-positive organisms. As ordered, obtain culture specimens from likely infection sites (wounds, I.V. lines, and respiratory, GI, and urinary tracts). In a patient with a nasotracheal or nasogastric tube, consider the sinuses a potential infection source.

Additional studies, such as chest and abdominal X-rays, sputum cultures, and computed tomography scans can also help identify the infection source. Once the organism and its source have been determined, the doctor will order specific antibiotic therapy. With sepsis from abscess or necrotic tissue, the patient may need surgery.

Other interventions for septic shock include:
- providing nutritional support
- maintaining adequate body temperature through cooling or warming measures
- providing comfort, rest, and emotional support.

Complications. Disseminated intravascular coagulation and respiratory failure (adult respiratory distress syndrome [ARDS]) most commonly complicate septic shock. (However, some researchers believe ARDS reflects a septic lung effect rather than a septic complication.)

Multisystemic failure—most notably acute renal failure, decreased myocardial contractility, and hepatic failure—develops if sepsis can't be controlled.

Continued on page 72

Septic shock: A therapy update

Various investigational therapies studied within the last 5 years may stop hyperdynamic (warm) septic shock from progressing to the more critical hypodynamic (cold) stage. These therapies include:

- *naloxone* (Narcan). A narcotic antagonist, this drug helps reverse hypotension associated with increased circulating beta-endorphins. Naloxone's mechanism of action remains unclear, but researchers believe it may block endorphin-mediated vasodilation by displacing endogenous opiates from receptor sites.
- *diphenhydramine* (Benadryl). This drug blocks histamine release.
- *lidocaine* (Xylocaine). This common antiarrhythmic may help stabilize endothelial cells in blood vessel walls.
- *indomethacin* (Indocin). This drug helps block prostaglandin $F_2\alpha$ synthesis, thereby reducing pulmonary vasoconstriction and improving pulmonary blood flow. Some patients improve from acetylsalicylic acid (aspirin) therapy, which has the same effect.
- *prostacyclin.* Low prostacyclin levels contribute to platelet aggregation in septic shock. Administering prostacyclin increases cyclic adenosine monophosphate levels, reduces cellular damage, and dilates renal vessels.
- *Anti-LPS (antiendotoxin) serum.* This hyperimmune human serum binds antibodies and inactivates and ingests endotoxins from bacteria killed by antibodies.
- *imidazoles.* In animal experiments, these drugs have reversed hypotension in septic shock.

Vascular Problems — 72 Shock

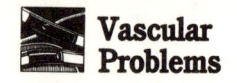

Obstructive shock: impeded blood flow

In obstructive shock, impeded blood flow causes decreased tissue perfusion, eventually impairing cellular function. Conditions that impede blood flow through the heart or great vessels (but that don't involve the heart valves or myocardium) may lead to shock through reduced cardiac output. Obstruction may affect the right ventricle (by reducing venous return) or the left ventricle (by impeding pulmonary artery flow).

For example, in pericardial tamponade, which impairs venous return, blood or fluid accumulates in the pericardial sac. Vena caval constriction results, reducing venous return to the right heart and blood flow into the left ventricle. If cardiac output drops by about 25%, inadequate perfusion—and ultimately shock—develop.

Primary pulmonary hypertension can cause a similar effect. Right ventricular ejection decreases from increased resistance to blood flow through the pulmonary vascular bed. Shock can also arise from obstructed pulmonary artery blood flow into the left ventricle, which reduces cardiac output, as in massive pulmonary embolism.

Distributive Shock

Septic shock—continued

Evaluation

Base your evaluation on the expected outcomes listed on your nursing care plan. To determine if the patient's improved, ask yourself these questions:
- Does the patient show signs of adequate tissue perfusion?
- Does he require less support to maintain adequate perfusion?
- Can he maintain urine output of at least 30 ml/hour?
- Can he maintain a normal level of consciousness?
- Does he have adequate blood pressure?

The answers to these questions will help you evaluate your patient's care and determine his future needs. Keep in mind that these questions stem from the care plan on page 70. Your questions may differ.

Self-Test

1. In shock's middle stage, the patient may have:
a. widened pulse pressure **b.** narrowed pulse pressure **c.** decreased diastolic pressure **d.** increased systolic pressure

2. If your patient's in hypovolemic shock, his hemoglobin and hematocrit values will initially:
a. increase from hemoconcentration **b.** decrease from hemoconcentration **c.** increase from hemodilution **d.** decrease from hemodilution

3. Which of the following should you consider the major development in cardiogenic shock?
a. cardiac output of 4.5 liters/minute/m² **b.** cardiac output of 8.5 liters/minute/m² **c.** cardiac index of 2 liters/minute/m² **d.** cardiac index of 4.5 liters/minute/m²

4. Anaphylaxis signs and symptoms most commonly stem from:
a. histamine release **b.** release of slow-reacting substance of anaphylaxis (SRS-A) **c.** release of eosinophil chemotactic factor of anaphylaxis (ECF-A) **d.** all of the above

5. Classic signs and symptoms of neurogenic shock include:
a. hypotension with tachycardia **b.** hypotension with bradycardia **c.** hypertension with tachycardia **d.** hypertension with bradycardia

Answers (page number shows where answer appears in text)
1. **b** (page 9)   2. **a** (page 27)   3. **c** (page 44)   4. **a** (page 57)
5. **b** (page 64)

Vascular Problems

73 Hypertension

Hypertension: Disturbed Blood Pressure Regulation

Barbara Milne, Assistant Professor at the University of British Columbia School of Nursing in Vancouver, wrote this chapter. Ms. Milne earned her BSN and MSN at the University of Toronto.

Hypertension, commonly known as high blood pressure, poses a national public health problem. Untreated, it's a major contributor to heart disease, stroke, and renal failure and a leading cause of disability and death. Because it's usually asymptomatic, hypertension can wield its pathologic effects insidiously until the patient experiences symptoms of target organ damage or until his elevated blood pressure becomes apparent during a routine medical checkup or hypertension screening program.

The World Health Organization's Expert Committee on Hypertension defines hypertension as systolic pressure of 160 mm Hg or higher, and/or diastolic pressure (fifth phase) of 95 mm Hg or higher. For comparison, normal adult blood pressure refers to systolic pressure of 140 mm Hg or lower and diastolic pressure of 90 mm Hg or lower. Consider pressures between these values and the hypertension values described above as borderline. From age 15 on, men have higher blood pressures than women. However, beginning at about age 55, women show higher pressures. (Because blood pressures in youth can help predict later hypertension, always measure blood pressure whenever you examine a child or adolescent to help identify patients at risk.)

In this chapter, we'll review the mechanisms that regulate blood pressure, hypertension's pathophysiologic process, and the assessment, planning, and intervention guidelines that will help you identify and manage hypertension and prevent its complications.

Pressure-regulating mechanisms. Hypertension reflects impaired regulation of blood pressure—the pressure exerted on blood vessels by blood flowing through them. Blood pressure depends on:
- *blood volume.* The heart affects blood volume by regulating cardiac output (the blood volume ejected each minute from the left ventricle into the aorta). The main determinant of systolic blood pressure, cardiac output depends in turn on heart rate and stroke volume (the blood volume the heart ejects with each beat). The kidneys help control blood volume by regulating sodium and water levels. Sodium and water conservation increases blood volume, thereby raising blood pressure. If pressure rises too high, the kidneys excrete sodium and excess water, and blood pressure drops to normal levels.

Continued on page 74

Classifying blood pressure

Diastolic blood pressure (mm Hg)	Systolic blood pressure (mm Hg)		
	BELOW 140	140 TO 159	160 OR GREATER
Below 85	Normal blood pressure	Borderline isolated systolic hypertension	Isolated systolic hypertension
85 to 89	High normal blood pressure	Borderline isolated systolic hypertension	Isolated systolic hypertension
90 to 104	Mild hypertension	Mild hypertension	Mild hypertension
105 to 114	Moderate hypertension	Moderate hypertension	Moderate hypertension
115 or greater	Severe hypertension	Severe hypertension	Severe hypertension

Pressures are based on the average of two or more measurements on two or more occasions.
Source: *Report of the Joint National Committee on Detection, Evaluation and Treatment of High Blood Pressure,* National Heart, Lung, and Blood Institute

Vascular Problems

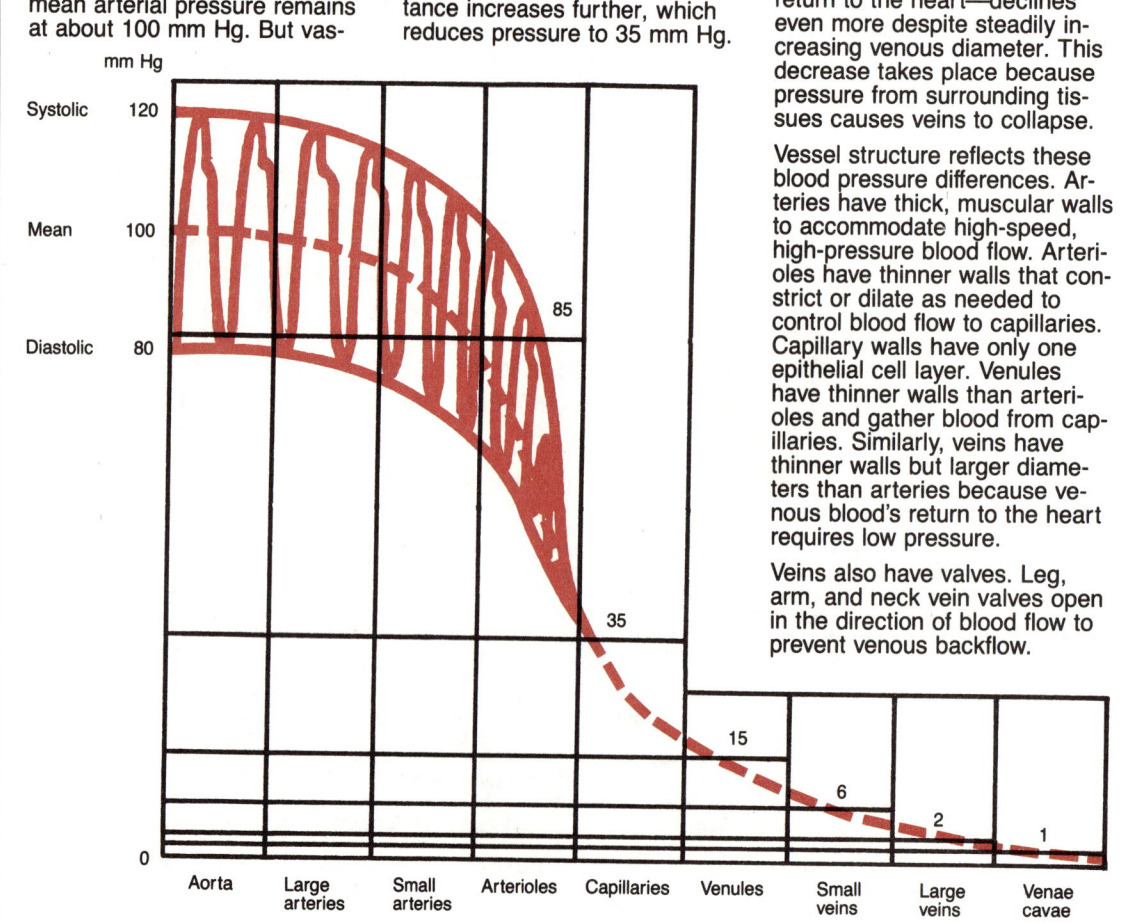

74 Hypertension

Hypertension

Continued

- *vascular resistance.* The major determinant of diastolic blood pressure, vascular resistance depends mainly on arteriolar vascular resistance (the friction between moving blood and arteriolar walls), blood viscosity, vessel size, and vessel wall diameter.

Neural, hormonal, and physical mechanisms interact to control blood volume and vascular resistance, ensuring appropriate blood flow to the right body parts at the right time (see *Tracking pressure through blood vessels*).

Neural regulators include baroreceptors and chemoreceptors. *Baroreceptors,* nerve endings embedded in blood vessels, respond to vessel wall stretching. They're found in internal carotid artery walls (in the carotid sinuses just above the carotid bifurcation), in aortic arch walls, and in most large neck and thoracic arteries. When these vessel walls stretch in response to increasing blood volume, baroreceptors signal the central nervous system (CNS) to inhibit the medulla's vasoconstrictor center and to stimulate the

---

Tracking pressure through blood vessels

Blood coursing through the vascular system travels through five vessel types: arteries, arterioles, capillaries, venules, and veins. Aortic blood flow meets virtually no vascular resistance; mean arterial pressure remains at about 100 mm Hg. But vascular resistance increases enough in arterioles (much smaller in diameter) to reduce mean pressure to 85 mm Hg. When blood crosses arterioles to capillaries, vascular resistance increases further, which reduces pressure to 35 mm Hg.

Optimal nutrient and gas exchange in the capillary bed requires such low pressure.

Blood pressure—only about 15 mm Hg when blood begins its return to the heart—declines even more despite steadily increasing venous diameter. This decrease takes place because pressure from surrounding tissues causes veins to collapse.

Vessel structure reflects these blood pressure differences. Arteries have thick, muscular walls to accommodate high-speed, high-pressure blood flow. Arterioles have thinner walls that constrict or dilate as needed to control blood flow to capillaries. Capillary walls have only one epithelial cell layer. Venules have thinner walls than arterioles and gather blood from capillaries. Similarly, veins have thinner walls but larger diameters than arteries because venous blood's return to the heart requires low pressure.

Veins also have valves. Leg, arm, and neck vein valves open in the direction of blood flow to prevent venous backflow.

Vascular Problems

75 Hypertension

Hypertension

vagal center. This results in peripheral vasodilation, decreased heart rate, and less vigorous contractions, with a corresponding arterial blood pressure decrease. When baroreceptors detect decreasing blood volume, they induce peripheral vasoconstriction, increased heart rate, and more vigorous contractions, with a corresponding arterial blood pressure increase. Baroreceptors respond quickly to slight blood pressure changes, but they usually don't respond to higher pressure levels after 1 or more days. Thus, they don't effectively control arterial pressure changes in a patient with chronic hypertension.

Chemoreceptors, nerve endings in carotid artery walls, the aorta, and the medulla, respond to abnormally low blood levels of dissolved oxygen and carbon dioxide. Chemoreceptors stimulate sympathetic nervous system (SNS) activity and inhibit parasympathetic activity, causing a reflex arterial pressure increase.

Hormonal regulators include:
- norepinephrine and epinephrine, secreted by the adrenal glands
- renin, secreted by the kidney's juxtaglomerular cells, with subsequent angiotensin I and II formation
- antidiuretic hormone (ADH), secreted by the hypothalamus
- prostaglandins, secreted by various body tissues.

SNS stimulation causes the adrenal medulla to release *norepinephrine* and *epinephrine*. These hormones cause effects similar to direct SNS cardiovascular stimulation—increased heart rate, blood pressure, automaticity, and contractility. They achieve their effects by stimulating SNS alpha- and beta-receptors throughout the vasculature. Alpha stimulation causes vasoconstriction; beta stimulation, vasodilation.

Renin secretion depends on the perfusion rate of afferent renal arterioles. Reduced blood flow through the kidneys triggers renin secretion, which then acts on plasma protein angiotensinogen to produce *angiotensin I*. When blood containing this hormone reaches the lungs, an enzyme in small lung vessels catalyzes its conversion to *angiotensin II*. Angiotensin II constricts arterioles (raising arterial pressure) and veins (promoting venous return to the heart and providing additional blood to pump against arterial pressure). Angiotensin II also affects the kidneys, directly decreasing sodium and water excretion and causing the adrenal cortex to secrete *aldosterone*, which further reduces sodium and water excretion. This entire process usually expands blood volume and raises blood pressure (see *The renin-angiotensin-aldosterone feedback system*, page 76).

The hypothalamus responds to decreased blood pressure by secreting *ADH*. This substance acts on renal tubules to promote water retention, which in turn boosts plasma volume and thus increases peripheral resistance and blood pressure.

Various *prostaglandins*, hormonelike substances found in many body tissues, probably also affect blood pressure regulation. In general, prostaglandins A and E dilate arteries and veins. (Prostaglandin E_2 probably acts as a vasodilator in the kidney, inhibiting the renin-angiotensin-aldosterone system.) Prostaglandin F constricts veins.

Physical blood pressure regulators include vascular stress-relaxation and capillary fluid shift. These mechanisms take longer than neural

Continued on page 76

Hypertension

The renin-angiotensin-aldosterone feedback system

An important homeostatic device, the renin-angiotensin-aldosterone system regulates blood pressure and sodium and water levels. Here's how:

Juxtaglomerular cells in the kidney's glomeruli secrete renin into the blood (see close-up, below left). Renin's secretion rate depends on the perfusion rate in afferent renal arterioles and on serum sodium levels. Low serum sodium levels and low perfusion pressure (as in hypovolemia) increase renin secretion; high serum sodium levels and high perfusion pressure decrease it.

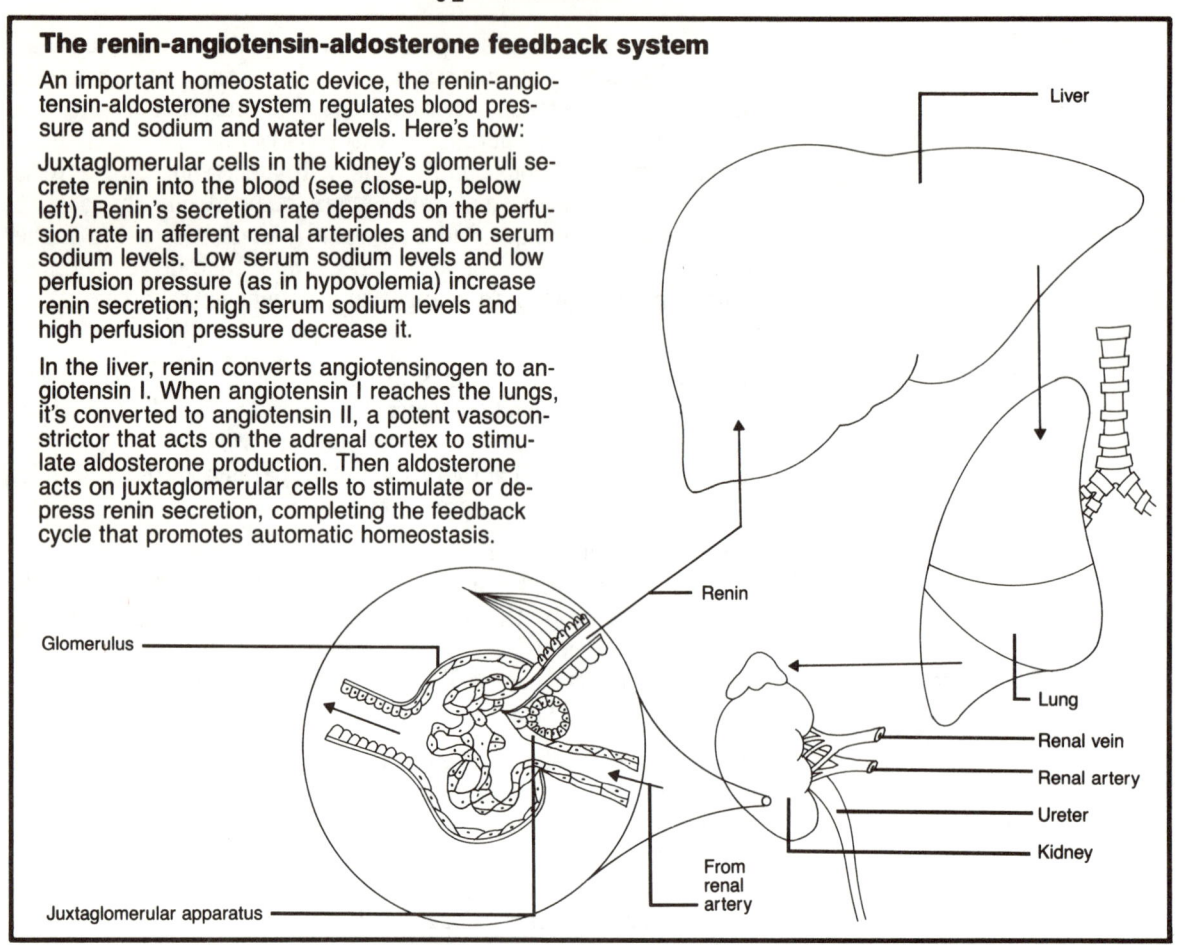

In the liver, renin converts angiotensinogen to angiotensin I. When angiotensin I reaches the lungs, it's converted to angiotensin II, a potent vasoconstrictor that acts on the adrenal cortex to stimulate aldosterone production. Then aldosterone acts on juxtaglomerular cells to stimulate or depress renin secretion, completing the feedback cycle that promotes automatic homeostasis.

Continued

or hormonal regulators to exert their full effects. *Stress-relaxation* allows a blood vessel to compensate for sudden volume and pressure shifts by adjusting its diameter without prolonging diameter and tension changes. Rapid volume and pressure increases lead to distention but only a transient tension increase; rapid volume and pressure reductions cause vessel shortening but only a transient tension decrease.

A compensatory mechanism, *capillary fluid shift* regulates fluid exchange across capillary membranes in response to arterial pressure changes. With a sharp pressure rise, capillary hydrostatic pressure increases, making fluid shift into interstitial spaces. With less fluid circulating, blood pressure drops. With a sharp pressure decrease, capillary hydrostatic pressure falls, leading to increased circulating volume and a corresponding blood pressure elevation.

Hypertension risk factors. In most cases, hypertension's cause remains unknown. However, certain factors can predispose a patient to hypertension. These include:
- *heredity.* Hypertension falls under genetic influences.
- *obesity.* In early adulthood (ages 20 to 30), obesity creates a potent risk factor for subsequent hypertension.
- *sodium, potassium, and calcium imbalances.* Excessive sodium in-

Hypertension

How hypertension damages blood vessels

Vascular injury begins with alternating areas of dilation and constriction in the arterioles. Increased intraarterial pressure damages the endothelium. Independently, angiotensin induces endothelial wall contraction, allowing plasma to leak through interendothelial spaces. Eventually, plasma constituents deposited in the vessel wall cause medial necrosis.

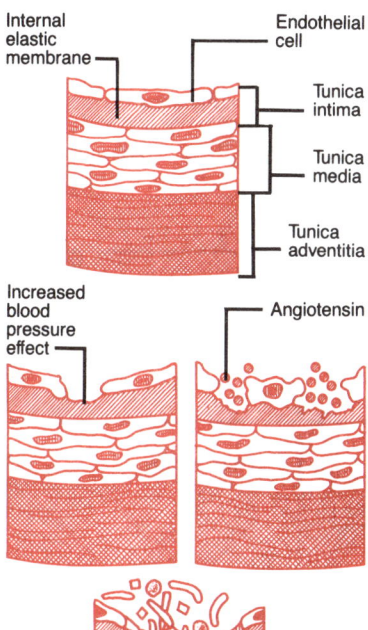

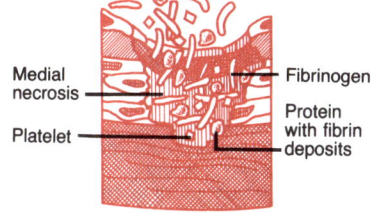

take may trigger hypertension in a genetically susceptible person. Potassium levels help regulate arterial tone. Calcium affects smooth muscle contractions; some researchers theorize that defective vascular metabolism of calcium underlies the abnormal vasoconstriction seen in hypertensive patients.

- *excessive alcohol use.* This may progressively increase systolic and diastolic pressures.
- *race.* Blacks have twice the hypertension risk of whites. And the disease frequently develops earlier in blacks, takes a more severe course, and causes more deaths at a younger age.

Note: Because the word *hypertension* suggests nervous tension, some people believe that stress predisposes a person to hypertension. Although acute physical or emotional stress may elevate blood pressure briefly, no one has proven a direct relationship between sustained stress and primary hypertension. The link between the nervous system and blood pressure remains uncertain.

Classifying hypertension. Hypertension can take one of two basic forms—primary (essential) or secondary. (A third type, malignant, or accelerated, refers to severe, progressive hypertension.)

Primary (or essential) hypertension—persistently elevated blood pressure with an unknown cause—accounts for at least 90% of all cases. Characterized by a progressive blood pressure increase over many years, it usually causes no symptoms. Blood pressure may be labile (fluctuating between normal and abnormal levels) before becoming fixed at a high level.

Although primary hypertension has no known cause, some experts theorize that it reflects several different defects. Genetic influence may increase susceptibility, but experts don't know how heredity and environment interact to produce hypertension. Most well-defined blood pressure control systems don't show any marked abnormality in hypertensive patients, although such patients may have an exaggerated SNS stress response. One study shows a link between increased noise exposure and sustained blood pressure elevations.

Researchers agree that small arteries and arterioles hypertrophy in hypertensive patients, probably to maintain (and perhaps amplify) the initial blood pressure increase. However, this mechanism alone doesn't cause hypertension. Experts also agree that primary hypertension stems partly from a primary defect in vascular smooth-muscle cell membranes that makes membranes more permeable to ions such as sodium and calcium. These changes increase cellular excitability, making cells more responsive to environmental stimuli. Cellular contraction intensifies, leading to increased total peripheral resistance. Resistance vessels undergo structural hypertrophy, which perpetuates (and possibly augments) this heightened pressor response.

Secondary hypertension describes elevated blood pressure with a known cause. It accounts for at most 10% of all cases and occurs much more commonly in children. Unlike primary hypertension, it has known, frequently correctable causes. (For details on some causes, see *Secondary hypertension: Reviewing common causes*, page 78.)

Continued on page 79

Vascular Problems

78 Hypertension

Hypertension

Secondary hypertension: Reviewing common causes

Various conditions can cause secondary hypertension. We'll review a few common causes below. Less common causes include pregnancy; increased intracranial pressure; advanced collagen disease; and use of such drugs as oral contraceptives and other estrogens, corticosteroids, sympathetic stimulators, monoamine oxidase inhibitors, appetite suppressants, and antihistamines. *Note:* Once the cause has been treated, secondary hypertension usually disappears.

Cause	How diagnosed	Treatment
Renovascular hypertension (RVH) The most common cause of secondary hypertension, RVH affects children and adolescents more frequently than adults. It usually results from renal artery stenosis caused by atherosclerosis or arterial wall fibromuscular dysplasia. Renal ischemia results, leading to reduced kidney perfusion that triggers the renin-angiotensin-aldosterone system. RVH produces few signs or symptoms. Suspect it in a patient with hypertension before age 25 (especially with diastolic pressure ≥ 110 mm Hg); sudden onset of labile or uncontrollable hypertension; hypertension onset before age 45 in a woman not taking oral contraceptives; recent hypertension onset after age 50; rapid acceleration of previously well-controlled hypertension; Grade III or IV Keith, Wagener, Barker funduscopic changes (hypertensive retinopathy); or a systolic or diastolic bruit in the upper abdomen or flank.	• Rapid-sequence I.V. pyelogram (IVP) • Plasma renin activity (PRA) test • Renal vein renin concentration • Renal angiography • Renal scan • Pharmacologic angiotensin blockade test	• Dietary sodium and calorie restriction • Diuretics • Antihypertensive medications • Renal artery revascularization • Renal artery bypass graft • Percutaneous transluminal renal angioplasty • Nephrectomy (occasionally)
Coarctation of the aorta This aortic narrowing, most common at the aortic arch's lower end, usually has a congenital cause. Signs and symptoms include decreased blood pressure in legs compared to arms, pulsating intercostal arteries (from enlargement of arteries carrying collateral blood flow around the coarctation), and diminished or absent femoral pulses.	• Physical examination • Chest X-ray • Aortography	• Surgical repair
Pheochromocytoma This disorder stems from a chromaffin tumor, usually in the adrenal medulla but occasionally elsewhere. The tumor manufactures and secretes excessive epinephrine and norepinephrine; this leads to hypertension and other effects. When the tumor secretes continuously, persistent high blood pressure occurs. When it secretes intermittently, signs and symptoms include sudden hypertensive episodes, severe headache with palpitations, accelerated metabolism, excessive sweating, heat intolerance, and anxiety.	• Vanillylmandelic acid test • Urine catecholamines • Computed tomography (CT) scan	• Tumor removal
Hyperaldosteronism This condition may result from primary aldosteronism (Conn's syndrome) caused by adrenal tumor or hyperplasia; from secondary aldosteronism stemming from conditions that stimulate aldosterone production; or from pseudoaldosteronism resulting from excessive licorice intake. Excessive aldosterone secretion by the adrenal cortex leads to excessive sodium reabsorption, which increases intravascular fluid volume and thus blood pressure. Signs and symptoms include mild or moderately elevated blood pressure, muscular weakness, polyuria, nocturia, polydipsia, tetany, paresthesia, and headache.	• Serum aldosterone test • Urine aldosterone test • PRA test • CT scan	• Tumor removal • Spironolactone (Aldactone) therapy • Treatment of underlying cause
Cushing's syndrome This condition results from adrenal cortex tumor or hyperplasia causing excessive glucocorticoid secretion. Signs and symptoms include central or girdle obesity, buffalo hump, purplish abdominal striae, hirsutism, moon face, edema, and mild hypertension.	• Physical examination • Plasma cortisol test • Urine 17-hydroxycorticosteroid test • PRA test • Dexamethasone suppression test	• Tumor removal
Renal parenchymal disease This condition usually stems from an immune system response to infection, such as chronic glomerulonephritis or pyelonephritis. Inflammatory changes take place in the kidneys' glomeruli and interstitia; consequently, the kidneys can't excrete sodium (which stimulates the renin-angiotensin-aldosterone system). Signs and symptoms include edema, oliguria, orthopnea, dyspnea, and hypertension.	• IVP • Renal angiography	• Depends on cause

Hypertension

Continued

Assessment

Your assessment technique will depend on whether your patient has known hypertension. If you discover hypertension during your assessment, focus on confirming it, determining possible causes (primary or secondary), and identifying any target organ damage. For a patient with known hypertension, find out if he's complying with prescribed therapy, determine therapeutic effectiveness, and check for possible target organ damage or complications of hypertension or therapy.

Nursing history. Begin your assessment with the nursing history. Establish a rapport with the patient and listen carefully as he responds to your questions. Ask open-ended questions and observe his nonverbal behavior carefully.

Chief complaint. Ask your patient why he's seeking medical care, and document his answer in his own words. If he can't identify a single chief complaint, ask a more specific question, such as "What made you seek medical care at this time?" His chief complaint may or may not relate to high blood pressure. A patient with known hypertension may not have any specific symptomatic complaint. A patient previously unaware of his hypertension may initially seek medical care for an unrelated problem or for hypertension-related symptoms (see *Hypertension findings: What to expect*). In this case, you may not discover hypertension until you've measured his blood pressure.

Present illness. As you gather additional information relevant to the chief complaint, your questions will vary, depending on whether your patient has a history of hypertension. If he has newly discovered hypertension, find out if he's had any related symptoms. Ask him how long he's had the symptom and how it affects his daily routine, when it began, and whether he has any other associated symptoms. Also ask about the location, duration, radiation, and intensity of any pain and about any precipitating, exacerbating, or relieving factors. Let the patient describe the problem in his own words. Avoid leading questions. When possible, use familiar expressions rather than medical terms.

If the patient has a history of hypertension, ask questions concerning his compliance with therapy, therapeutic effectiveness, and any associated symptoms.

Past medical history. For a patient with newly discovered hypertension, the past medical history should include general questions designed to uncover possible causes. Ask the patient if he's had similar symptoms before. If so, did he see a doctor? What was the medical diagnosis and treatment, if any? Has he had any major acute or chronic illnesses requiring hospitalization? (If he has, note the course of the illness, its treatment, and any consequences.) Does he use alcohol, tobacco, or caffeine? Does he take any prescription, over-the-counter, or recreational drugs? Make sure to document drug use carefully; certain drugs may raise blood pressure or reduce the effectiveness of antihypertensive therapy.

Find out if your patient has allergies to any foods, drugs, or other agents. If so, have him describe the reaction he's had. Ask a female

Continued on page 80

Hypertension findings: What to expect

Although most patients with mild to moderate hypertension lack signs and symptoms and seem surprised when told of their problem, a patient with *severe* hypertension may have any of the following signs and symptoms:

- **Headache.** This typically occurs occipitally and worsens when the patient wakes up in the morning. He may report awakening during the night with a severe occipital headache that improves after standing and walking for a few minutes. Cerebrospinal fluid (CSF) pressure increases when the patient's supine, causing a headache; when he resumes an upright position, CSF pressure drops and the headache disappears. (For comparison, a tension headache usually occurs frontally and worsens during the day.)
- **Cerebrovascular signs and symptoms.** Dizziness, syncope, blackouts, one-sided numbness or weakness, and blurred vision may result from hypertension alone or may indicate cerebrovascular atherosclerosis.
- **Cardiovascular signs and symptoms.** Chest pain, palpitations, dyspnea, and peripheral edema usually develop only with coronary artery disease, which causes heart failure. Intermittent claudication indicates leg atherosclerosis.
- **Renal signs and symptoms.** Peripheral edema may occur from increased sodium and water retention. Fatigue, weakness, nocturia, and excessive urinary sediment may also indicate renal involvement.
- **Epistaxis.** When this disorder develops secondary to hypertension, blood pressure recorded at its onset is almost always elevated. Epistaxis may be a safety mechanism that relieves severe hypertension and thus helps prevent cerebral hemorrhage.

Hypertension

Continued

patient about any pregnancies and find out if she's begun menopause. Does she use oral contraceptives or estrogens? Has she ever had pregnancy-induced hypertension?

Also ask about cardiovascular risk factors, such as a history of cardiac or vascular disease, diabetes mellitus, hyperlipidemia, congenital heart defects, rheumatic fever, or syncope. Ask about a history of renal disease or obesity. Note whether the patient's currently overweight.

For a patient with known hypertension, the past medical history should include general history information and questions that will update his status. For example, find out what medications he takes and how much caffeine, alcohol, or tobacco he uses.

Family history. Your patient's family history may suggest genetic or environmental factors that may affect his current health problems and needs. Determine if any blood relatives have had such diseases as hypertension, heart or kidney disease, diabetes mellitus, or stroke. This information's particularly important if your patient has newly discovered hypertension. If he's a known hypertensive, you'll need this information to update his record.

Social history. Obtain information about your patient's occupation, educational background, living arrangements, daily activities, and family relationships. Explore any potentially stressful circumstances. Also ask about his diet. Does he eat at fast-food restaurants frequently? If so, his salt and cholesterol intake may be excessive. Does he eat much licorice? This may lead to pseudoaldosteronism, causing secondary hypertension.

Ask about his sleep habits. Because blood pressure normally falls during sleep, insomnia may make blood pressure hard to control. If the patient works at night and sleeps during the day, his medication schedule may need readjustment. Also ask about his exercise habits, which may influence his blood pressure. And find out if he's had any sexual dysfunction. Some men complain of impotence after beginning antihypertensive medication.

Throughout your history-taking session, note the appropriateness of the patient's responses, his speech clarity, and his mood so you can identify any later changes. Also assess his cognition and comprehension levels to help determine his health education needs.

Physical examination. After completing the health history, perform a thorough physical examination. Include the important steps described below.

Blood pressure measurements. Determining arterial blood pressure with a sphygmomanometer and stethoscope detects and diagnoses hypertension and helps evaluate therapeutic effectiveness in a patient with known hypertension. Take two or more blood pressure measurements with the patient supine or seated and two or more measurements with the patient standing. Make sure to measure pressures with the recommended technique (see *How to measure blood pressure accurately*). Measurement variations frequently stem from the widely varying techniques health care professionals use.

Continued on page 82

Hypertension

How to measure blood pressure accurately

To ensure accurate blood pressure measurement—essential to proper hypertension assessment—follow the guidelines described below.

For an adult:
Seat your patient comfortably, with his arm slightly flexed and his forearm supported at heart level on a smooth surface. Blood pressure increases with the arm below heart level, decreases with the arm above heart level—in both cases, by as much as 10 mm Hg for both systolic and diastolic pressures.

For the initial examination, measure and record pressure in both arms. For subsequent examinations, use the arm with higher initial pressure.

To ensure accurate results, take blood pressure readings with your patient in a quiet room at a comfortable temperature. Because anxiety, food intake, tobacco use, bladder distention, pain, and talking can affect blood pressure, try to control or eliminate these stimuli during measurement. If possible, instruct the patient to avoid exposure to cold, exertion, smoking, and eating for 30 minutes before measurement and to avoid postural changes for 5 minutes beforehand. Make sure his arm's not constricted by clothing or other material.

Use the correct pressure cuff bladder width for your patient's arm diameter. If the bladder's too narrow, the reading will be falsely high; too wide, falsely low. The bladder width should be 40% of the circumference of the patient's arm at midpoint (or 20% wider than the diameter). Bladder length also affects measurement accuracy. Make sure it's approximately twice the recommended width. Choose a cuff based on the patient's *size*, not his age.

Palpate the brachial artery and place the stethoscope's bell over it firmly so that its complete circumference contacts the skin. (The bell amplifies low-frequency sounds better than the diaphragm.) With the stethoscope in place, raise the pressure about 30 mm Hg above the point at which the pulse disappears, then release the pressure at a rate of 2 to 3 mm Hg per second.

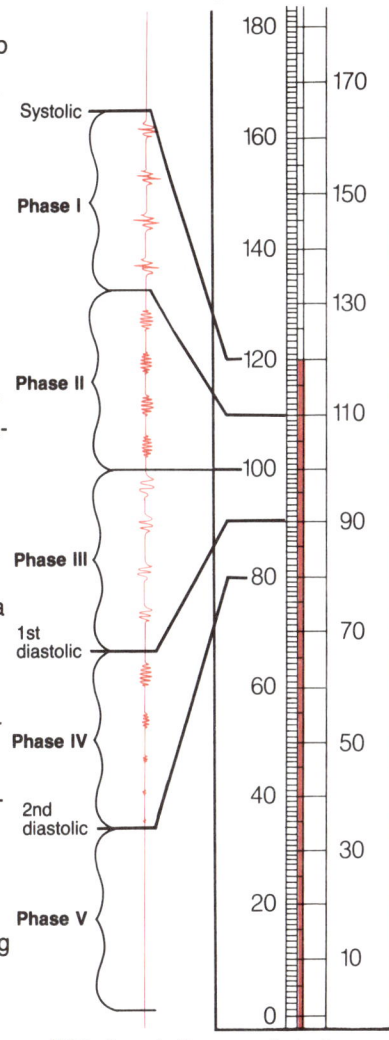

With the stethoscope's bell over the brachial artery, listen for Korotkoff's sounds (produced by blood movement and vessel vibration) as you deflate the cuff. As pressure declines, listen for:
• *Phase I*, marked by the first faint, clear, tapping sounds of gradually increasing intensity
• *Phase II*, marked by a murmur or swishing sound
• *Phase III*, marked by increased sound intensity and crispness
• *Phase IV*, marked by distinct, abrupt muffling of sounds that gives them a soft, blowing quality
• *Phase V*, marked by disappearance of sounds.

Note: Some hypertensive patients may have an *auscultatory gap*—premature, temporary disappearance of sounds late in Phases I and II. Sounds disappear as pressure drops and reappear at a lower pressure level. Because this gap may cover a range up to 40 mm Hg, you may seriously underestimate systolic pressure or overestimate diastolic pressure unless you exclude the gap by first palpating for radial pulse disappearance as you increase cuff pressure.

Record systolic pressure as the point when you hear the initial tapping sound (Phase I). Record diastolic pressure as the point at which sounds disappear (Phase V).

In some circumstances, you may measure blood pressure in the thigh instead of the arm. If so, use a larger, wider cuff. Expect the thigh's systolic pressure to exceed the arm's by 10 to 40 mm Hg; diastolic pressure remains essentially the same.

For an infant or a child:
For auscultatory blood pressure measurement, use either the largest cuff that snugly fits the child's arm or a cuff with a bladder that's 40% of arm circumference. The inflatable bladder within the cuff should completely or nearly encircle the arm.

Use the same auscultatory technique as described for adults. However, record diastolic pressure as the onset of muffling (Phase IV), rather than the disappearance of sounds (Phase V). In a child, the sounds may not disappear.

In some infants, auscultatory sounds may be too faint to hear. If you can't obtain an auscultatory blood pressure, use an ultrasonic device (such as a Doppler device), which accurately measures systolic pressure. If you don't have a Doppler device, measure blood pressure by the *flush method*. Place the cuff on the infant's wrist or ankle. Then elevate his arm or leg and compress it by wrapping it firmly with an elastic bandage. Then, when compression's complete, lower the limb to heart level and rapidly inflate the cuff to 200 mm Hg. Remove the bandage and gradually lower manometer pressure by no more than 5 mm Hg per second. Mark the point at which you note skin flushing distal to the cuff. Record this pressure, which reflects *mean*, not systolic, pressure.

Hypertension

Continued

Patient preparation and position, hearing and visual acuity differences among observers, and use of different end points as the diastolic pressure can affect measurement and diagnosis.

Keep in mind that a single elevated reading doesn't indicate hypertension. If your patient has an elevated blood pressure measurement, determine whether it's an isolated elevation that will probably disappear on remeasurement (requiring only follow-up) or sustained hypertension (requiring closer observation, evaluation, and therapy). (See *Hypertension follow-up criteria*.)

Height and weight measurement. Measure the patient's height and weight carefully to provide baseline data, determine obesity, and help identify possible hypertension causes.

Funduscopic examination. This can identify arteriolar narrowing, arteriovenous compression, hemorrhages, exudates, and papilledema—possible signs of hypertension. Grade hypertensive retinopathy from I to IV (mild to increasing severity):
- Grade I—arterial narrowing or spasm
- Grade II—arteriovenous nicking
- Grade III—hemorrhages and exudates
- Grade IV—papilledema.

Grade III indicates accelerated hypertension; Grade IV, malignant hypertension (see *Reviewing retinal funduscopic examination*).

Neck examination. Check your patient's neck for carotid bruits, distended veins, and an enlarged thyroid gland. Note your findings carefully—they may help determine hypertension's cause and identify possible complications.

Heart examination. Inspect, palpate, and auscultate for increased heart rate and size, precordial heave, murmurs, dysrhythmias, and

Hypertension follow-up criteria

Diastolic blood pressure (mm Hg)	Systolic blood pressure (mm Hg)		
	BELOW 140	**140 TO 199**	**200 OR GREATER**
Below 85	Recheck within 2 years*	*First occasion* Confirm within 2 months	Evaluate or refer for care within 2 weeks
85 to 89	Recheck within 1 year	*Second occasion* Evaluate or refer promptly for care	
90 to 104	*First occasion* Confirm within 2 months *Second occasion* Evaluate or refer promptly for care		
105 to 114	Evaluate or refer for care within 2 weeks		
115 or greater	Evaluate or refer immediately for care		

Criteria refer to asymptomatic individuals age 18 and older. Values reflect the average of two or more measurements taken on two occasions.
*Rechecking within 1 year is recommended for individuals at increased risk (those with a positive family history or obesity, blacks, oral contraceptive users, and those who consume excess alcohol).
Source: *Report of the Joint National Committee on Detection, Evaluation and Treatment of High Blood Pressure*, National Heart, Lung, and Blood Institute

Hypertension

Reviewing retinal funduscopic examination

Examining the retina—the only site where arteries can be seen without invasive techniques—reliably indicates hypertension's severity. Evidence of retinal blood vessel damage signals similar damage to vessels elsewhere. The doctor will use the Keith, Wagener, Barker method to grade retinal damage from hypertensive vascular disease.

Grade I: Mild sclerosis or arteriolar narrowing, associated with mildly elevated blood pressure.

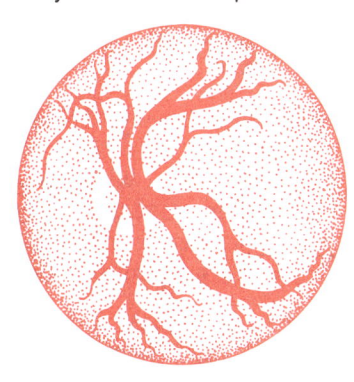

Grade II: Marked retinal changes with increased light reflexes and vein compression at crossings, indicating progressive, sustained hypertension. Overt cardiac or renal complications don't accompany these changes.

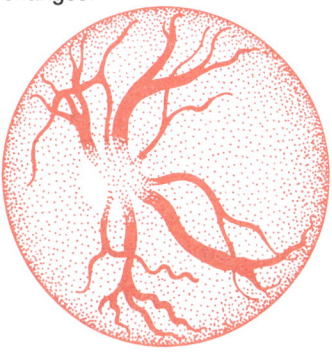

Grade III: Angiospastic retinitis and sclerotic arteriolar changes, possibly with edema. This indicates severe, sustained hypertension, possibly associated with evidence of cardiac and renal complications, such as dyspnea on exertion, EKG changes, nocturia, proteinuria, hematuria, headache, and vertigo.

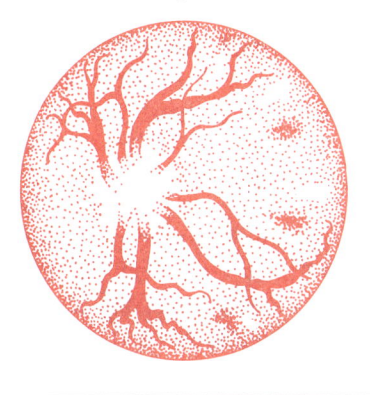

Grade IV: Papilledema with exudates and extensive hemorrhages. Disk edema associated with severe arteriolar narrowing and diffuse retinitis characterizes this grade. These changes indicate malignant hypertension.

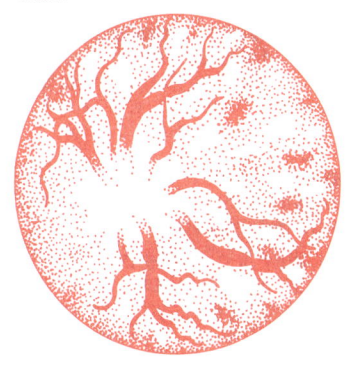

third (S_3) or fourth (S_4) heart sounds. If the point of maximal impulse occurs downward and laterally, suspect heart enlargement. If you hear an S_4, suspect a rigid left ventricle from hypertrophy. S_3 usually arises as an early sign of congestive heart failure.

Abdominal examination. Check for bruits, enlarged kidneys, and aortic dilation. Auscultate over the epigastrium—a continuous bruit commonly occurs here with renal artery stenosis, which may indicate renovascular hypertension.

Arm and leg examination. Check for edema and signs of peripheral vascular disease, such as skin discoloration, temperature changes,

Continued on page 84

Vascular Problems — 84 Hypertension

Hypertension
Continued

and weak or absent peripheral pulses. These may provide clues to hypertension's cause and alert you to complications. Inspect the patient's skin closely for café-au-lait spots (common with pheochromocytoma).

Neurologic examination. Perform a general neurologic assessment, including level of consciousness, Glasgow Coma Scale score, pupil reaction, muscle strength, gait, coordination, and speech. Your findings may help detect complications and determine if hypertension's progressed.

Respiratory examination. Perform a general respiratory assessment. Although your findings usually won't provide clues to hypertension's cause, they can suggest complications. Wheezes and crackles, for example, may indicate congestive heart failure. (See *Secondary hypertension: Reviewing common causes*, page 78, for other signs and symptoms suggesting secondary hypertension.)

Diagnostic studies. The doctor usually diagnoses hypertension from repeated blood pressure measurements. However, he may order diagnostic studies to help determine hypertension's cause, to detect any complications, and to obtain baseline data before initiating therapy. Diagnostic tests may include:
- complete blood count
- urinalysis
- serum chemistries (particularly serum potassium, creatinine, sodium, uric acid, glucose, and cholesterol [both total and high-density lipoprotein])
- electrocardiogram (EKG)
- chest X-ray.

If the doctor suspects secondary hypertension, he may order other diagnostic studies to confirm his suspicions. However, he'll usually order these more expensive tests only if the patient particularly risks secondary hypertension, as in these circumstances:
- the patient's younger than age 20 or older than age 50
- his hypertension had a rapid onset (especially if he has no family history of hypertension)
- his hypertension suddenly worsens
- he doesn't respond to antihypertensive therapy
- he develops an abdominal bruit.

Planning
Before determining your nursing care plan, develop the nursing diagnosis by identifying the patient's problem or potential problem, then relating it to its cause. Possible nursing diagnoses for a patient with hypertension include:
- noncompliance; related to denial of the disease
- knowledge deficit; related to inadequate health teaching
- sexual dysfunction; related to adverse effects of antihypertensive medications
- self-concept, disturbances in; related to chronic illness diagnosis
- family dynamics, alterations in; related to disease
- anxiety; related to chronic illness
- coping, ineffective; related to chronic illness
- tissue perfusion, alteration in; related to vascular damage.

Automatic blood pressure monitors
Automatic blood pressure monitors come in several varieties. We'll review two types.

Continuous automatic blood pressure monitor. Besides air hoses and a pressure cuff, the continuous monitor has these essential features:
- mean arterial pressure (MAP) readout
- heart rate and minutes elapsed since the last cuff inflation
- systolic arterial pressure readout
- diastolic arterial pressure readout
- switches for setting the time interval between cuff inflations
- a switch for an immediate blood pressure readout
- a switch for setting high and low MAP alarm limits.

To use the monitor, apply the blood pressure cuff as you would for a manual reading. Then turn on the machine and set the MAP limits and the time interval between cuff inflations (1 to 160 minutes).

When the preset time interval has elapsed, air passes through the hoses and automatically inflates the cuff to 160 mm Hg. The machine then deflates the cuff in increments of about 6 mm Hg. During deflation, the cuff detects brachial artery pulsations. A precalibrated transducer inside the monitor translates the pulsations into electric impulses, which appear on various readouts. The next cuff inflation will reach a pressure 35 mm Hg higher than the previous systolic reading, and then the whole cycle repeats.

This highly sensitive system can detect blood pressures 2 to 6 mm Hg higher than you can palpate or auscultate. However, sometimes this sensitivity can cause problems. For example, if your patient flexes his arm while the cuff's deflating, you'll see an inaccurately high reading. To guard against this, make sure you take a baseline pressure reading when you first set up the monitor.

A patient's positional change can cause a blood pressure rise with the next readout. Try to keep the patient in the same position he was in when you obtained baseline pressure. If you get a suspi-
Continued

Vascular Problems

85 Hypertension

Automatic blood pressure monitors
Continued

ciously high reading, always consider the patient's position.

Keep these other important points in mind when using a continuous monitor:
- Check cuff position periodically. Use a proper size cuff. A cuff that slips from the proper position will cause an inaccurately low reading; a cuff that's too small, an inaccurately high reading.
- When you take manual blood pressure measurements to double-check monitor accuracy, always use the same arm to which the monitor was attached.
- If your patient's attached to an EKG machine that shows a higher pulse rate than the monitor, check the patient for cardiac dysfunction. The monitor detects only peripheral pulsations; it won't detect dysrhythmias such as frequent premature ventricular contractions.
- Remember that although the machine's sensitive and reliable, it's no substitute for your expert nursing skills. Assess your patient frequently and intervene as necessary.

Ambulatory continuous automatic blood pressure monitor. This monitor permits you to assess your patient's blood pressure fluctuations as he performs his daily activities. Besides a blood pressure cuff, the system includes these essential features:
- a lightweight, portable monitor that contains a microprocessor to record pressure measurements
- a random access memory (RAM) data pack to store measurements
- a portable operating system for home analysis
- an analysis station for hospital analysis
- a detachable battery pack.

To use this system, the patient attaches the monitor to his belt or a shoulder strap and slips the blood pressure cuff into place. Then the microprocessor records the patient's blood pressure at 6- to 60-minute intervals, depending on doctor's orders. It displays digital readings on its miniscreen and stores them in the RAM data pack. After the prescribed monitoring period (usually 24 hours), blood pressure readings will be evaluated for trends, plotted on a graph, and printed out.

Hypertension

The sample nursing care plan below shows expected outcomes, nursing interventions, and discharge planning for one nursing diagnosis listed above. However, you'll want to tailor each care plan to fit the patient's needs.

Intervention

The hypertensive patient requires treatment to avoid illness caused by prolonged high blood pressure. The doctor will order measures aimed at reducing blood pressure enough to minimize cardiovascular risk. Although many clinical studies show that therapy can help, the doctor's decision to begin therapy for a particular patient depends on hypertension's severity and whether the patient has complications or other risk factors. Treatment may be nonpharmacologic, pharmacologic, or a combination of both.

Nonpharmacologic therapy. The doctor may order nonpharmacologic measures for a patient with mild hypertension or as an adjunct in a patient with more severe hypertension who's receiving pharmacologic therapy. These measures may help reduce drug dose requirements, potentiate beneficial drug effects, and diminish adverse effects.

Major nonpharmacologic therapies include:
- dietary intervention (weight reduction, sodium restriction, increased potassium intake, and other measures)
- exercise
- behavior modification.

Weight reduction forms an integral part of therapy for an obese hypertensive patient. Body weight and blood pressure correlate strongly, as do body weight and blood pressure increases—partic-

Continued on page 86

Sample nursing care plan: Hypertension

Nursing diagnosis	Expected outcomes
Noncompliance; related to denial of disease	The patient will: • show compliance with therapy. • show he understands the disease and its process. • show he understands his treatment and care plan.

Nursing interventions	Discharge planning
• Discuss disease and its process with patient and his family. Answer any questions they may have. • Discuss treatment and care plan with patient and his family. • Discuss with patient the need to comply with therapy. • Discuss with patient and his family methods he can use at home to remember his medications (for example, cuing techniques, such as placing his pill container beside his denture cup). • Discuss with patient and his family nonpharmacologic techniques to reduce blood pressure (for example, a low-sodium diet, weight reduction, and relaxation and biofeedback techniques). • Encourage patient to participate in his care planning and to express his feelings about the disease.	• Teach patient about his medications, if indicated. • Reinforce patient's treatment and care plan. • Teach patient and his family how to take home blood pressure measurements. • Reinforce cuing techniques, if indicated. • Arrange for follow-up medical care, as needed. • Reinforce the need for follow-up care and therapeutic compliance. • Inform patient and his family about community referral agencies and refer him, if needed. • Provide patient with support materials, as needed. • Tell patient when to seek medical care.

Hypertension

Continued

ularly among children and young to middle-aged adults. Frequently, weight reduction leads to a substantial blood pressure decrease, even if the patient can't reach his ideal body weight.

If your hypertensive patient needs to lose weight, help him maintain his commitment to dieting by encouraging him and by urging his family and other support persons to encourage him, too. To help motivate him, stress the benefits of weight loss.

Moderate sodium restriction (to 2 g or less per day from the average of 3 to 5 g per day) can also help reduce blood pressure. Virtually all patients benefit from moderate sodium restriction, which may enhance diuretic therapy and reduce associated potassium wastage. However, compliance with sodium restriction can prove a challenge even for a highly motivated patient. Almost all processed food (which accounts for more than half the typical American diet) contains sodium. So simply telling your patient to limit his salt intake may not help much. But you can encourage compliance by arranging for dietary counseling and by giving him detailed information about the salt content of various foods.

Preliminary evidence suggests that increased potassium intake (independent of decreased sodium intake) helps lower blood pressure. No one's discovered the underlying mechanism and current studies aim to substantiate these findings (see *How increased potassium intake may reduce blood pressure*). If the doctor orders this for your patient, arrange for dietary counseling and teach the patient about foods with a high potassium content.

Other dietary considerations that help control hypertension include reducing alcohol consumption and dietary fat. Again, provide or arrange for dietary counseling as appropriate. If your patient smokes, advise him to stop. Nicotine raises arterial pressure acutely, although no definitive evidence proves that prolonged nicotine use increases the hypertension risk. However, smoking does increase cardiovascular risk.

Exercise plays a controversial role in routine hypertension treatment. Some studies suggest that regular isotonic (dynamic) exercise, such as jogging, walking, or swimming, may reduce blood pressure. Because exercise also contributes to weight loss, encourage your patient to incorporate it into his weight control program. However, warn him to start any exercise program *gradually*, after appropriate medical evaluation, and to avoid isometric (static) exercise, which markedly increases systolic and diastolic pressures.

The doctor may also recommend a behavior modification program. Some researchers theorize that increased SNS activity promotes primary hypertension. Thus, modifying the SNS response to stress through behavior modification could reduce blood pressure. A behavior modification program trains the patient to voluntarily lower his metabolic rate, creating a state of decreased SNS arousal in which his heart rate, oxygen consumption, respiratory rate, and blood pressure decline. The patient can achieve this state through various relaxation techniques. He can also learn to voluntarily control autonomic nervous system functions (including blood pressure) through biofeedback. Various relaxation and biofeedback therapies may reduce your patient's blood pressure substantially. Such

---

How increased potassium intake may reduce blood pressure

Preliminary evidence suggests that increased potassium intake helps lower blood pressure. Researchers studying how potassium intake affects blood pressure regulation theorize four probable mechanisms:
• Potassium promotes weight loss and increases serum creatinine levels, leading to reduced extracellular fluid volume—presumably from a direct effect on the kidneys.
• Potassium improves baroreceptor function.
• Potassium prevents the plasma norepinephrine increase that usually accompanies sodium restriction.
• Potassium intake improves compliance with a low-sodium diet (few people add salt to high-potassium foods, such as fruits).

Vascular Problems

87 Hypertension

Hypertension

Using the stepped-care approach

Step 1
For a patient requiring antihypertensive medication, the doctor will initially order less than a full dose of a thiazide-like diuretic or a beta blocker (such as atenolol, metoprolol, or propranolol). Then he'll proceed to a full dose, if necessary and desirable. If the patient doesn't achieve good blood pressure control, he'll proceed to the next step.

Step 2
The doctor will add a small dose of an adrenergic inhibiting agent (for example, clonidine, guanabenz, methyldopa, reserpine, or a beta blocker). Or he'll add a small dose of a thiazide-like diuretic. He'll increase the dose to maximum, as necessary and desirable. He may make additional substitutions at this point by adding an angiotensin-converting enzyme inhibitor or a slow-channel calcium blocker. (*Note:* He may also substitute an angiotensin-converting enzyme inhibitor at Steps 1, 3, or 4.) If these measures don't control blood pressure, the patient will proceed to the next step.

Step 3
The doctor will add a vasodilator (such as hydralazine or minoxidil) or a slow-channel calcium blocker. If the patient responds poorly, he'll move to the next step.

Step 4
The doctor will add guanethidine.

reductions particularly help a patient with mild hypertension but also help a patient with more severe hypertension when combined with pharmacologic therapy.

Pharmacologic therapy. Experts disagree as to when drug therapy should begin and what patients it can help. Initially, such therapy aims to achieve and maintain diastolic pressure below 90 mm Hg (if feasible), then to achieve the lowest diastolic pressure consistent with the patient's safety and medication tolerance.

For a patient whose diastolic pressure persists above 95 mm Hg, or in one who has lower pressure but other risk factors (such as target organ damage, diabetes mellitus, or major cardiovascular risk factors), drug therapy's benefits seem to outweigh any known risks. For a patient whose diastolic pressure ranges from 90 to 94 mm Hg and who's otherwise at low risk, the doctor may order aggressive nonpharmacologic measures along with careful blood pressure monitoring. If diastolic pressure remains above 90 mm Hg despite nonpharmacologic measures, the doctor may start antihypertensive medications. However, drug therapy for a patient with pressure in this range could have long-term adverse effects (for example, hypokalemia, hyperglycemia, and decreased high-density lipoprotein cholesterol), which could minimize or negate drug therapy's short-term benefits. The doctor may delay specific drug therapy for this patient if the pressure doesn't *consistently* rise above 94 mm Hg and if the patient shows no signs of target organ damage or cardiovascular risk factors.

The doctor tailors drug therapy to each patient's needs, carefully considering all possible benefits and adverse effects. Until recently, doctors tried various drugs or drug combinations until they hit on something that worked. However, in the early 1970s, they began using the *stepped-care approach.* This calls for a single, mild antihypertensive drug initially, followed by an increased dose of that drug. Then the doctor adds or substitutes one drug after another in gradually increasing doses, as needed, until the patient achieves a predetermined blood pressure goal, experiences intolerable adverse effects, or reaches the maximum dose of each drug. (See *Using the stepped-care approach*, at left, and *Guide to common antihypertensive drugs*, pages 88 and 89, for details on drug therapy.) *Note:* Because tranquilizers and sedatives don't lower blood pressure effectively, the doctor won't order them as primary therapy.

The patient on stepped-care therapy requires regular blood pressure monitoring. Depending on the results, the doctor may adjust the patient's therapy as appropriate by stepping the regimen up or down. With some exceptions, therapy must continue for life. After the patient's maintained good blood pressure control for more than 3 months, the doctor will step his therapy down if this won't compromise control. If the patient's on a single drug and his diastolic pressure remains consistently below 80 mm Hg, the doctor will probably stop the medication temporarily to see if the patient can maintain normal pressure. Of course, the patient will need regular follow-up care to make sure his pressure doesn't increase again.

Here's how the stepped-care regimen works:
• *Step 1.* The patient receives a thiazide-like diuretic (or, in some cases, a beta blocker) as initial therapy (barring any contraindi-

Continued on page 89

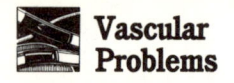

Hypertension

Guide to common antihypertensive drugs

Drug	Description and action	Common adverse effects
VASODILATORS		
hydralazine (Apresoline)	Peripheral vasodilator that directly relaxes vascular smooth muscle	Postural hypotension, headaches, tachycardia, nausea, vomiting, palpitations, fatigue, lupus syndrome (incidence less than 1%; occurs with high doses and prolonged therapy)
minoxidil (Loniten)	Extremely potent peripheral vasodilator given to patients resistant to traditional antihypertensive therapy	Hypertrichosis, fluid retention, weight gain, precipitation of angina, cardiac tamponade, EKG changes, tachycardia
prazosin (Minipress)	Originally thought to directly relax vascular smooth muscle; recent studies suggest vasodilatory effect	Syncope with first dose, postural hypotension, palpitations, dizziness, lack of energy, weakness
ANGIOTENSIN-CONVERTING ENZYME INHIBITOR		
captopril (Capoten)	A specific inhibitor of angiotensin I—converting enzyme, which interrupts the renin-angiotensin-aldosterone system	Cutaneous rash, taste impairment, proteinuria, leukopenia
DIURETICS		
chlorothiazide (Diuril)	Increases renal excretion of sodium chloride and water, mainly by inhibiting sodium reabsorption in the early distal tubules; initial antihypertensive effect caused by volume reduction and lowered cardiac output	Hyponatremia, hypokalemia, hyperuricemia, hypercalcemia, hyperglycemia
chlorthalidone (Hygroton, Thalitone)	See *chlorothiazide*	Hyperglycemia, hyperuricemia, hypercalcemia, hyponatremia, hypokalemia
hydrochlorothiazide (Oretic, Esidrix, HydroDIURIL)	See *chlorothiazide*	Hyperglycemia, hyperuricemia, hypercalcemia, hyponatremia, hypokalemia
metolazone (Zaroxolyn, Diulo)	Primarily inhibits sodium reabsorption at the cortical diluting site and in the proximal convoluted tubule	Hyperglycemia, hyperuricemia, hypercalcemia, hyponatremia, hypokalemia, azotemia
bumetanide (Bumex)	Primarily inhibits reabsorption of sodium chloride and water in the ascending loop of Henle; also exerts a weak diuretic effect in the proximal tubules	Hyperglycemia, hyperuricemia, hypochloremia, hyponatremia, hypokalemia, fluid and electrolyte imbalance
ethacrynic acid (Edecrin)	Primarily inhibits reabsorption of sodium chloride and water in the ascending loop of Henle; also exerts a weak diuretic effect in the proximal and distal tubules	Hyperuricemia, hyperglycemia, hyponatremia, hypochloremia, hypokalemia, gastrointestinal symptoms in large doses, fluid and electrolyte imbalance
furosemide (Lasix)	See *ethacrynic acid*	Hyperglycemia, hyperuricemia, hypochloremia, hyponatremia, hypokalemia, fluid and electrolyte imbalance, mild diarrhea, deafness (in large doses)
amiloride (Midamor)	A potassium-conserving drug with weak natriuretic and antihypertensive activity	Nausea, anorexia, diarrhea, vomiting, hyperkalemia
amiloride, 5 mg, and **hydrochlorothiazide**, 50 mg (Moduretic)	See *chlorothiazide* and *amiloride*	Electrolyte imbalance, elevated blood urea nitrogen level, hyperkalemia, mild skin rash
spironolactone (Aldactone)	Antagonizes aldosterone in the distal tubule, increasing excretion of sodium and water but sparing potassium	Gynecomastia, menstrual irregularity, amenorrhea, postmenopausal bleeding, hyperkalemia
spironolactone, 25 mg, and **hydrochlorothiazide**, 25 mg (Aldactazide)	See *chlorothiazide* and *spironolactone*	Gynecomastia, gastrointestinal symptoms
triamterene (Dyrenium)	Has a diuretic effect on the distal renal tubules to inhibit the reabsorption of sodium in exchange for potassium	Blood dyscrasia, photosensitivity, skin rash, hyperkalemia
triamterene, 50 mg, and **hydrochlorothiazide**, 25 mg (Dyazide)	See *chlorothiazide* and *triamterene*	Electrolyte imbalance, muscle cramps, rash, weakness, photosensitivity, gastrointestinal disturbances

Continued

Hypertension

Guide to common antihypertensive drugs—continued

Drug	Description and action	Common adverse effects
triamterene, 75 mg, and **hydrochlorothiazide,** 50 mg (Maxzide)	See *chlorothiazide* and *triamterene*	Electrolyte imbalance, muscle cramps, rash, weakness, photosensitivity, gastrointestinal disturbances
ADRENERGIC BLOCKERS		
clonidine (Catapres)	Centrally acting alpha-adrenergic agonist that decreases sympathetic cardioaccelerator and vasoconstrictor outflow from the central nervous system	Dry mouth, sedation, drowsiness, headaches, rebound hypertension
guanabenz (Wytensin)	See *clonidine*	Dry mouth, sedation, drowsiness, fatigue, impotence, withdrawal syndrome, dizziness
methyldopa (Aldomet)	Central action uncertain; an alpha-adrenergic receptor inhibitor with net effect being reduced peripheral resistance	Lassitude, drowsiness, dry mouth, mild orthostatic hypotension, positive Coombs' test (with high doses), positive rheumatoid and lupus erythematosus factors, impotence
labetalol (Normodyne, Trandate)	Nonselective beta-adrenergic receptor antagonist that also has an alpha-adrenergic blocking action	Dizziness, orthostatic hypotension, fatigue
nadolol (Corgard)	Nonselective beta-adrenergic receptor antagonist for available beta-receptor sites; it has little direct myocardial depressant activity	Bradycardia, dizziness, fatigue, bronchospasm
pindolol (Visken)	Nonselective beta-adrenergic antagonist with intrinsic sympathomimetic activity	Insomnia, muscle cramps, dizziness, fatigue, edema, nervousness
propranolol (Inderal)	Nonselective beta-adrenergic receptor blocker that competes with beta-adrenergic receptor stimulators for available receptor sites	Fatigue, dizziness, vivid dreams, depression, impotence; masks symptoms of hypoglycemia
timolol (Blocadren)	Nonselective beta-adrenergic receptor blocker that lacks significant intrinsic sympathomimetic and direct myocardial depressant activity	Fatigue, headaches, bradycardia, dizziness, pruritus, dyspnea
acebutolol (Sectral)	Beta$_1$-selective adrenergic receptor blocker that possesses weak intrinsic sympathomimetic activity	Bradycardia, development of antinuclear antibodies, back and joint pain, pruritus, anxiety, vomiting, abdominal pain
atenolol (Tenormin)	Beta$_1$-selective adrenergic receptor blocker without membrane-stabilizing or intrinsic sympathomimetic activities; lacks selectivity with high doses	Bradycardia, dizziness, postural hypotension, cold extremities, fatigue
metoprolol (Lopressor)	Beta$_1$-selective adrenergic receptor blocker, specifically of receptors in cardiac muscle; also inhibits beta$_2$-adrenergic receptors in bronchial and vascular muscle in higher doses	Fatigue, dizziness, depression, bradycardia

Continued

cations). In most patients with mild hypertension, a diuretic or a beta blocker alone controls blood pressure. Most thiazide-like diuretics and many beta blockers prove effective when taken once a day. The doctor will probably choose a diuretic if the patient's over age 50; black; or has peripheral vascular disease, asthma, or chronic pulmonary disease. Using the smallest effective diuretic dose minimizes adverse effects. If the patient's under age 50 (especially if he has a rapid resting pulse rate and a wide pulse pressure) or has ischemic heart disease, the doctor may choose a beta blocker initially. Beta blockers usually reduce blood pressure to the level achieved with diuretics.

Continued on page 90

Hypertension

Removing compliance barriers

As the first step in promoting patient compliance with hypertension treatment, identify and correct any problems that reduce your patient's compliance. Whenever possible, take these steps:
• *Reduce waiting time.* Your patient must visit the doctor regularly for lifelong blood pressure control. But the frustration brought on by long waiting times can deter him from keeping scheduled appointments. Minimize delay and maximize convenience by suggesting to the doctor that he provide individual appointment times convenient to the patient; that he contract with the patient, agreeing to see him promptly if he comes on time; and that he keep visits brief whenever appropriate.
• *Keep the regimen simple.* A complex regimen can deter compliance. If you suspect that a patient's poor compliance stems from a complex drug regimen, consider suggesting to the doctor that he reduce the frequency or number of prescribed medications.
• *Encourage the patient to participate in his care.* If appropriate, have him monitor his blood pressure at home. This helps transfer responsibility to the patient—especially important for the patient who resents the passive role he may be forced to take in a long-term therapeutic relationship. Home pressure measurement also provides the doctor with information about blood pressure during daily activities—an invaluable therapeutic aid.

If these measures don't prove effective, try to improve compliance with these additional steps:
• *If your patient misses an appointment, contact him promptly to make a new one.* If he consistently fails to keep appointments, consider arranging a visit through a public health agency. Alternatives include having blood pressures recorded at work or at a community screening program.
• *Increase supervision.* If poor compliance keeps your patient from achieving good blood pressure control, you may need to schedule more frequent visits or to recruit help from a family member. Also, focus attention directly on the therapeutic goal when talking to the patient.

Continued

Hypertension

Continued

If these drugs don't control the patient's blood pressure (or if adverse effects limit the use of other drugs), the doctor may add an angiotensin-converting enzyme inhibitor at this point or at Steps 2, 3, or 4.

• *Step 2.* If the patient doesn't respond to diuretic therapy, the doctor will add small doses of an adrenergic inhibiting agent (such as a beta blocker). Similarly, if the patient began therapy with a beta blocker but didn't respond, the doctor will add a diuretic or substitute a diuretic for the beta blocker. If these measures don't control blood pressure, he may order full doses of the Step 2 drug or may substitute another adrenergic inhibitor. Or, instead of increasing the Step 2 drug dose to maximum, he may add a vasodilator or substitute another drug, such as a slow-channel calcium blocker. Smaller doses of two drugs with different mechanisms of action may prove more effective than larger doses of a single drug. This approach frequently minimizes adverse effects without significantly reducing effectiveness.

• *Step 3.* If Step 2 drugs don't control blood pressure, the doctor will add a vasodilator or a slow-channel calcium blocker to the patient's regimen.

• *Step 4.* If the first three steps prove ineffective and if secondary hypertension has been ruled out, the doctor may add guanethidine or substitute this drug or another adrenergic inhibitor for a Step 2 drug.

Although any hypertensive patient can use the stepped-care program, the doctor may modify the regimen for a patient with a diastolic pressure of 115 mm Hg or higher. For instance, he may begin treatment with full diuretic and adrenergic inhibitor doses simultaneously to control blood pressure more rapidly. He may also decrease the intervals between regimen changes and increase the maximum dose of some drugs. (If the patient has an average diastolic blood pressure of 130 mm Hg or more, he'll need more urgent treatment.)

Patient compliance. For many hypertensive patients, therapeutic compliance presents a major problem. Encourage your patient to participate in his care as soon as the doctor's diagnosed primary hypertension and initiated therapy. To help your patient make the crucial decision to control his blood pressure, explain these important facts:
• His blood pressure exceeds normal limits.
• He needs long-term treatment and follow-up care.
• He still needs treatment even if he doesn't have symptoms.
• Treatment can control but not cure hypertension.
• Consistently following his treatment regimen can help ensure an excellent prognosis and a normal life-style.

Stress to your patient that although diagnosis and treatment remain the doctor's responsibility, the patient must make the critical decision to control his hypertension by adhering to the prescribed regimen.

To ensure successful intervention and follow-up, first assess your patient's willingness to participate in his care and modify his lifestyle, if necessary. When assessing his willingness to learn, con-

Hypertension

Removing compliance barriers
Continued

• *Provide reminders for his medication regimen.* Ask the patient to describe his normal routine, then tailor his regimen to incorporate his medication. For example, if he shaves each morning, suggest that he put his pill container near his razor and take his medication before shaving. Other reminders might be his toothbrush, coffee cup, eyeglasses, or hair dryer.

• *Praise the patient when he achieves blood pressure reduction.* Tell him his blood pressure at each visit, or, better still, have him log his blood pressure measurements and medication administration and bring the log at each visit. Praise him for complying with therapy and for achieving his blood pressure goal. Keep in mind that patient education may not improve compliance—but patient *motivation* frequently does.

Hypertension

sider his previous health practices and his compliance with other health care regimens. Also determine whether he's likely to adjust physically, mentally, and emotionally to the recommended changes. For example, if your patient needs long-term dietary changes, take into account his established eating habits, overall health, economic and educational status, and life-style when helping him plan these changes.

For best results, work together with the patient and other members of the health care team to monitor the patient's progress toward his blood pressure goal and to resolve potential problems. You can also make a crucial difference to the patient's progress by aiding communication, motivating him, and expressing sensitivity to cultural and individual concerns.

Once therapy begins, help your patient maintain good blood pressure control by following these guidelines during subsequent visits:

• Ask the patient if he's had any adverse effects since he started his medication. He may not associate certain symptoms with drug use and thus may not mention them unless you ask (for instance, some antihypertensive drugs can cause sexual dysfunction).

• Teach the patient how to deal with common nontoxic adverse drug effects.

• Provide feedback and reinforcement to motivate the patient to achieve his blood pressure goal. Suggest that he keep a graphic chart of his serial blood pressure readings as a visual aid.

• If he has other modifiable cardiovascular risk factors, such as hyperlipidemia or smoking, encourage him to minimize these and help him establish realistic goals (for example, through an individualized program).

• Suggest nonpharmacologic ways to enhance his drug therapy. These might include a stepped exercise program (incorporating patient preferences) supervised by the doctor; stress management techniques, such as progressive deep-muscle relaxation; a reduced-sodium, high-potassium diet; a weight-loss program; and reduced alcohol consumption (if needed).

• Be aware that hypertension's diagnosis and treatment can cause anxiety or provoke dependent behavior. Ask your patient how he feels about his condition and the life-style changes he thinks he should make. Then, with this knowledge, explain how hypertension will affect his daily activities, for example, by necessitating daily medication or dietary sodium restriction. Encourage him to continue his current social and recreational activities and to lead as normal a life as possible.

If the doctor wants the patient to lose weight, take medications, stop smoking, and/or reduce salt intake, keep in mind that the patient will need considerable information and support. Your patient's more likely to participate in an educational program if he's accepted his illness. He may progress through classic stages of psychosocial adaptation to illness—shock and disbelief, developing awareness, reorganization, resolution, and identity change. Give a newly diagnosed hypertensive patient time to accept his disease and assume responsibility for controlling it. During the first adaptation phase, he may not absorb everything you tell him. Discuss, in a well-focused manner, only the most essential information. Most patients in this phase adapt easily to their medication regimen because it doesn't alter life-style dramatically.

Continued on page 93

Hypertension

Hypertension and pregnancy

Hypertension can have serious consequences for a pregnant patient and her fetus. To prevent these consequences, you need to understand the vascular changes that normally accompany pregnancy so you can recognize abnormal changes.

In a normal pregnancy, blood volume increases by 30% to 50%. Both red blood cell and plasma components increase. The renin-angiotensin-aldosterone system accelerates (probably from increased estrogen production), resulting in elevated plasma levels of renin, angiotensin II, and aldosterone. Although the pregnant woman normally develops resistance to the pressor effect of angiotensin II, increased aldosterone encourages sodium reabsorption and water retention. This increases total body water and contributes to increased blood volume.

Blood volume expansion increases stroke volume, heart rate, and cardiac output. In a nonpregnant patient, this could result in hypertension. However, in a pregnant patient, arterioles dilate (probably from increased progesterone levels) and peripheral vascular resistance drops. As a result, blood pressure falls slightly (about 20 mm Hg diastolic) beginning in the first trimester and continuing through the second. Lowest between weeks 16 and 20, blood pressure rises toward the patient's baseline during the third trimester.

In some patients, however, blood pressure regulation goes awry. The patient may have *chronic hypertension*—blood pressure of 140/90 before pregnancy, or 140/90 before the 20th gestational week, possibly persisting indefinitely after delivery. She may develop *late,* or *transient, hypertension*—blood pressure that rises during labor or early postpartum but returns to normal within 10 days after delivery. Or she may develop *pregnancy-induced hypertension* (PIH)—the most serious blood pressure disorder in pregnancy.

Formerly known as toxemia of pregnancy, PIH falls into two categories—preeclampsia and eclampsia. PIH, whose cause remains unknown, involves vasospasm, causing arteriolar constriction and increased peripheral vascular resistance (in contrast to arteriolar dilation and decreased peripheral vascular resistance in a normal pregnancy). Vasospasm probably results from vascular sensitivity to vasopressors.

In preeclampsia, blood pressure rises to 140/90, or increases by 30 mm Hg systolic or 15 mm Hg diastolic over baseline, on two occasions at least 6 or more hours apart. The patient develops proteinuria and edema (generally limited to the face and hands, and appearing even after arising in the morning). Signs and symptoms arise after the 20th gestational week (proteinuria may not occur until late in PIH). Preeclampsia most commonly develops in women under age 20 or over age 35 and occurs almost exclusively during the patient's first pregnancy. Occasionally, it occurs in a woman with previous pregnancies who has vascular disease, chronic renal disease, or uterine overdistention (as with twins).

As preeclampsia worsens, the patient may have systolic pressure of 160 mm Hg or diastolic pressure of 110 mm Hg, even on bed rest. Proteinuria may increase. Cerebral or visual disturbances, such as altered consciousness, scotoma, or blurred vision, may also develop. Evidence of advancing disease includes epigastric or upper quadrant pain, thrombocytopenia, impaired liver function, hyperreflexia of deep tendon reflexes, and oliguria.

Treatment goals include preventing vital organ ischemia, preventing or minimizing complications, and ensuring safe infant delivery. The doctor will order treatment to stabilize the mother's condition until she can deliver a mature infant. The patient's blood pressure, the disease's severity and effects on the mother and fetus, and fetal gestational age determine which measures he'll choose. Treatment may include:
- antihypertensive medications
- a high-protein diet
- positioning the patient laterally (especially on her left side to avoid compressing the aorta and inferior vena cava)
- normal sodium and fluid intake.

Important: Don't advise the patient to restrict dietary sodium.

In severe preeclampsia, additional treatment may include hospitalization with bed rest in a quiet, darkened room (to avoid inducing seizure activity) and administration of magnesium sulfate and/or antihypertenisve medications.

Preeclampsia may progress to eclampsia, with more severe signs and symptoms, including seizures. Eclampsia may occur before labor, during labor, or within 48 hours after delivery. Treatment includes seizure interventions and administration of such medications as anticonvulsants and magnesium sulfate.

Uterus—supine position

Aorta
Inferior vena cava

Uterus—left-side lying position

Inferior vena cava
Aorta

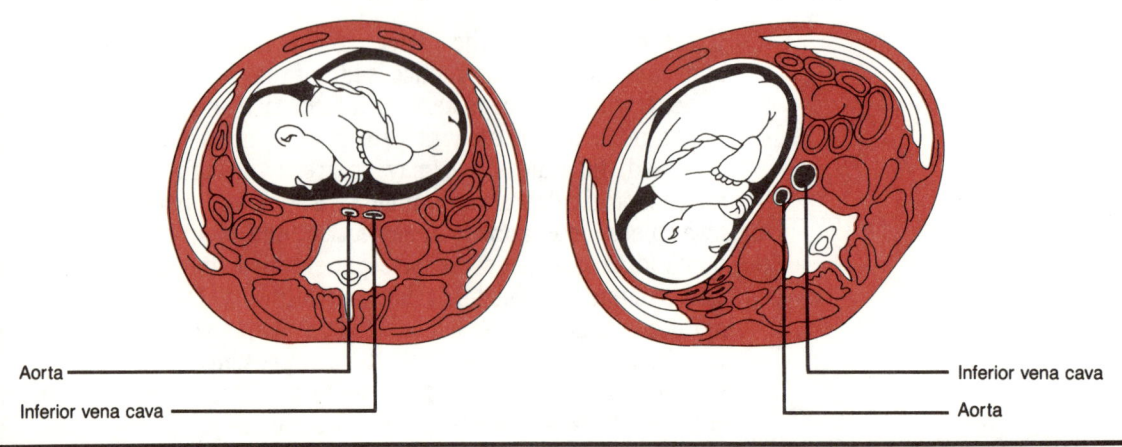

Hypertension

Continued

During the second adaptation phase, the patient develops an awareness of his disease and its personal meaning and implications. He'll have many questions that you must answer honestly—the rapport you establish early can facilitate a trusting attitude in this phase. As his interest increases, he's more likely to participate in a hypertension education program.

During the third adaptation phase—reorganization—the patient develops greater acceptance of his hypertension and greater flexibility in adapting and adjusting to his therapeutic regimen. You'll find clarifying and reinforcing teaching goals easier now. The patient

Continued on page 94

Hypertension in children

When providing care for any child over age 3, make sure to measure his blood pressure annually. Hypertension *can* occur in children, and early detection helps minimize the risks and ensure appropriate treatment.

The pediatric blood pressure grids shown below will help you determine the appropriate percentile based on the child's blood pressure, age, and sex. A child with blood pressure above the 95th percentile for his age and sex on three separate measurements needs further evaluation. Take a thorough family history and assess him for other cardiovascular risk factors. Ask the child and his parents about any signs or symptoms the child may have experienced. Most *asymptomatic* children and adolescents with elevated blood pressure are overweight and have a family history of hypertension; they usually have primary hypertension. Most *symptomatic* children and adolescents with elevated pressure have severe hypertension with an identifiable cause. These children need thorough evaluation for secondary hypertension.

By identifying high-risk children, you can help introduce nonthreatening interventions designed to reduce their risk factors. Avoid causing unnecessary anxiety or labeling an asymptomatic child as hypertensive, but *do* encourage the high-risk child and his family to take positive action to combat hypertension. As ordered and indicated, promote nonpharmacologic therapies, such as weight control, dietary sodium reduction, exercise, and stopping smoking. (These measures also help minimize cardiovascular risk factors.) In a patient with mild hypertension, these measures involve life-style changes but may eliminate the need for drug therapy. In a patient with more severe hypertension, they may be used along with drug therapy.

Doctors don't know how long-term antihypertensive drug use affects children. If your patient needs drug therapy, expect the doctor to use the stepped-care approach, with emphasis on minimal effective doses of appropriate drugs.

Pediatric blood pressure grids

Boys

Girls

Source: High Blood Pressure Information Center

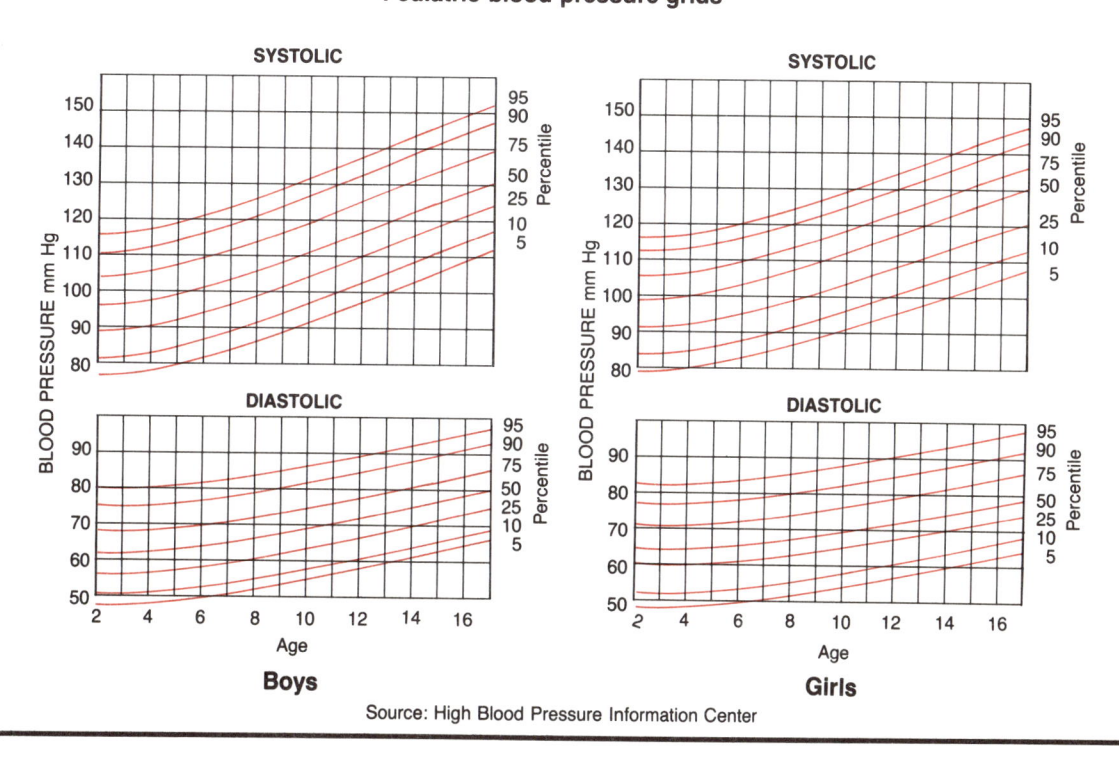

Isolated systolic hypertension

Isolated systolic hypertension (systolic pressure of 160 mm Hg or higher and diastolic pressure below 90 mm Hg) commonly occurs in elderly patients and increases the risk of cardiovascular disease. Usually, the doctor will treat this disorder with nonpharmacologic measures. However, if systolic pressure consistently remains above 160 mm Hg, he'll consider drug therapy.

Hypertension
Continued

may begin to take responsibility for reducing his risk factors and may be more receptive to suggestions for incorporating his treatment plan into his life.

During the last two adaptation phases, expect him to readily acknowledge his disease, comply with his medication regimen, and attend regularly scheduled medical appointments.

Throughout your patient's adaptation and continuing care, boost his motivation by making him feel that he's an active participant in his overall health care plan.

Complications

Sustained, untreated hypertension can lead to complications ranging from target organ damage (from serious heart and vascular damage) to malignant hypertension and hypertensive crisis. You can play a major role in preventing or minimizing complications by assessing all patients for hypertension and by encouraging hypertensive patients to comply with therapy.

Target organ damage. Hypertension forces the left ventricle to work harder than normal to raise left ventricular pressure above aortic pressure. In response to the chronically increased work load, muscle fibers hypertrophy and ventricle walls thicken, resulting in left ventricular hypertrophy. When hypertrophy reaches its limits but blood pressure remains elevated, the left ventricle dilates to maintain normal stroke volume. But ventricular hypertrophy and dilation have limits. If blood pressure increases (or if coronary circulation decreases from atherosclerotic coronary vessels), the left ventricle can't maintain normal stroke volume. This leads to congestive heart failure—five times more common in hypertensive patients than in normotensives.

Hypertension can cause characteristic atherosclerotic plaques in the aorta and large and medium-sized arteries, with corresponding problems. Coronary artery disease—twice as common in hypertensives as in normotensives—may bring on angina pectoris or myocardial infarction. Atherosclerosis of the carotid arteries and circle of Willis results in various forms of cerebrovascular accident (CVA)—three times more common in hypertensives. Leg artery involvement causes peripheral arterial occlusive disease—more than twice as common in hypertensives. Atherosclerotic renal artery narrowing can worsen hypertension and impair renal function.

Dissecting aortic aneurysm can also occur, probably from degenerative or destructive processes in the aorta's medial lining. With prolonged stretching from long-term, severe hypertension, medial fibers may rupture. In a hypertensive patient, this usually accompanies severe atheromatous lesions.

Hypertension also leads to characteristic small blood vessel damage. Kidney arterioles may thicken, causing impaired renal function. Retinal vascular changes can result in central retinal artery occlusion or retinal vein thrombosis. In the brain, cerebral hemorrhage can arise from aneurysm rupture in a tiny cerebral artery. Such aneurysms may stem from elevated blood pressure alone, independent of any atheromatous cerebral arterial lesion.

Hypertension

Malignant hypertension. This disorder—severe, fulminant hypertension—develops in about 7% of patients with primary hypertension. Blood pressure elevation becomes progressive and severe; diastolic pressure usually hovers near 130 mm Hg or higher. Accompanying changes may include retinal hemorrhage and papilledema. Vessel necrosis can lead to renal failure.

Hypertensive crisis. In this rare disorder, sometimes referred to as hypertensive encephalopathy, arterial blood pressure rises rapidly and severely, threatening the patient's life by compromising his cerebral, cardiovascular, or renal function. (Keep in mind that hypertensive crisis describes a clinical state, not a particular blood pressure level.) Causes include:
* abnormal renal function
* intracerebral hemorrhage
* acute left-sided heart failure
* abrupt withdrawal of antihypertensive medications such as clonidine (Catapres)
* myocardial ischemia
* eclampsia
* pheochromocytoma
* monoamine oxidase (MAO) inhibitor interactions.

Hypertensive crisis produces severe and widespread signs and symptoms, possibly including severe headache; blurred vision; nausea and vomiting; progressive impairment of consciousness, ranging from mild to severe confusion to convulsions and, eventually, coma; leg and arm numbness or tingling; azotemia; chest pain; oliguria; dyspnea; and retinal hemorrhagic exudates and papilledema.

Review these findings carefully—this emergency requires thorough but fast evaluation of the patient's blood pressure and clinical status. Take special care to rule out CVA, which calls for different treatment. The doctor will try to lower blood pressure *rapidly* if your patient has hypertensive crisis; *gradually*, if your patient's suffered CVA. (*Note:* Suspect CVA if your patient shows focal or lateralizing neurologic signs rather than generalized ones and if he develops neurologic deficits suddenly rather than progressively.)

Hypertensive crisis gravely theatens your patient by rapidly and severely compromising four important target organs—the brain, eyes, heart, and kidneys.

Although no one knows exactly how hypertensive crisis affects the brain, some researchers theorize that it causes severe vasoconstriction, which may lead, in turn, to cerebral ischemia and tissue damage. Other researchers propose that blood-brain barrier disturbances associated with acute hypertension allow fluid accumulation in brain tissue. Increasing edema then causes signs and symptoms of hypertensive encephalopathy (severe headache, visual disturbances, nausea and vomiting, decreasing level of consciousness progressing to convulsions and coma, and arm or leg numbness and tingling).

In the eyes, severe vasoconstriction affects the retinal arteries. On funduscopic examination, these arteries may appear thready and one-third to one-fourth their normal size—or you may not see them at all. (*Note:* If your patient had accelerated or malignant hyper-

Continued on page 96

Hypertension

Continued

tension before the crisis, you may also see Grade III or Grade IV retinopathy.)

Hypertensive crisis affects the heart by increasing heart wall stress. As blood pressure increases, less blood flows to the heart's subendocardial layer. The wall becomes ischemic, resulting in decreased left ventricular compliance that raises left ventricular end-diastolic (filling) pressure. Rising pressure and ischemia cause inefficient pumping. As the heart begins to fail, blood backs up into the lungs, leading to pulmonary edema. This results in acute dyspnea.

In the kidney, hypertensive crisis may cause severe arteriolar vasoconstriction. Impaired renal circulation causes proteinuria, microscopic hematuria, and renal insufficiency, leading to renal failure.

To prevent or minimize these severe effects, the doctor must lower blood pressure quickly but carefully, usually with I.V. medications titrated to the patient's response. (However, some doctors now combine parenteral and oral drugs for initial treatment because this combination lowers blood pressure more effectively and allows earlier transition to long-term oral therapy.) Although your patient's in crisis, the doctor will usually begin treatment with a low drug dose. Then he'll evaluate the patient's response before proceeding. This lessens the chance for extreme vasodilation and dangerous hypotension.

Expect the doctor to order any of the following common antihypertensive drugs for a patient in hypertensive crisis:
• *nitroprusside* (Nipride), a vasodilator that acts directly on smooth muscle of resistance arterioles within seconds, decreasing peripheral resistance and arterial blood pressure and increasing venous capacity. Nitroprusside also decreases preload and afterload, reducing myocardial oxygen demands.
• *diazoxide* (Hyperstat), a vasodilator that acts within 3 to 5 minutes to dilate arteriolar smooth muscle, reducing peripheral vascular resistance and blood pressure. Reflex SNS activity results in increased heart rate, stroke volume, cardiac work load, and cardiac output. (*Note:* Serial low-dose I.V. injections reduce blood pressure more gradually than a single large bolus and pose less danger of stroke or myocardial infarction.) Diazoxide produces marked sodium and water retention and temporary hyperglycemia.
• *hydralazine* (Apresoline), a vasodilator that acts directly on arteriolar smooth muscle within 15 minutes (I.V.) or within 30 minutes (I.M.). Reflex SNS activity leads to increased heart rate, stroke volume, cardiac work load, and cardiac output. Hydralazine also increases renal blood flow.
• *trimethaphan* (Arfonad), a ganglionic blocking agent that acts within 1 to 2 minutes to block SNS and parasympathetic impulses, causing arteriolar and venous dilation. The resulting blood pressure drop depends largely on the patient's position, so maximize the drug's effect by raising the head of the bed 4″ to 6″. Trimethaphan also reduces preload and afterload.
• *phentolamine* (Regitine), an alpha-adrenergic blocking agent that acts within seconds to produce vasodilation. It's especially useful for hypertensive crisis associated with excess catecholamine release from pheochromocytoma or from food or drug interactions with MAO inhibitors.

Hypertension

Other drugs used to treat hypertensive crisis include I.V. nitroglycerin; I.M. reserpine (Serpasil); labetalol (Normodyne, Trandate) via I.V. bolus followed by infusion; or I.V. methyldopa (Aldomet).

If the doctor orders an I.V. drug, expect him to gradually increase the infusion rate until the patient's blood pressure begins to drop. Then he'll order a maintenance infusion rate. When blood pressure stabilizes at the desired level (which may take days), the doctor will begin the transition from I.V. to oral medications. Make sure to measure blood pressure just before and after each medication change. Assess the patient frequently for hypotension and for signs and symptoms of heart failure, myocardial infarction, or stroke.

Evaluation

Base your evaluation on the expected outcomes listed on your nursing care plan. To determine if the patient's improved, ask yourself the following questions:
- Does the patient comply with his therapy?
- Has he maintained an acceptable blood pressure?
- Does he understand the disease process?
- Does he understand his treatment plan?
- Has he expressed his feelings about the disease?
- Has he accepted his disease?

The answers to these and other questions will help you evaluate your patient and his care. Keep in mind that these questions stem from the sample care plan on page 85. Your questions may differ.

Self-Test

1. According to the World Health Organization, hypertension's defined as:
a. systolic blood pressure of 160 mm Hg or higher and/or diastolic blood pressure of 95 mm Hg or higher **b.** systolic blood pressure of 160 mm Hg or higher and/or diastolic blood pressure of 95 mm Hg or lower **c.** systolic blood pressure below 160 mm Hg and/or diastolic blood pressure of 95 mm Hg or higher **d.** systolic blood pressure below 160 mm Hg and/or diastolic blood pressure of 95 mm Hg or lower

2. In the stepped-care approach to controlling hypertension, the doctor may order:
a. a thiazide-like diuretic **b.** a beta blocker **c.** an angiotensin-converting enzyme inhibitor **d.** all of the above

3. For a patient experiencing a hypertensive crisis, the doctor may order all of the following except:
a. nitroprusside **b.** hydralazine **c.** dopamine **d.** diazoxide

4. Which of the following will you hear during Phase IV of Korotkoff's sounds?
a. faint, clear tapping sounds **b.** distinct, abrupt muffling sounds **c.** a murmur or swishing sound **d.** disappearance of sounds

Answers (page number shows where answer appears in text)
1. **a** (page 73)   2. **d** (page 87)   3. **c** (page 96)   4. **b** (page 81)

Vascular Problems

98 Peripheral Vascular Disease

Patient Evaluation: Assessment Techniques

Roseann Prader Hendrickson, who wrote this chapter, is a Staff Nurse in the Emergency Department at Underwood-Memorial Hospital, Woodbury, N.J. She received her RN from the Presbyterian University of Pennsylvania Medical Center School of Nursing, Philadelphia.

Peripheral vascular disease (PVD) encompasses various blood vessel abnormalities that can affect arteries, veins, or both. Usually degenerative, PVD has become more common as more people live longer. PVD can be acute or chronic, can affect the arms or legs, and can threaten life or limb.

When evaluating a patient with suspected PVD, try to determine if the disorder's arterial or venous. Even if the affected vessels seem obvious, you'll still need to obtain a thorough history and perform a careful physical examination.

In this chapter, we'll review general techniques used to evaluate any PVD type. For details on specific disease processes, causes, and evaluation techniques, read Chapters 7 through 9.

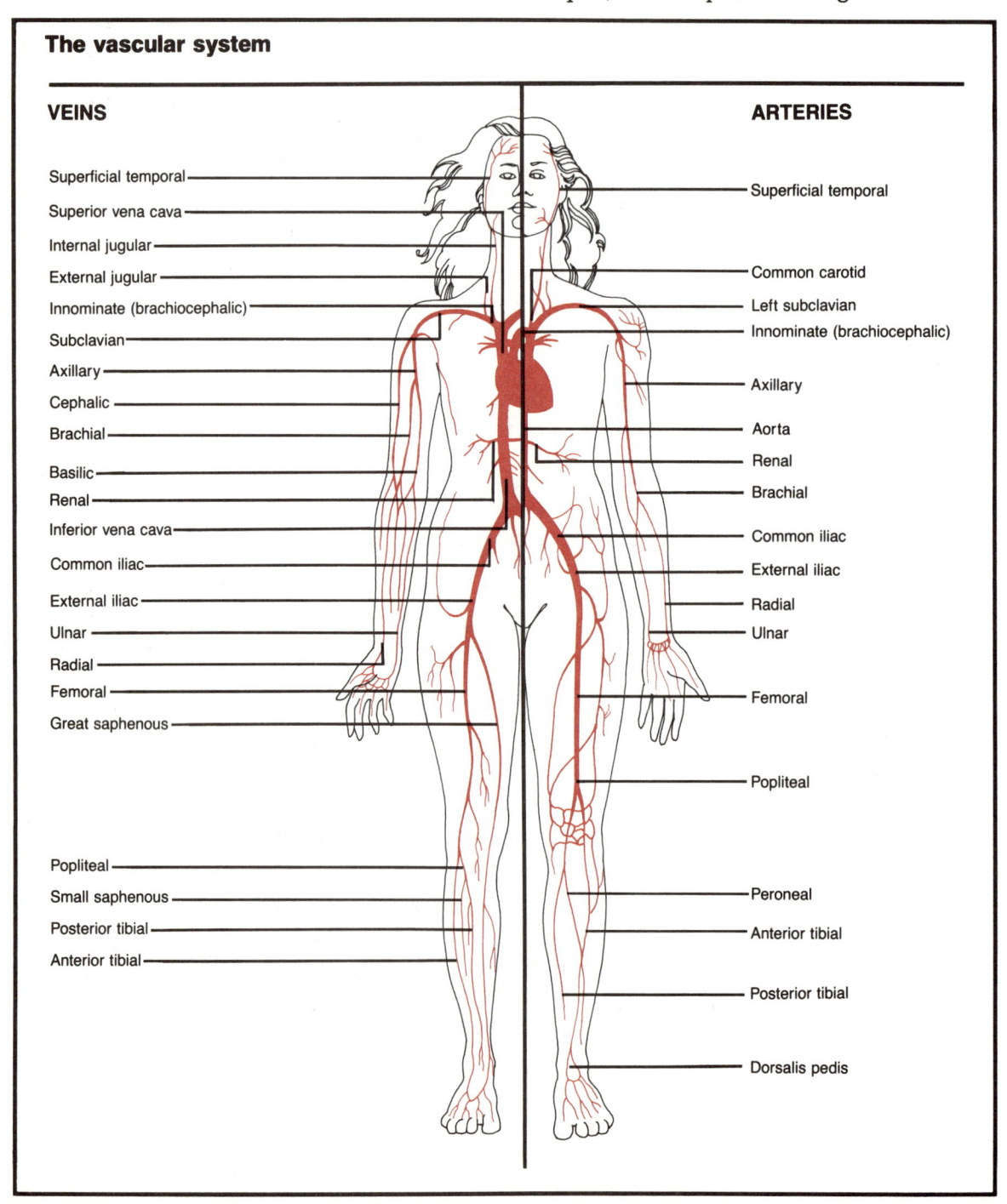

The vascular system

VEINS
- Superficial temporal
- Superior vena cava
- Internal jugular
- External jugular
- Innominate (brachiocephalic)
- Subclavian
- Axillary
- Cephalic
- Brachial
- Basilic
- Renal
- Inferior vena cava
- Common iliac
- External iliac
- Ulnar
- Radial
- Femoral
- Great saphenous
- Popliteal
- Small saphenous
- Posterior tibial
- Anterior tibial

ARTERIES
- Superficial temporal
- Common carotid
- Left subclavian
- Innominate (brachiocephalic)
- Axillary
- Aorta
- Renal
- Brachial
- Common iliac
- External iliac
- Radial
- Ulnar
- Femoral
- Popliteal
- Peroneal
- Anterior tibial
- Posterior tibial
- Dorsalis pedis

Vascular Problems

99 Peripheral Vascular Disease

Patient Evaluation

Acute peripheral arterial occlusion: The five Ps

If you suspect your patient has acute peripheral arterial occlusion, be sure to check for the five *P*s:

Pain. Does the patient complain of arm or leg pain?

Pallor. Does one limb look paler than the other? Discolored? Mottled?

Pulselessness. Can you detect all pulses?

Paresthesia. Does the patient report abnormal arm or leg sensations?

Paralysis. Does he experience paralysis?

Another *P, poikilothermy* (body temperature that varies with environmental temperature), may also suggest peripheral arterial occlusion. To assess for this, compare limb temperatures on both sides.

The nursing history

Begin your assessment with a complete nursing history. Put your patient at ease by establishing a rapport with him early. This will make his hospital stay more pleasant and will promote better therapeutic compliance during what could be a long recovery period.

Ask open-ended questions and document the patient's answers in his own words. Closely observe his nonverbal behavior and assess his cognition and comprehension levels to help determine his health teaching needs. If you believe he's in immediate danger, identify his problem quickly. Otherwise, don't rush through the history. Hurrying the patient (especially an elderly patient) may make him confused, frustrated, and even uncooperative. If you must perform an abbreviated assessment, get whatever initial information you need; then tell the patient you'll return to complete the interview.

Chief complaint

To begin the health history, identify the patient's chief complaint by asking him to tell you why he's seeking medical care. Because PVD's typically chronic, pinpointing the patient's chief complaint can prove essential.

Avoid leading questions, such as, "How long has your leg been swollen and painful?" If he's had swelling for a long time, he may be seeking help for a different reason. A more effective question might be, "What troubles you most at this time?"

Present illness

This part of the nursing history describes information relevant to the chief complaint. To identify the course of the symptom's development, find out about its onset, duration, quality, severity, and location. Have him point with one finger to the troublesome site. Also ask about alleviating and/or precipitating factors. Does anything relieve the symptom or make it worse? To find out about associated symptoms, ask if anything else bothers him when he has the symptom.

Past medical history

Find out if the patient has any contributing factors for vascular disorders by asking him if he's sought treatment for any other current or past medical problems. Has he had any major illnesses (acute or chronic) requiring hospitalization or prolonged bed rest? Also ask about:
• medications. Record all prescribed and over-the-counter medications the patient has taken, noting their dose and frequency. Also find out if he uses recreational drugs.
• allergies or sensitivities. Has he experienced reactions to any foods, drugs, or other agents? Have him describe the reaction and make sure to record his responses.
• diet. Ask about his normal eating patterns. Does he eat many high-fat foods? If he's overweight, to what degree and for how long?
• habits. Does the patient drink alcohol or caffeinated beverages? How much? Does he smoke? Does he exercise regularly? Ask him to describe his exercise routine.

Family history

The patient's family history may suggest environmental or genetic illnesses that may relate to his current health problem and needs.

Continued on page 100

Vascular Problems

Peripheral Vascular Disease

Patient Evaluation

The nursing history—*continued*

Because vascular disorders may stem partly from genetic factors, ask if any blood relatives have been treated for a vascular or cardiac disorder, diabetes mellitus, hypertension, or hypothyroidism.

Social history
The patient's psychological and sociologic status can profoundly affect his health. Prolonged stress, in particular, may increase his PVD risk. To help determine if stress has contributed to the problem, have the patient describe his occupation and sleep habits.

Key symptoms

Defining the patient's key symptoms can help you recognize and evaluate a specific disorder and determine whether PVD's arterial or venous. The following key symptoms require further investigation.

Pain
Patients with PVD (especially arterial occlusion) most frequently complain of pain. Carefully note how the patient describes his pain to help you recognize characteristic patterns.

Acute arterial occlusion. This causes pain that usually begins suddenly and peaks rapidly. The patient may report severe pain, then weakness. If he was standing when it began, the pain may have forced him to sit down immediately. Or perhaps it caused his leg to give way so that he crumpled to the ground. The pain may subside quickly and completely after the initial vasospasm, depending on the severity of any remaining ischemia and the effectiveness of collateral channels.

Chronic arterial occlusion. This can lead to one of two characteristic pain patterns: intermittent claudication or ischemic rest pain. *Intermittent claudication* occurs in a muscle after exercise (such as climbing stairs, running, or walking) and is relieved by rest. During exercise, the muscle cramps from inadequate oxygen (caused by PVD, which reduces the muscle's blood supply). With rest, however, the muscle's oxygen needs decrease and its oxygen supply increases. Pain subsides presumably as the body eliminates accumulated metabolites. Document the degree of claudication in terms of how far your patient can walk before pain forces him to rest. However, be aware that collateral circulation can mask claudication somewhat. The patient may experience pain only after much exercise if collateral channels supply enough oxygen.

Only rest relieves intermittent claudication. Gait and postural changes don't affect the pain. To help rule out other pain types that could originate from the involved area, consider these distinctions: nerve pain (such as sciatica) causes a shooting pain unrelieved by rest; orthopedic pain (such as from shin splints) usually stems from trauma; and arthritis pain involves joints, not muscles.

Ischemic rest pain typically occurs at night as severe, diffuse foot pain, distal to the metatarsal bones. Typically, the patient awakens from pain and must walk around, rub his foot, or take an analgesic for relief. These measures relieve the pain promptly but accidentally: as the patient moves from a horizontal to an upright position, gravity improves perfusion pressure to distal tissues. The patient may begin

101 Peripheral Vascular Disease

Patient Evaluation

sleeping with his foot dependent (below heart level), for example, by dangling it over the bedside or by sleeping in a comfortable chair.

Venous disease. This disease causes pain less frequently than do arterial syndromes. A patient with varicose veins usually feels diffuse leg fatigue or heaviness but occasionally may have a well-localized burning, tingling, pricking, or pulling sensation. Leg elevation (which facilitates blood flow return) relieves these symptoms, although tingling and burning commonly worsen briefly before subsiding.

Venous thrombosis in the leg or foot may cause little or no pain. However, if it's accompanied by marked inflammation, it may cause localized tenderness along the vein. A patient with early or late postphlebitic syndrome may report swelling with moderate aching and a tight or heavy sensation.

Swollen arm or leg

Swelling (edema) usually arises from a systemic disorder, trauma, lymphatic insufficiency or obstruction, or deep-vein valvular incompetence or obstruction.

Usually, the valved venomotor pump mechanism helps reduce pressure, thus helping to relieve swelling. Extravasated protein returns to the central circulation via the lymphatic system. But if this system's clearance capacity diminishes (from lymphangitis or outflow obstruction), protein-rich lymph accumulates in the tissues, causing swelling.

Increased peripheral venous pressure (the most common cause of arm or leg swelling) may stem from a cardiac disorder, an intrinsic venous obstruction, or extrinsic compression. Increased pressure most frequently develops from continuous, unopposed gravitational pressure (in an upright position) accompanied by incompetent valves (in the deep and communicating veins).

When trying to determine swelling's cause, check for the clues described in *Chronic leg swelling: Differentiating the causes,* page 102. If you don't detect any obvious skin changes but the edema pits easily with pressure, suspect a central or systemic cause. Such swelling (also called orthostatic edema) has diffuse distribution that's greatest peripherally; it always involves the foot.

With peripheral venous disease, edema doesn't pit readily. When chronic, this disease leads to frankly brawny edema and skin changes typically seen in chronic venous hypertension. The characteristic reddish brown discoloration stems from breakdown of extravasated red blood cells (RBCs). Along with increased interstitial fluid fibrin, RBC breakdown causes subcutaneous tissue inflammation and fibrosis. The patient's feet may be affected less than his ankles and lower legs because the incompetent perforating veins that transmit venous hypertension to the superficial veins occur in the leg's lower third (the "gaiter" area).

Lymphedema, also diffusely distributed, always appears greater distally, from the toes upward. Neither pitting nor brawny, this edema feels firm and spongy and rebounds immediately when pressure's withdrawn.

Continued on page 102

Peripheral Vascular Disease

Patient Evaluation

Chronic leg swelling: Differentiating the causes

Swelling characteristic	Orthostatic disorder	Lipedema	Lymphatic disorder	Venous disorder
Process	Edema from prolonged sitting or standing	Fatty leg deposits	Lymphatic obstruction	Deep venous obstruction or valvular incompetence
Consistency	Soft; pits on pressure	Doesn't compress (fat)	Spongy; may become hard and nonpitting	Soft; pits on pressure; brawny in later stages
Effect of elevation	Complete relief	Minimal relief	Mild relief	Depends on valvular competence
Location	Diffuse; greatest in distal regions	Greatest in ankles and legs; none in feet	Diffuse; greatest in distal regions	Mostly in ankles and legs; none in feet
Skin changes	Shiny; mild pigmentation, no trophic changes	None	Hypertrophy, thickening, hardening	Atrophy and pigmentation, ulceration, subcutaneous fibrosis
Pain features	Little or no pain	Dull aching, cutaneous sensitivity	Heavy aching or no pain	Heavy aching, tight or bursting sensation
Symmetry	Bilateral but may be unequal	Bilateral	Frequently bilateral	Usually unequal but may be bilateral
Appearance				

Key symptoms—continued

Lipedema most commonly affects women who have chronically swollen legs. On questioning, such a patient may reluctantly report that she's always had thick ankles. This patient has poorly distributed fat with excessive peripheral deposition, which predisposes her to superimposed orthostatic edema. Lipedema causes a dull ache and overlying skin sensitivity. Swelling, which develops symmetrically and doesn't affect the feet, persists despite leg elevation or diuretic use.

Peripheral pulse changes

Check your patient's peripheral pulses and note their rate, amplitude (volume index), and rhythm. Keep in mind that a peripheral arterial pulse reflects a pressure wave extending from the left ventricle to the aortic root, then to peripheral vessels. Be sure to compare right and left pulses for symmetry.

Peripheral pulse changes can indicate various conditions. A normal artery feels soft and pliable; a sclerotic vessel usually feels hard and cordlike. Atherosclerosis may make the artery feel beaded and tortuous. In a patient with arterial occlusion, expect an absent or diminished pulse distal to the occlusion. Venous disorders rarely affect peripheral pulses.

Skin temperature and appearance changes

These usually result from vascular changes. If the patient's skin feels cool or looks markedly pale, suspect peripheral vasoconstriction from reduced blood supply (as in arterial occlusion). Warm skin

Peripheral Vascular Disease

Patient Evaluation

Reviewing pulse characteristics

Evaluate your patient's pulses for rate, amplitude (volume), rhythm, and symmetry. Record pulses as: 0 absent; 1+ weak, thready, and hypokinetic; 2+ normal; or 3+ bounding and hyperkinetic. *Note: Pulse deficit* means that cardiac contractions exceed palpable pressure waves at the peripheral pulse point.

Pulse type	Description
Normal (2+)	Easily palpated but may disappear with pressure. A single pulsation's waveform rises in systole, peaks, then descends more slowly in diastole. A slight secondary rise associated with aortic valve closing (dicrotic notch) occurs on the downward slope.
Small, weak (1+)	May be hard to palpate; easily obliterated by finger pressure (a thready pulse means a weak pulse with variable amplitude)
Large, bounding (3+)	Easily palpable; won't fade with finger pressure (also called hyperkinetic or strong)
Pulsus alternans	Alternates between strong (large amplitude) and weak (small amplitude) pulsations; rhythm usually remains normal
Bigeminal pulse	Amplitude alternates from beat to beat; results from premature contraction (with abnormally small amplitude) after a normal pulsation
Water-hammer pulse	Abnormally large amplitude; rapidly rises to a narrow peak, then descends suddenly (also known as a *collapsing pulse*)
Pulsus bisferiens	Has two primary peaks: percussion wave (probably reflecting pulse pressure) and tidal wave (reverberation from the periphery); best detected by carotid artery palpation
Pulsus paradoxus	Amplitude decreases dramatically (more than 10 mm Hg) during inspiration, increases during expiration.

reflects local inflammation (as in thrombophlebitis). Reddish brown discoloration (rubor) that develops with a dependent leg position results from damaged, dilated vessels (as in arterial occlusive disease). Bluish discoloration (cyanosis) occurs with insufficient blood oxygenation.

You may also note other skin changes resulting from an arterial occlusive disorder that leads to prolonged ischemia or poor perfusion; for example, dryness, scaling, and atrophy. Check the patient's nails for thickening or brittleness. Also ask the patient about any recent hair loss. Severe prolonged ischemia causes tissue decay and necrosis and may lead to gangrene.

If you suspect a venous disorder, check for signs of infection and ulceration. Stagnant blood pooling from blood stasis in the arms and legs provides a medium for bacteria growth and subsequent infection and ulceration.

Leg ulcers

The most common leg ulcer types include ischemic, stasis, and neurotrophic ulcers.

Ischemic ulcers typically stem from arterial insufficiency. They usually cause considerable pain, including nocturnal ischemic rest pain in the foot (relieved by dependency). In the early stages, these ulcers may have irregular edges; chronic ulcers usually appear "punched out." Occasionally, ischemic ulcers develop pretibially, but in most cases, they appear distally over the upper foot or toe surface.

Continued on page 104

Vascular Problems

Peripheral Vascular Disease

Patient Evaluation

Assessing common leg ulcers

Features	Ischemic ulcer	Neurotrophic ulcer	Stasis ulcer
Typical location	Upper foot or toe surface (distally)	Over pressure points	On leg's lower third ("gaiter" area)
Appearance	Poor granulation tissue with an irregular edge	"Punched out" with deep sinus; chronic inflammation may surround ulcer	Granulating base; shallow, irregular shape with rounded edges
Manipulatory effects	Little to no bleeding	Brisk bleeding	Venous oozing
Pain	Severe (especially at night); relieved by dependent leg position	None	Mild (relieved by leg elevation)
Associated findings	Trophic changes associated with chronic ischemia	Neuropathy	Surrounding stasis dermatitis

Key symptoms—*continued*

Poorly developed, grayish granulation tissue typically forms the ulcer base; surrounding skin may appear pale or mottled.

Stasis ulcers (frequently resulting from chronic venous insufficiency) develop on the leg's lower third, typically near the medial malleolus. Although irregularly outlined, like early ischemic ulcers, stasis ulcers usually appear shallower and larger, with a moist granulating base and surrounding stasis dermatitis.

Neurotrophic ulcers (most common in patients with long-standing diabetes and neuropathy) bleed with manipulation but don't cause pain. Deep and indolent, they're usually surrounded by chronic inflammation and thickened skin and typically occur over pressure points. (For more information on ulcers, see Chapter 9.)

Physical examination

Your physical findings can help determine whether your patient's PVD stems from an arterial or a venous problem. Usually diffuse, arterial disease involves several body regions. Venous disease typically remains localized—most commonly in the legs.

On the following pages, we'll describe findings for both arterial and venous disorders. When examining a patient with known or suspected PVD, try to use a room with a temperature of about 74° F. (23.3° C.) to avoid promoting vasodilation or vasoconstriction. Expect fibrotic vessels (pipelike and hard) in an older patient with PVD. Prone to orthostatic hypertension, this patient may adapt poorly to temperature changes. Be prepared to support him when he stands and be sure to keep him warm.

Provide privacy and drape the patient so you can see both legs from the groin down. During the examination, keep his history in mind, especially any complaint of pain or leg or arm swelling. Remember—if he has an arterial problem, he'll probably have limb pain, intermittent claudication or ischemic rest pain, and little or no swelling. If his problem's venous, expect limb swelling and a

Vascular Problems

105 Peripheral Vascular Disease

Patient Evaluation

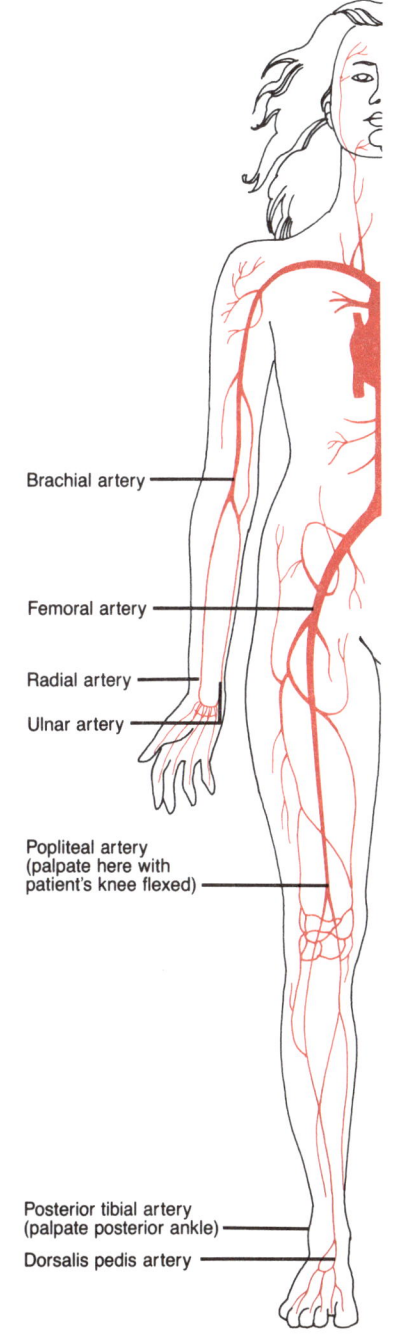

complaint of deep muscle pain. These clues can help you focus the physical examination on either the arterial or venous system.

Inspection
Check your patient's arms and legs for the following signs of *peripheral arterial disease*:
- atrophy or no limb size change (with acute or chronic disease)
- thin, shiny, dry, hairless skin (with chronic disease)
- thickened nails (with chronic disease)
- pallor (with acute disease)
- pallor with limb elevation and rubor with limb dependency (with chronic disease).

Also check his arms and legs for these signs of *peripheral venous disease*:
- edema or swelling
- skin mottling
- varicose veins
- ulceration (especially on the leg's lower third)
- reddish brown discoloration (from postphlebitic syndrome).

Palpation
Palpate for peripheral pulses and skin temperature (using the back of your hand). Cool skin over the affected area usually reflects peripheral arterial disease. Warm or hot skin suggests a venous disorder (however, with severe edema, the limb may feel cool). Be sure to compare the left and right sides for skin temperature changes.

Assess peripheral pulses for rate, amplitude, rhythm, and symmetry. (See *Palpating pulse points*.) Findings suggesting peripheral arterial disease include:
- diminished or absent pulses distal to the occlusion site
- a beaded and tortuous (atherosclerotic) vessel
- a hard, cordlike (sclerotic) vessel that resists occlusion.

Percussion
You'll skip this step when examining a patient for PVD.

Auscultation
To assess for peripheral arterial disease, listen for bruits (blowing sounds) over arteries. Caused by increased blood flow turbulence, a bruit may indicate such problems as an aneurysm or arteriovenous fistula. A Doppler device can enhance auscultation.

Next, measure the patient's blood pressure in both arms while he sits, stands, and lies supine. Compare right and left measurements: a 20 to 30 mm Hg difference can mean subclavian artery stenosis. Also measure arterial pressure over the leg and ankle; normally, ankle pressure equals or slightly exceeds arm pressure while the patient lies supine. (For details on ankle pressure measurement, see page 110.)

Reviewing other body systems

Although you'll focus on the vascular system when assessing a patient with known or suspected PVD, stay alert for these findings from other systems that may aid your assessment.

Continued on page 106

Palpating pulse points

Begin your assessment of the patient's peripheral pulses by palpating the most distal pulse point. If you palpate normal dorsalis pedis and posterior tibial artery pulses, assume no blood flow disruption to that leg. Expect a weak or absent pulse distal to an obstruction. If you suspect PVD, examine all superficial pulse points.

The illustration below shows where to palpate the arms and legs for best results.

- Brachial artery
- Femoral artery
- Radial artery
- Ulnar artery
- Popliteal artery (palpate here with patient's knee flexed)
- Posterior tibial artery (palpate posterior ankle)
- Dorsalis pedis artery

Vascular Problems

106 Peripheral Vascular Disease

Patient Evaluation

Assessing for carotid artery stenosis and abdominal aortic aneurysm

Although peripheral vascular disease most frequently affects the arms and legs, it can affect vessels anywhere. Take special care to evaluate your patient's head and neck for carotid artery stenosis and his abdomen for abdominal aortic aneurysm.

Carotid artery stenosis. To assess carotid artery patency, ask the patient if he's experienced the following:
• dizziness, sudden unexplained falls, or blackouts
• numbness, tingling, or weakness in the face, arms, or legs
• facial drooping
• disturbed vision, speech, or verbal comprehension.

Signs and symptoms of carotid stenosis always occur hemispherically: *ipsilateral* eye symptoms (right carotid = right eye) and *contralateral* extremity symptoms (right carotid = left arm and leg). For example, stenosis of the *left* internal carotid might produce fleeting blindness in the *left* eye but causes weakness or numbness in the *right* arm or leg. Dominant hemisphere involvement can affect speech.

Find out how long the patient's had symptoms. A transient ischemic attack produces symptoms lasting 24 hours or less; a reversible ischemic neurologic deficit causes symptoms lasting from a few days to a week. Deficits persisting after a week indicate an evolving or completed stroke.

Palpate the common carotid pulse (between the trachea and the sternocleidomastoid muscle) and the temporal and facial pulses. You can't palpate the internal carotid artery (supplying the brain), but you can palpate the external carotid at various points along its branches (the temporal and facial arteries). To listen for a carotid bruit, place your stethoscope over the bifurcation and ask the patient to hold his breath. If you hear a bruit, verify its carotid artery origin by moving the stethoscope toward the clavicle. Diminishing sound implicates the carotid artery; intensifying sound suggests the heart or subclavian artery. If you can't detect a previously documented bruit, suspect total occlusion. Report this and any new bruits immediately.

Abdominal aortic aneurysm. To assess your patient for this, auscultate the abdominal aorta for a bruit. Then, find out if he's had pain in his abdomen, lower back, or sides, or if he feels bloated after meals.

Next, gently palpate the abdominal aorta for an expansible, pulsatile mass that bulges to the sides. If you suspect an aneurysm, be sure to notify the doctor immediately.

(For more information on these disorders, see Chapters 7 and 8.)

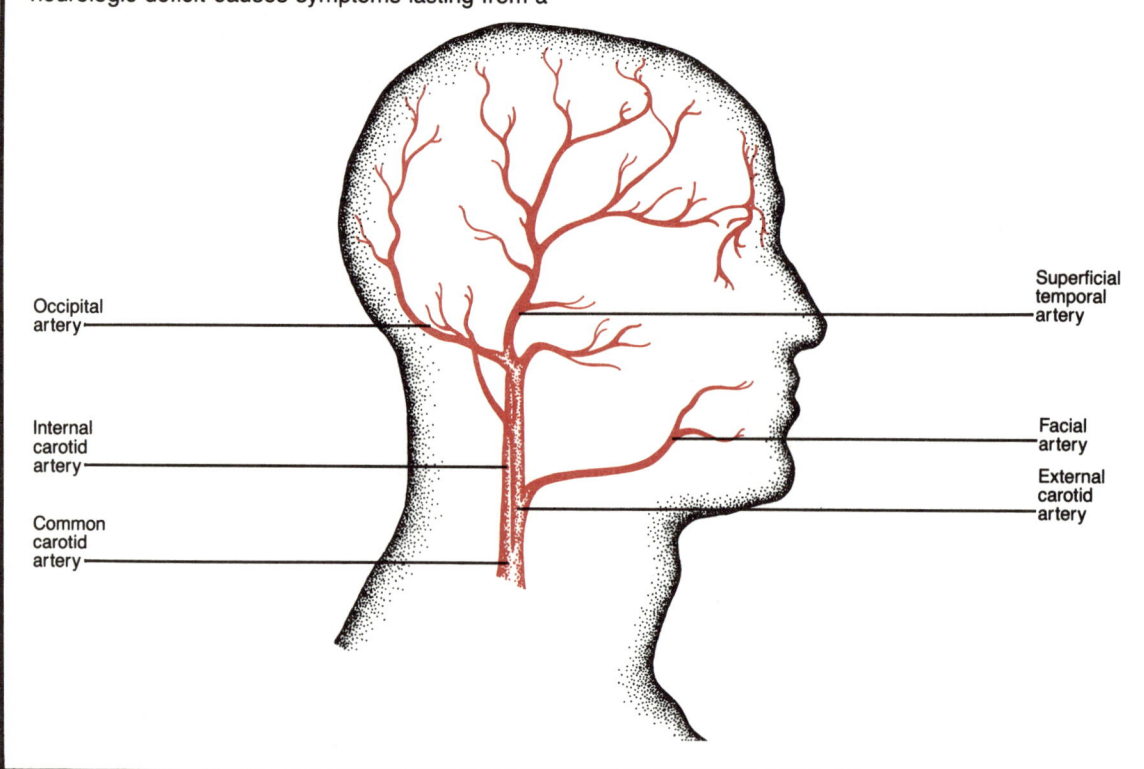

- Occipital artery
- Internal carotid artery
- Common carotid artery
- Superficial temporal artery
- Facial artery
- External carotid artery

Reviewing other body systems—*continued*

• Neurologic system: dizziness; numbness, tingling, or weakness in the face, arms, or legs, suggesting a transient ischemic attack or cerebrovascular accident (CVA), possibly from carotid artery stenosis; speech or language comprehension changes, suggesting carotid artery stenosis

Vascular Problems

107 Peripheral Vascular Disease

Patient Evaluation

- Ophthalmologic system: vision disturbance, suggesting carotid artery stenosis
- Cardiovascular system: history of coronary artery disease or hypertension, suggesting peripheral arterial disease
- Gastrointestinal system: epigastric pain or pulsatile abdominal mass, suggesting an abdominal aortic aneurysm.

Diagnostic studies

The doctor will choose diagnostic studies based partly on whether he suspects arterial or venous disease. Test results may help confirm the diagnosis and indicate the disease's extent or severity.

On the next few pages, we'll review diagnostic studies commonly ordered for a patient with known or suspected PVD. For information about tests that help evaluate a specific disorder, see the relevant chapter.

Doppler ultrasonography
This transcutaneous detection technique, which helps evaluate blood flow in peripheral arteries and veins, may involve continuous-wave (most common) or pulsed flow detection. (Either type may be directional.) A probe (transducer) will be placed on the patient's skin over an artery or a vein at about a 60° angle. An acoustic water-soluble gel serves as a coupling agent. The probe contains two piezoelectric crystals; the first emits a low-intensity ultrasound beam toward a blood vessel. Sound waves strike the moving RBCs and reflect back to the second (receiving) crystal. The probe detects and amplifies the resulting frequency shift (known as the Doppler effect), which occurs in direct proportion to RBC flow velocity.

Arteries normally produce a high-pitched, crisp sound; veins, a blowing sound that varies with respiration. A directional Doppler detector can also reveal whether a vessel's blood flows toward or away from the probe. Further analysis comes from a recording device that translates the reading into a paper tracing showing flow velocity and direction. (See *Doppler ultrasonography*, page 108.) Doppler techniques also help evaluate segmental systolic arm and leg pressures, blood flow through bypass grafts, the carotid and major peripheral arteries, and most superficial veins. However, they can't assess deep veins.

A *duplex scan* takes advantage of sophisticated Doppler techniques to provide sound samples for analysis and ultrasonic imaging.

Plethysmography
This procedure measures fluid volume variations in an organ or body region. Arterial measurements correspond to cardiac cycle stages; venous measurements, to respirations (or Valsalva's maneuver). Waveform tracings of these changes can also be obtained.

Plethysmography techniques include volume displacement (using air or water); impedance; straingauge (mercury-in-Silastic); photoelectric; and ocular.

Volume displacement plethysmography. In this technique, arm or leg pressure is measured after inflation of a pneumatic air cuff (similar to a blood pressure cuff) wrapped around the limb. The pressure, obtained indirectly, reflects the limb's volume changes.

Continued on page 108

Peripheral arterial and venous disease: Comparing assessment findings

Peripheral arterial disease
Pain: sharp, cramplike
- *Occurrence:* walking (intermittent claudication); horizontal (sleeping) position (ischemic rest pain)
- *Precipitating factors:* cold temperatures, exercise
- *Relieving factors:* standing, stopping to rest (intermittent claudication); leg dependency (ischemic rest pain)

Pulses: diminished, weak, or absent

Integumentary changes
- *Edema:* none or mild
- *Appearance:* thin, shiny, dry skin; thickened nails; no hair growth
- *Skin temperature:* usually cool
- *Skin color:* pale, especially on elevation; dusky red when leg's dependent

Ulcers: may develop on toes or on foot trauma points

Peripheral venous disease
Pain: deep muscle pain
- *Occurrence:* standing
- *Precipitating factor:* dependent leg position (as when standing)
- *Relieving factor:* leg elevation

Pulses: normal (any edema may make palpation difficult)

Integumentary changes
- *Edema:* frequently marked (brawny)
- *Appearance:* stasis dermatitis; veins may be visible
- *Skin temperature:* warm (but may be cool with marked edema)
- *Skin color:* normal or cyanotic when leg's dependent; possible reddish brown ankle discoloration

Ulcers: may involve leg's lower third ("gaiter" area)

Peripheral Vascular Disease

Patient Evaluation

Periorbital ultrasound examination

This Doppler technique assesses the carotid artery by evaluating blood flow to the forehead—normally supplied by the internal carotid artery (through the ophthalmic branch) and the external carotid artery (through the superficial temporal artery).

Normally, test results show blood flowing from the orbit toward the forehead. With superficial temporal artery compression, the external carotid can't contribute to forehead flow. To compensate, ophthalmic artery flow increases. With advanced internal carotid stenosis, ultrasound testing may reveal reversed flow in the frontal or supraorbital branches. Superficial temporal artery compression, which reduces or eliminates the flow signal in periorbital branches, can confirm this finding. Facial artery compression also helps evaluate blood flow.

This examination can also help detect turbulent flow in stenotic carotid arteries. The examiner places the flow probe along the common carotid artery at three sites: above the clavicle, at the neck's midsection, and at the jaw angle (carotid bifurcation). Changed sound quality signifies stenosis.

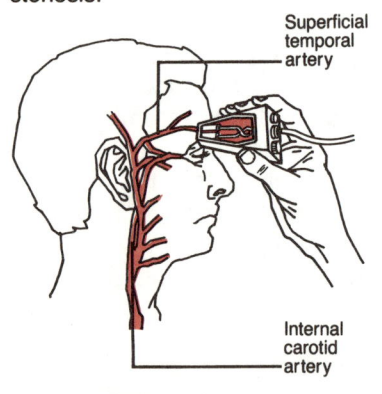

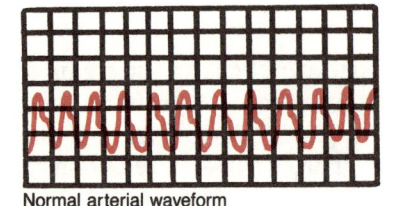

Superficial temporal artery
Internal carotid artery
Normal arterial waveform

Doppler ultrasonography

A Doppler *arterial* study normally produces a waveform with three phases reflecting flow (as shown in the waveforms below):
- forward flow produced by systole, which appears as an upward stroke
- reverse flow during diastole, which has a downward stroke
- returning forward flow in late diastole, which has an upward swing.

(A Doppler *venous* study normally shows a phasic signal when the patient breathes quietly. Respiratory patterns, which affect venous flow, partly determine waveform shape.)

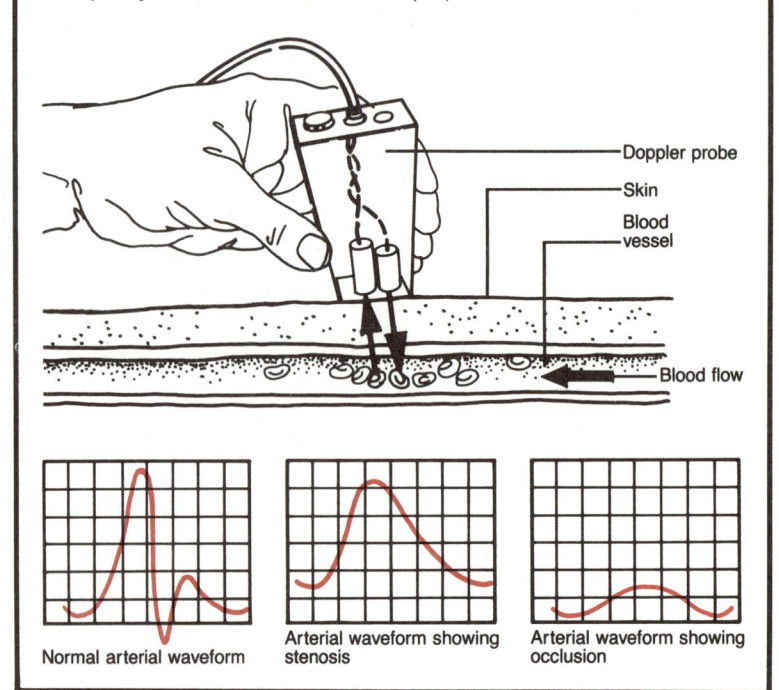

Doppler probe — Skin — Blood vessel — Blood flow

Normal arterial waveform | *Arterial waveform showing stenosis* | *Arterial waveform showing occlusion*

Diagnostic studies—*continued*

Impedance plethysmography. Using electrodes placed on the patient's legs, impedance plethysmography records electrical resistance (impedance) changes caused by blood volume variations. It can also reflect velocity changes. This technique's usually used to detect venous thrombosis.

Straingauge (mercury-in-Silastic) plethysmography. In this technique, thin Silastic tubing filled with mercury encircles the patient's arm or leg, permitting measurement of volume changes at the encircled level. A voltage change across a gauge connected to the tubing relates proportionally to the gauge length and reflects volume changes.

Photoelectric plethysmography. This method (also called photoplethysmography) uses an infrared, light-emitting diode and a photosensor. It works on the principle that whole blood's more opaque to red and near-infrared light than the surrounding tissue; therefore, the degree of light attenuation relates proportionally to blood volume. Of the two basic photoplethysmograph types, one can be used only for thin, relatively transparent organs because it requires sandwiching the tissue between the light source and the sensor. Another version uses reflected light from a probe with a light source and sensor mounted side-by-side. This probe easily attaches to any body part with clear double-stick tape. Photoplethysmography particularly helps evaluate finger and toe pulses.

Vascular Problems
Peripheral Vascular Disease

Patient Evaluation

Ocular pneumoplethysmography (OPG). This study indirectly measures internal carotid artery pressure by gauging pressure in the ophthalmic artery (the first major branch of the internal carotid artery's intracranial portion). An internal carotid artery lesion decreases carotid artery pressure and, in turn, ophthalmic artery pressure. The resultant pulsatile blood flow through the ophthalmic artery produces phasic eye volume changes, which OPG detects and measures.

The most common OPG tests include the Kartchner-McRae and the OPG-Gee tests. Because both studies use plastic cups placed on the eye, the patient receives anesthetic eye drops. The Kartchner-McRae test monitors pulse arrival time at both eyes (through a saline-filled system attached to the cups) and at the earlobe (through sensors). A delay in pulse arrival time at the eye (through the internal carotid) compared to the earlobe (through the external carotid) suggests marked internal carotid artery stenosis.

In the OPG-Gee test, the patient wears air-filled cups on both sclera. Attached to a calibrated vacuum unit, the cups directly measure systolic ophthalmic artery pressure (which reflects internal carotid pressure). When suction draws the sclera into the cup, intraocular pressure rises. When intraocular pressure exceeds systolic ophthalmic artery pressure, the eye pulse trace disappears. Releasing

Continued on page 110

Carotid phonoangiography

Using an extremely sensitive electronic stethoscope, carotid phonoangiography (CPA; also called carotid audiofrequency analysis) helps evaluate the carotid artery. The stethoscope detects bruits (turbulence from stenosis) that appear as a pattern on an oscilloscope screen. This technique can reveal mild internal carotid stenosis that Doppler ultrasound devices or ocular pneumoplethysmography can't detect. It can also help differentiate cervical bruits localized to the carotid bifurcation from those transmitted from the aortic arch or heart.

For reliable results, the test must take place in a quiet room—even slight noises can alter the tracing. To avoid muscle twitching that could produce a turbulent tracing, the patient lies on his back with his neck relaxed. Then, as the camera photographs the pattern, he stops breathing for a moment to prevent respiratory sounds that could interfere with the tracing.

The CPA records patterns just above the clavicle, high in the neck, and at midneck over the carotid bifurcation. Normally, tracings contain a first and second heart sound without turbulence. Stenosis produces bruits after the first heart sound; the bruit's duration depends on the degree of stenosis. Bruits caused by carotid bifurcation stenosis sound most intense in the middle and upper neck regions.

Ocular pneumoplethysmography

These ocular pneumoplethysmography (OPG) tracings (from a patient with left internal carotid artery stenosis) show left OPG pressure recordings that fall more than 4 mm Hg below those of the contralateral side. This disparity indicates occlusion that significantly affects blood flow.

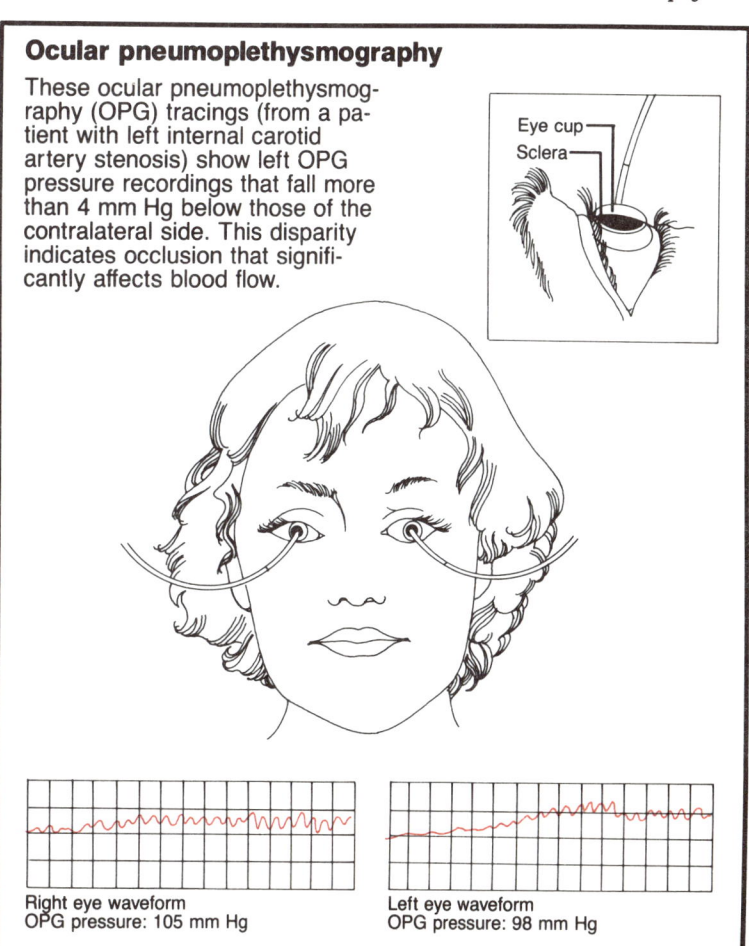

Right eye waveform
OPG pressure: 105 mm Hg

Left eye waveform
OPG pressure: 98 mm Hg

Patient Evaluation

Diagnostic studies—continued

the vacuum allows pulsations to return. Eyeball pressure recordings for each eye (correlating directly with internal carotid pressure on that side) can then be compared.

If your patient requires an OPG test, explain that he'll feel mild pressure on the eye surface. Assure him that although this may cause discomfort and a momentary vision loss, it probably won't cause residual effects (except for scleral reddening that disappears in a few hours).

The required scleral contact makes this test risky for any patient with a history of retinal detachment, eye trauma, recent eye surgery, untreated or unstable glaucoma, conjunctivitis, or allergy to topical anesthetic.

Segmental limb pressure (SLP)

Measuring SLP (for example, from the thigh, calf, and ankle) helps determine arterial occlusion's location and severity. Using pneumatic cuffs and a Doppler probe as a stethoscope, this technique records pressure for each limb segment, starting at the most distal cuff. After locating the pulse below the cuff, the doctor inflates the cuff until the pulse disappears, then deflates it. The manometer reading when the pulse returns indicates systolic pressure. Sequential readings permit determination of the pressure differential, or gradient, between levels. For example, thigh pressure normally measures no more than 20 mm Hg below brachial systolic pressure (BSP); consequently, a gradient above 20 mm Hg between leg segments suggests a lesion in the intervening artery. (However, this interpretation doesn't apply to high pressure readings caused by incompressible vessels, as in a patient with diabetes mellitus.) Because systemic systolic pressure affects SLP, the pressures obtained provide a useful index of arterial occlusion. For example, the ankle brachial index (ABI) may be evaluated by dividing ankle systolic pressure (ASP) by BSP (expressed as ABI = ASP/BSP). In an occlusion-free leg, expect an ABI of 1 or higher. With occlusion, expect an index below 1.

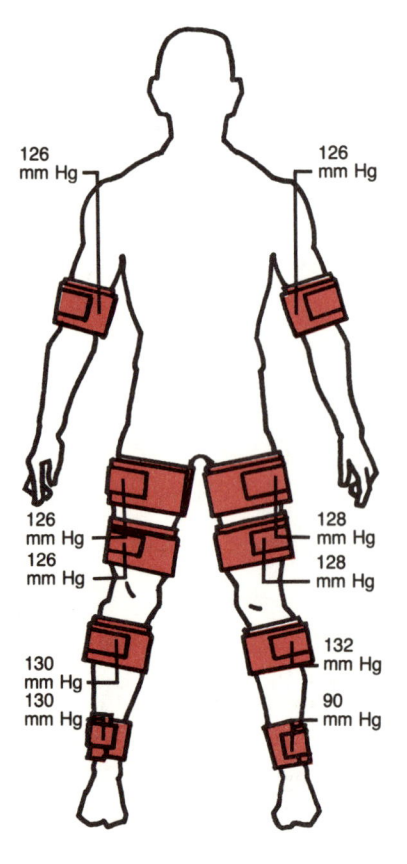

Pulse volume measurements

These measurements show pressure changes as waveforms. They supplement SLP findings and permit perfusion assessment in areas not easily evaluated by a Doppler probe (for example, the foot and toes). Measurements may be taken just before or after SLP readings, using the same pressure cuff placement and sequence. A pressure transducer records pressure changes on cuff inflation and deflation. During the cardiac cycle, leg volume variations produce proportional changes in the inflated cuff. A normal waveform tracing has a characteristic rapid upstroke (peaking and declining abruptly), with a downstroke broken by a small diastolic wave. As arterial occlusion progresses, the diastolic wave initially disappears, then the waveform broadens. Eventually, wave amplitude disappears.

Exercise (treadmill) test

Evaluating the patient's ABI after exercise helps identify arterial occlusive disease and differentiate intermittent claudication from neuromuscular disorders. First, the doctor records the patient's at-rest ABI. Then, the patient exercises mildly by walking for about

---

Segmental limb pressure

The illustration below shows typical differences in segmental limb pressure readings for a patient with left tibial occlusion.

- 126 mm Hg
- 126 mm Hg
- 126 mm Hg
- 126 mm Hg
- 128 mm Hg
- 128 mm Hg
- 130 mm Hg
- 130 mm Hg
- 132 mm Hg
- 90 mm Hg

Vascular Problems

111 Peripheral Vascular Disease

Patient Evaluation

Pulse volume measurements

The waveforms shown below include a normal pulse volume tracing and tracings indicating mild, moderate, and severe arterial stenosis.

Note how increasing stenosis causes progressive waveform flattening and lengthening.

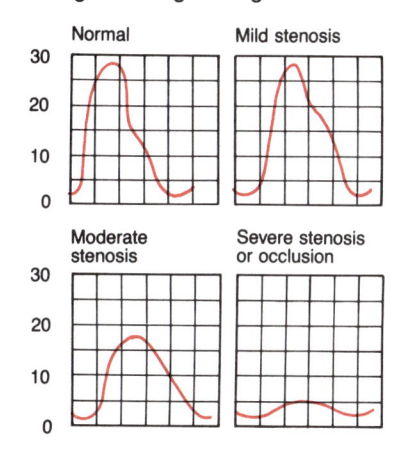

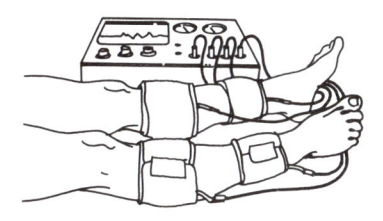

5 minutes at a rate of 1.5 miles/hour on a treadmill with a 10% incline (or until signs or symptoms of intolerance, such as claudication or shortness of breath, develop). At this point, the doctor takes new ankle pressure, pulse volume, and BSP readings and compares them to baseline pressures. Normal postexercise results show a total limb volume increase but little or no ABI change. With major arterial occlusion, ABI markedly decreases and the pulse volume waveform changes. The pressure drop results from increased blood flow across a stenotic vessel and from blood flow diversion to higher-resistance collateral vessels in leg muscles.

Angiography

During this study, a radiopaque contrast dye injected into a vessel makes the vessel visible on X-ray (moving and/or still pictures). Angiography can be classified by the vessel type under examination: arteriography (for arterial examination) or venography (for venous examination).

Arteriography. This procedure helps identify the extent and location of an arterial disorder, such as an aneurysm or occlusion. It requires hospitalization and postprocedure care because it poses risks. The risks include:
- hemorrhage at the needle puncture site
- dye-induced allergic reactions
- thrombosis of the punctured artery
- emboli from dislodged plaques, a clot, or air in the catheter.

After arteriography, check the patient for complications every hour for at least 6 hours (early complications usually appear during this period). Assess his general appearance and mental status (particularly after a cerebral study), heart rate, blood pressure and peripheral pulses, and hematocrit level (if you note hemorrhage signs). Also check the puncture site for signs of infection or bleeding. The patient may also report a burning sensation or irritation (usually at the puncture site) caused by the radiopaque dye.

Arteriography's potential complications include:
- dehydration from dye-induced diuresis (to prevent this, ensure adequate hydration for 12 to 24 hours)
- renal deterioration from diuresis and nephrotoxic contrast dye (especially in a patient with diabetes mellitus or chronic renal insufficiency)
- neurologic deficits (which may lead to a CVA if persistent)
- hemorrhage
- diminished pulses (indicating partial or complete arterial obstruction)
- false aneurysm
- infection.

Venography. Used primarily to diagnose leg deep-vein thrombosis, venography also gives the most accurate evaluation of subclavian-vein thrombosis in a patient with acute arm pain and swelling. It also helps define venous anatomy before deep-vein valve reconstruction or venous bypass.

Risks and complications include allergic reactions, thrombophlebitis (from the contrast dye), and dye extravasation at the puncture site (for leg studies, the dye's usually injected on the upper foot surface).

Continued on page 112

Patient Evaluation

Diagnostic studies—continued

After the procedure, have the patient walk or perform foot pump exercises (if he has a normal venogram) to contract the calf muscles and drain the dye from deep veins. If he has a positive venogram, maintain bed rest with leg elevation and, as ordered, administer systemic heparinization to clear the dye.

Digital subtraction angiography (DSA). This study allows direct arterial visualization but avoids direct arterial puncture and its complications. Combining arteriography and computerized fluoroscopy, DSA uses a peripheral vein rather than a peripheral artery. After injection of a contrast medium into an antecubital vein (or into a catheter guided through an antecubital vein into the superior vena cava), a fluoroscope takes serial images at 1.5-second intervals. A computer subtracts early images from later ones, eliminating unwanted images of other soft tissues and bone and leaving only the dye-filled artery. Enhanced images can be displayed on video monitors, stored on videotape, or converted to hard-copy arteriograms.

Other radiographic studies. Ultrasonography and computed tomography also evaluate arteries and veins.

Radionuclide studies

Tests such as radionuclide angiography can help confirm peripheral arterial insufficiency, predict therapeutic results, monitor the patient's response to therapy, and provide long-term follow-up evaluation. These tests can also:
• detect arterial injury and determine patency of grafts and major arteries
• verify and quantify arteriovenous shunts
• determine skin perfusion pressure
• predict healing potential after surgical amputation
• assess regional perfusion distribution at the microcirculation level under various stresses
• predict an ischemic ulcer's healing potential by measuring its relative perfusion.

Current radionuclide techniques for studying peripheral arterial circulation involve measuring various circulation times, local tissue clearances, or regional blood flow distribution. Radioactive tracers used include several technetium 99m–labeled substances.

Studies that help evaluate peripheral venous disorders (especially deep-vein thrombosis) include:
• iodine-125–fibrinogen uptake test, which identifies areas of increased radioactivity at active leg or arm venous thrombosis sites
• radionuclide phlebography (venography), which provides dynamic venous scintiphotographs and yields images similar to contrast venograms
• thrombus scintigraphy, which produces static radioisotope images of intravascular thrombi.

Vascular Problems

113 Peripheral Vascular Disease

Aortic Disorders: Aneurysm, Dissection, and Other Problems

A disorder affecting the aorta, the body's largest artery, can disrupt the entire arterial system. In this section, we'll discuss aortic aneurysms and other aortic problems. Although other arteries can develop aneurysms, the aorta's the most common aneurysm site. To provide the best possible care for a patient with an aortic disorder, take the time to review aortic function and structure by reading *Inside the aorta*, page 114.

Thoracic/abdominal aortic aneurysms

A localized, abnormal blood-vessel dilation, aneurysm usually results from atherosclerosis. This vascular disease causes degenerative effects in the tunica media—the arterial wall's middle layer—that make the wall less elastic. (For more information on atherosclerosis, see the NURSEREVIEW section on "Cardiac Problems.") Once the tunica media weakens, the tunica intima (inner wall layer) and tunica adventitia (outer wall layer) stretch, forming the aneurysm. As the aneurysm grows, its outer layer becomes hyperplastic, with a thick, tough, fibrous coat that strengthens the weakened

Continued on page 115

John and Sharon VanRiper wrote this chapter. John, who received his BSN from Wayne State University, Detroit, is an Intensive Care Nurse in the Cardiac Catheterization Laboratory at the University of Michigan Medical Center, Ann Arbor. Sharon, who received her MS from the University, is Assistant Head Nurse at the Medical Center. She has also earned her CCRN.

Common aneurysm sites

In the aorta, aneurysms most frequently develop in the aorta's abdominal section, just below the renal arteries (infrarenal) or in the descending aorta just below the subclavian artery to the diaphragm. Occasionally, aneurysms develop in the ascending thoracic aorta or aortic arch.

In peripheral arteries, aneurysms most commonly develop in the popliteal or femoral artery. Most peripheral artery aneurysms are *false*. Peripheral *atherosclerotic* aneurysms, now rare, may gain a higher incidence as the elderly population increases.

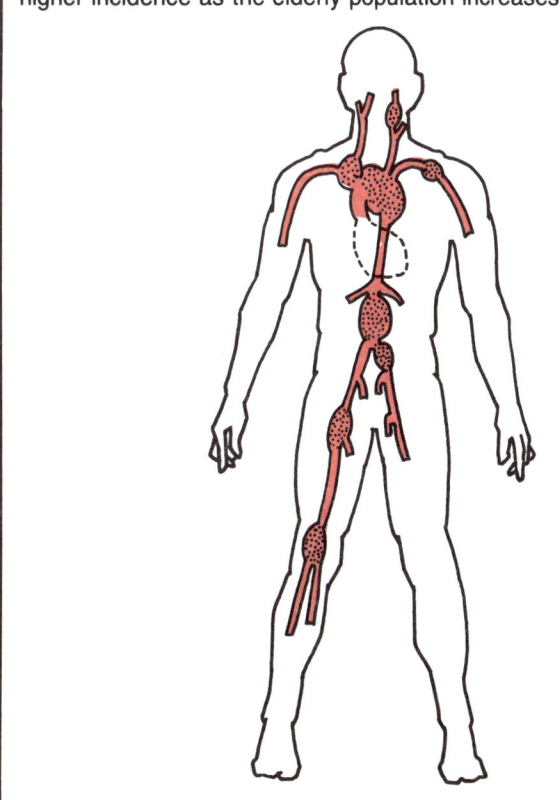

Vascular Problems

Peripheral Vascular Disease

Aortic Disorders

Inside the aorta

The body's largest artery, the aorta has thoracic and abdominal sections. Three segments make up the thoracic aorta:
• the ascending thoracic aortic segment
• the aortic arch
• the descending thoracic aortic segment.

In a normal adult, the *ascending thoracic aortic segment* lies just right of midline, with its proximal region in the pericardial cavity. It measures about 3 cm (1⅛″) wide at its origin from the heart's base and extends 5 to 6 cm (2″ to 2⅜″).

The *aortic arch*—the starting point for all brachiocephalic vessels—travels leftward in front of the trachea.

The aorta continues beyond the arch as the *descending thoracic aortic segment.* This segment rests left of the vertebral column in the posterior mediastinum, passing in front of the column as it descends. It lies behind the esophagus and passes through the diaphragm (usually at the 12th thoracic vertebral level).

The aortic arch and descending thoracic aorta join at the *aortic isthmus*—the typical aortic coarctation site. The ascending thoracic aorta and arch (the aorta's mobile portions) become relatively fixed here. The aorta's most likely to suffer trauma at the isthmus.

The *abdominal aorta,* a thoracic aorta extension, begins at the diaphragm and ends in the aortic bifurcation (where the iliac arteries begin) at the 4th lumbar vertebral level. An adult's aorta normally measures about 2 cm (¾″) in diameter at the celiac axis level, narrowing as it nears the bifurcation.

The aortic wall has three layers. The inner layer—the *tunica intima*—contains endothelial cells that provide a smooth surface for blood passage, reducing turbulence. The intima's easily traumatized.

The thick middle layer—the *tunica media*—gets its strength from laminated, intertwined elastic tissue sheets arranged spirally. The media contains little smooth muscle (however, some smooth muscle links with collagen between the elastic membranes). Elasticity also proves vital for circulatory function.

The outer layer, the *tunica adventitia,* consists of connective tissue that supports and protects the aorta. Composed mainly of collagen, the adventitia also contains the vasa vasorum, lymphatics to nourish the aortic wall, and nerve fibers.

The aorta's thickness necessitates a network called the vasa vasorum to carry its blood supply. A microscopic collection of tiny arteries, veins, and sympathetic nerve fibers, the vasa vasorum weaves through the arterial wall to deliver nutrients and oxygen to the media and adventitia and to remove waste. The intima and most of the media receive nutrients by diffusion from circulating blood. Vasa vasorum loss weakens the muscle wall and may allow atherosclerosis and similar diseases to progress.

The aorta helps circulate blood from the heart. With ventricular systole, part of the contracting ventricle's force changes into potential energy stored in the aortic wall as it stretches with blood. With diastole, this potential energy transforms into kinetic energy as the aorta decompresses. The force created acts against blood within the lumen, further propelling blood distally into the arterial bed. The pulse wave travels along the aorta to the periphery at about 5 m/second—faster than intraluminal blood, which travels only 40 to 50 cm/second.

Aortic systolic pressure results from:
• the blood volume ejected into the aorta
• the aorta's compliance (stretch)
• the resistance to blood flow.

The aorta also helps control heart rate and systemic vascular resistance. Pressure-sensitive receptors in the ascending aorta and aortic arch relay afferent signals to the brain stem's vasomotor center via the vagus nerve. Increased aortic pressure leads to reflex reduction of systemic vascular resistance and bradycardia. Decreased pressure speeds the heart rate.

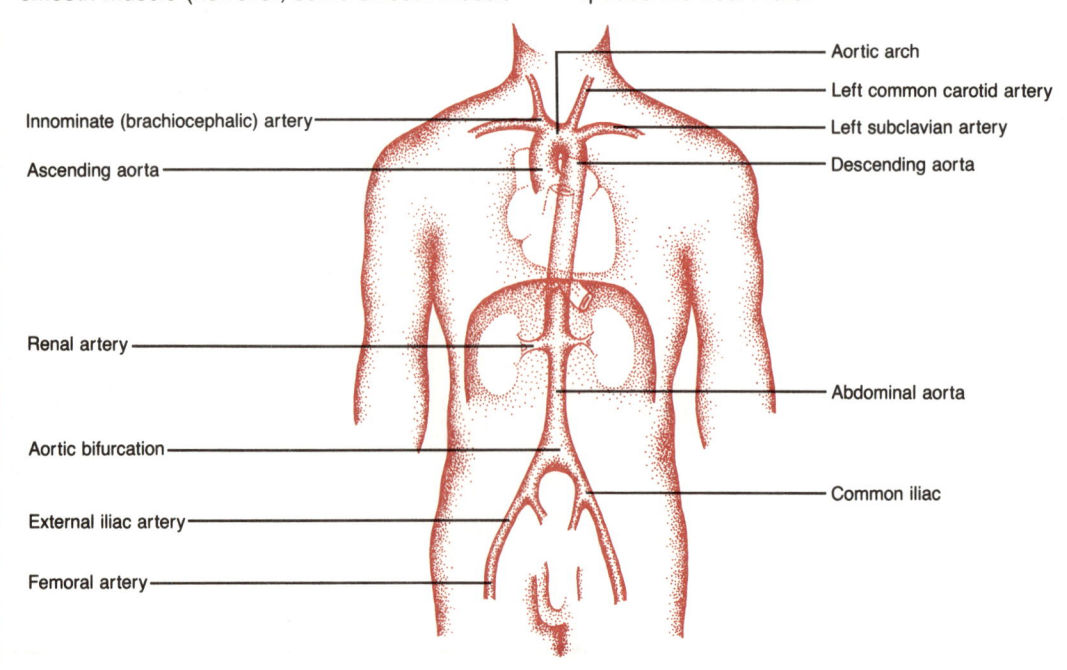

Aortic Disorders

Thoracic/abdominal aortic aneurysms—continued

vascular wall. Plaques accumulate and mural thrombi form on the wall, obstructing the lumen. These thrombi, which may break off and lodge in distal vessels, narrow the lumen and may markedly impair blood flow.

An aneurysm can be acquired or congenital. Besides atherosclerosis, causes of acquired aneurysm include infection, inflammatory or autoimmune disease, aging, trauma, and hypertension. By speeding medial degeneration or by damaging the vessel lining, hypertension can further injure the artery. It also decreases blood flow into the vasa vasorum, reducing the media's nutrient supply and leading to ischemia and vessel wall weakening. Recent studies show that the left ventricle's ejection velocity exerts a major shearing stress on the aortic wall, promoting aortic aneurysm dissection.

A congenital aneurysm can result from a congenital arterial defect or an inherited connective tissue disorder (for example, cystic medial necrosis associated with Marfan's syndrome). Mechanical stress from systemic arterial flow that exacerbates congenital or acquired vessel wall weakness can also cause an aneurysm.

Although an aneurysm can be true or false, it's usually classified by location. Aneurysms reviewed in this chapter include:
- *thoracic aortic*—those involving the ascending and descending aortic sections and the aortic arch
- *thoracoabdominal aortic*—thoracic aneurysms extending into the abdominal aorta
- *abdominal aortic*—those limited to the abdominal aorta. Because these aneurysms share many features, we'll review them together, pointing out their differences where appropriate.

About 25% of atherosclerotic aneurysms involve the thoracic aorta, with dilation arising anywhere along the thoracic aorta (but most common in the arch and descending portions).

Saccular aneurysms develop more commonly than fusiform aneurysms in the thorax. (See *Classifying aneurysms* for more on these aneurysm types.)

A thoracic aortic aneurysm's less likely to rupture without warning than an abdominal aortic aneurysm; compression of surrounding structures usually produces signs and symptoms that signal thoracic aortic aneurysm growth.

About 75% of atherosclerotic aortic aneurysms occur within the abdominal aorta, with most located between the renal arteries and aortic bifurcation. An abdominal aortic aneurysm usually arises as a fusiform aneurysm, rarely saccular. Vessel wall tension increases with aortic widening, accelerating the aneurysm's growth and further increasing tension. This vicious cycle commonly causes rapidly progressive dilation.

A clinically significant aneurysm measures at least 4 cm (1 5/8″) in diameter. As it grows, the aneurysm may compress adjacent structures. Where blood stagnates within the aneurysm, thrombi may develop. If thrombotic and atherosclerotic debris embolize distally,

Continued on page 116

Classifying aneurysms

True aneurysm. This aneurysm type involves all three arterial wall layers (intima, media, and adventitia). The elastic medial layer weakens, allowing the layers to stretch and bulge. A true aneurysm can be fusiform, saccular, or dissecting.

A *fusiform aneurysm,* the most common, typically encompasses the aorta in a spindlelike shape involving the artery's total circumference. X-ray or angiography identifies its characteristic bulging.

A *saccular aneurysm,* the type most likely to rupture, bulges unilaterally from the main arterial segment. Classically, this aneurysm has a narrow neck and a balloon shape.

A *dissecting aneurysm,* the most dangerous type, involves a separation or tear between the arterial wall layers. This creates a false channel that appears on angiography.

False aneurysm. Commonly called a pulsating hematoma, this aneurysm's the remnant of a leak that's resulted in a large blood clot contiguous with the artery's outer wall. Angiography reveals a normal or near-normal arterial lumen. X-rays show a classic arterial aneurysm's outpouching.

Aortic Disorders

Thoracic/abdominal aortic aneurysms—*continued*

they may compromise tributary circulation and eventually lead to aneurysmal rupture. Rupture nearly always takes place retroperitoneally and commonly results in death within 24 hours. A few aneurysms rupture into the peritoneal cavity, with exsanguination rapidly causing death.

Assessment
The patient with a thoracic/abdominal aortic aneurysm may report symptoms (such as abdominal or back discomfort) resulting from the aneurysm's effect on surrounding tissues and organs. Because the aneurysm may displace, erode, compress, or adhere to these structures, signs and symptoms vary with the aneurysm site. However, he'll probably lack symptoms until dissection occurs. The typical aneurysm patient—a mildly obese, sedentary man over age 60 who smokes—has hypertension and evidence of other vascular disorders, such as carotid artery disease. He may also have diabetes.

Remember—an aortic aneurysm reflects one potential atherosclerosis outcome. Therefore, consider aneurysm possible in any patient with a history of atherosclerotic disease.

If your patient has a history of aneurysm, assess him for aneurysm enlargement. An aneurysm smaller than 4 cm calls for frequent evaluation to detect any growth, leakage, or rupture or to investigate any signs or symptoms. An aneurysm between 4 cm and 6 cm (1⅝" and 2⅜") should be resected. Aneurysm detection usually comes about accidentally during assessment for another complaint—usually stemming from aneurysmal pressure on adjacent structures.

Physical examination. Because the abdominal segment's usually the only palpable aortic region, you'll more frequently detect an abdominal aortic aneurysm than a thoracic or thoracoabdominal aortic aneurysm (unless an extensive abdominal segment's involved). Up to 80% of abdominal aneurysms can be palpated.

Physical findings may include a pulsatile abdominal mass, an abdominal bruit, or abdominal distention. If you suspect an abdominal aortic aneurysm, palpate the abdomen cautiously, especially with a tender mass. Tenderness may indicate rapid aneurysm growth or imminent rupture. Palpable abdominal aneurysm pulsations in a man of medium build and average height suggest an aneurysm measuring 5 cm to 6 cm (2" to 2⅜").

Diagnostic studies. With a symptomatic patient, the doctor may diagnose a thoracic/abdominal aortic aneurysm from the history and physical findings. Diagnostic studies help confirm the diagnosis and detect possible complications. With an asymptomatic patient, diagnostic studies may give the first clue to an aneurysm.

Expect the doctor to order any of these tests:
• chest X-ray, which may show mediastinal widening and/or aneurysm wall calcification
• abdominal X-ray, which may also show aneurysm wall calcification
• arteriography

Thoracic/abdominal aortic aneurysm: Assessment findings

The following signs or symptoms suggest a thoracic/abdominal aortic aneurysm:
• abdominal bruit (from intraaortic turbulence or renal blood flow disruption)
• claudication (from arterial blood flow interference)
• dysphagia (from pressure on the esophagus)
• dyspnea (from pressure on the lungs)
• hemoptysis (from aortopulmonary fistula)
• hoarseness (from pressure on the recurrent laryngeal nerve)
• low back pain (from pressure on the lumbar nerves)
• lower GI bleeding (from aortoduodenal fistula)
• pulsatile abdominal mass (from turbulent abdominal aortic blood flow)
• scapular pain (referred pain from aneurysmal pressure)
• sensation of abdominal fullness (from pressure on the duodenum)
• steady, boring (penetrating) epigastric pain (from intestinal angina or impending aneurysm rupture)
• tracheal displacement (from aneurysmal pressure).

Peripheral Vascular Disease

Aortic Disorders

Assessing abdominal aortic aneurysm: Some tips

Keep these important points in mind when assessing a patient for an abdominal aortic aneurysm.
- Because the aortic bifurcation lies at the umbilical level, you'll palpate most aneurysmal masses at or above the navel.
- Don't mistake a tortuous aorta for an aneurysm. Usually lying entirely left of midline, a tortuous aorta's much more movable than an aortic aneurysm. By contrast, with an aneurysm, you can palpate both expansile borders, particularly the one right of midline.
- If you palpate transmitted pulsations, don't assume they're from an aneurysm. Retroperitoneal tumors (for example, pancreatic tumors) transmit pulsations that mimic an aneurysm's. However, such tumors don't feel expansile.
- If your patient's thin, lordotic, hyperthyroid, or hypertensive, you may feel marked aortic pulsations in the anterior abdominal wall. Don't mistake these for an aneurysm.

- computed tomography (CT) scan, ultrasonography, and digital subtraction angiography, which help determine the aneurysm's extent and size
- Doppler ultrasonography, which helps evaluate arterial blood flow
- plethysmography, which helps assess peripheral vessel compromise.

Planning

Before determining your nursing care plan, develop the nursing diagnosis by identifying the patient's actual or potential problem, then relating it to its cause. Possible nursing diagnoses for a patient with a thoracic/abdominal aortic aneurysm include:
- tissue perfusion, alteration in; related to aortic clamping during surgery
- injury, potential for (infection); related to surgery
- cardiac output, alteration in (decreased); related to aneurysm rupture
- comfort, alteration in (pain); related to dissecting aneurysm
- anxiety; related to emergency hospitalization
- injury, potential for (graft occlusion); related to postoperative emboli.

The sample nursing care plan below shows expected outcomes, nursing interventions, and discharge planning for one nursing diagnosis listed above. You'll want to individualize each care plan, however, to fit your patient's needs.

Continued on page 118

Sample nursing care plan: Aortic aneurysm

Nursing diagnosis	Expected outcomes
Tissue perfusion, alteration in; related to aortic clamping during surgery	The patient will: • maintain adequate tissue perfusion, as shown by adequate blood pressure and urine output of at least 30 ml/hour. • appear awake, alert, and oriented. • maintain adequate leg circulation as indicated by palpable dorsalis pedis and/or posterior tibial pulses; warm, normally colored legs and feet; and normal motor and sensory function. • maintain normal bowel function.
Nursing interventions • Assess and record patient's vital signs (including level of consciousness) on admission to unit, every 30 minutes until stable, then every 2 to 4 hours. • Mark and record pedal pulse presence and quality. Notify doctor of any changes. • Assess and record leg temperature, color, and motor and sensory functions on admission to unit, then every 30 to 60 minutes. Notify doctor if decrease occurs. • Monitor and record urine output every hour; if output's less than 30 ml/hour, notify doctor. • Assess for bowel sounds every 4 hours. Once bowel sounds return, monitor for stool passage. • Check for increasing abdominal girth by taking measurements every shift.	**Discharge planning** • Assess patient's level of understanding and willingness to learn. • Discuss postoperative care instructions with patient and family. • Advise patient when to seek medical care, such as after a bowel or bladder habit change, leg temperature or color change, leg pain, or abdominal pain or enlargement. • Arrange for follow-up medical care.

Aortic Disorders

Thoracic/abdominal aortic aneurysms—continued

Intervention

For a thoracic, thoracoabdominal, or abdominal aortic aneurysm, aneurysmectomy remains the preferred treatment (see *Aneurysmectomy* for details on this procedure).

In some cases, such as those involving major arteries to other organ systems (such as the kidneys, spinal cord, and bowel), the doctor cuts a "window" in the graft material, then patch-grafts the affected arteries into the window, using original aortic tissue. As an alternative, he may use a segmental graft bypass of the affected arteries.

With a thoracic or thoracoabdominal aortic aneurysm, the patient's survival odds depend on the aneurysm's size. Thoracic aneurysms greater than 6 cm and those causing signs or symptoms rupture more commonly than smaller, asymptomatic ones. Because a thoracic aneurysm usually stems from severe generalized atherosclerosis, many patients die from atherosclerotic complications before the aneurysm ruptures.

Experts recommend excision for an ascending or descending thoracic aortic aneurysm measuring 6 cm or more. However, a smaller aneurysm that produces symptoms should also be resected, depending on the patient's general condition.

The aneurysm type dictates the surgical procedure. Sometimes the doctor can excise a saccular aneurysm directly without resecting the aorta. The favored method for resecting a fusiform aneurysm in the ascending or descending thoracic aorta replaces the aneurysm with a prosthetic tubular sleeve. Removal of an ascending aortic aneurysm requires total cardiopulmonary bypass. Resection of a

---

Aneurysmectomy

To repair a thoracic/abdominal aortic aneurysm, the doctor resects the involved segment (see left illustration, below). He then places biologically neutral graft material (Dacron or a derivative) over the diseased section (see middle illustration). After cleaning it by removing any plaques or clotted blood, he sutures this section around the implanted graft (see right illustration). The cleansed section then covers the graft.

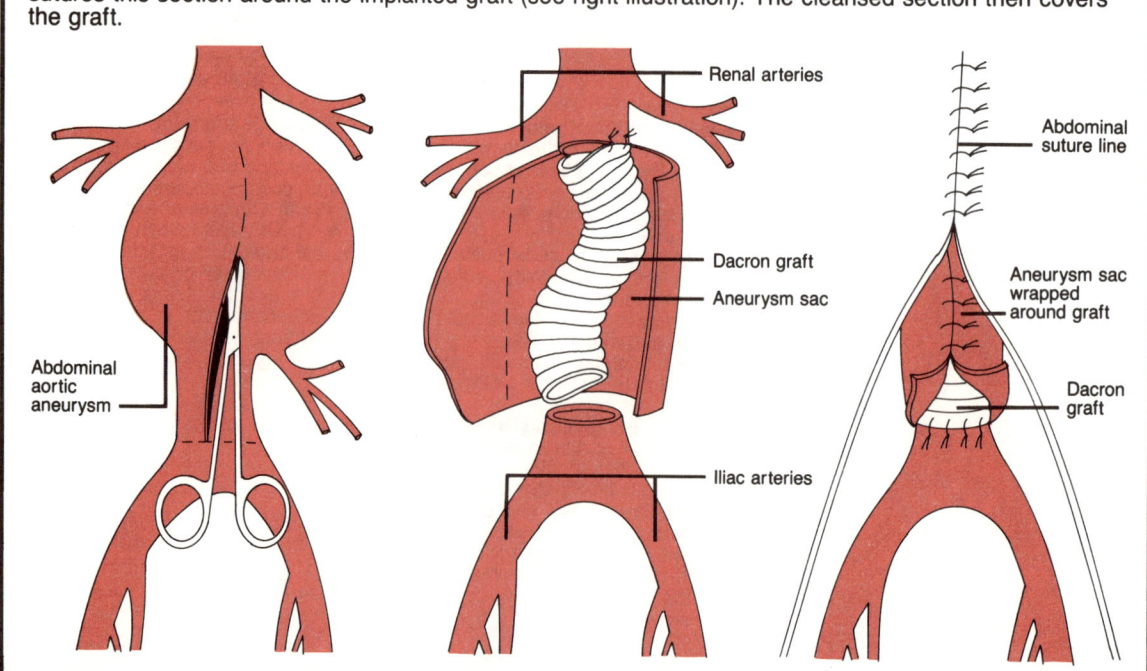

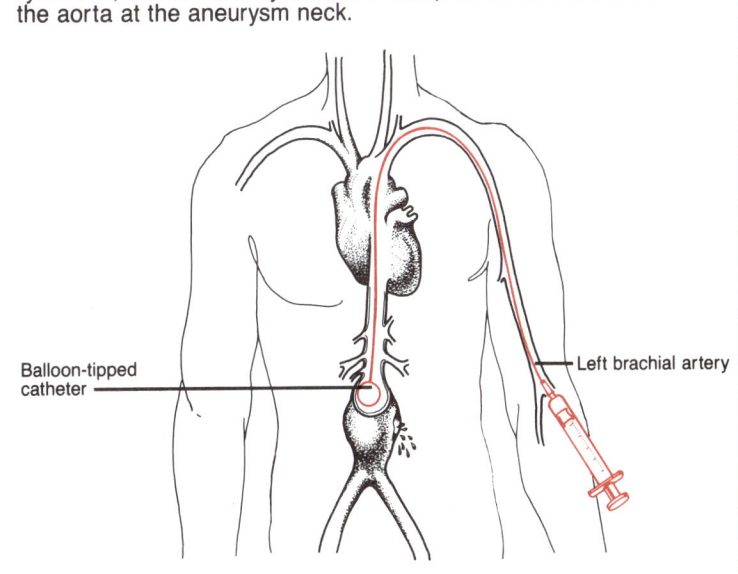

Aortic Disorders

Traumatic aneurysm

Although the term traumatic aneurysm usually refers to a false aneurysm, a traumatic *true aneurysm* can also occur. A true aneurysm develops after trauma from partial arterial wall weakness or disruption that permits vessel distention beneath the adventitia.

Most traumatic aneurysms caused by penetrating trauma arise from gunshot or stab wounds. Most aneurysms from blunt trauma stem from blunt chest impact, such as from a deceleration injury.

A traumatic aneurysm may also result from an invasive procedure. For example, femoral artery catheterization may produce a traumatic femoral artery aneurysm. Intraaortic balloon pump insertion may produce a thoracic aortic or femoral artery aneurysm.

Traumatic aneurysms fall into three categories. *Acute traumatic pulsatile hematoma* results from a penetrating arm or leg wound that causes full-thickness arterial wall disruption. Although contained by surrounding tissues or organs, the hematoma grows until it ruptures freely or until a chronic fibrous wall develops.

Chronic traumatic aneurysm forms when a periarterial hematoma inside the containing sac liquefies and becomes absorbed, leading to surrounding tissue fibrosis. Progressive dilation of a weakened arterial wall can also cause chronic traumatic aneurysm if the adventitia remains intact.

Saccular dilation, a false traumatic aneurysm, may accompany chronic arteriovenous fistula.

Assessment. If you detect a pulsatile mass in any patient with a history of trauma (especially penetrating trauma), suspect a traumatic aneurysm. On auscultation, expect to hear a systolic bruit over the mass. Angiography, X-rays, ultrasonography, and computed tomography scans help confirm the diagnosis. Treatment usually involves surgical repair.

descending thoracic aortic aneurysm may require partial bypass to support circulation distal to the aneurysm. The doctor may use a temporary shunt from the proximal aorta to the region beyond the aneurysm to divert blood around the aneurysm site during the procedure. Surgical excision for a fusiform aortic arch aneurysm carries a high risk because it necessitates brachiocephalic vessel excision and reimplantation.

Half of all abdominal aortic aneurysms greater than 6 cm rupture within a year. Doctors now recommend surgery for such aneurysms unless other medical problems make surgery too risky. Up to 20% of smaller aneurysms rupture within a year of diagnosis. In a good surgical candidate, the doctor will resect an aneurysm as small as 4 cm. A poor-risk patient with an aneurysm measuring 4 cm to 6 cm requires close monitoring. He'll need immediate surgery if signs of aneurysm growth or impending rupture appear.

Surgery involves aneurysm resection and prosthesis insertion. Sometimes a simple tube graft suffices, although complete excision usually requires extension into one or both iliac vessels. With a large aneurysm, the doctor may leave most of the aneurysm wall in place. This reduces the need for extensive dissection, consequently decreasing aortic cross-clamping time and making postoperative sexual dysfunction less likely.

Complications

Complications of a thoracic/abdominal aortic aneurysm may include rupture, vascular insufficiency, distal embolization, and death.

Besides the usual postoperative complications (such as atelectasis or infection), surgical aneurysm repair can lead to graft occlusion,

Continued on page 120

Balloon tamponade

If your patient has a ruptured aortic aneurysm, the doctor may use balloon tamponade to help establish hemostasis before surgery. He inserts a Fogarty balloon-tipped catheter through the left brachial artery and passes it to the aortic arch, where he partially inflates it. After aortic blood flow carries the balloon to the aneurysm site, the doctor fully inflates it and pulls it back to occlude the aorta at the aneurysm neck.

Aortic Disorders

Other aneurysms

Infected (mycotic) aneurysm. Infection can cause fusiform or saccular aneurysmal dilation or false aneurysm. In some cases, infection develops within an existing aneurysm. Typical causative pathogens include *Staphylococcus aureus* and *Salmonella* organisms. As an infected aneurysm grows, its wall thins, leading to eventual rupture.

A vessel can become infected by any of the following:
• septic emboli from bacterial endocarditis or diffuse bacteremia that infect normal or diseased tissue
• infection that spreads from an adjacent abscess, infected lymph node, or empyema
• infection introduced from an external source, such as trauma, I.V. injection, or surgery (more common in peripheral arteries than in the aorta).

An infected aneurysm leads to marked temperature elevation and chills. Localized growth of an infected aneurysm can also cause signs and symptoms such as dysphagia from esophageal compression and pain in adjacent regions. A palpable infected aneurysm nearly always feels tender to the patient.

To confirm the diagnosis, the doctor may order angiography, ultrasound, or gallium or computed tomography scans.

Treatment involves surgical excision and adjunctive antibiotic therapy. Major arterial involvement usually calls for prosthetic tube graft insertion.

Anastomotic aneurysm. A patient who's had a surgically placed vascular graft may subsequently develop an anastomotic aneurysm. This stems from partial or total anastomotic separation between the artery and the graft. Separation may result from suture line disruption, graft infection, or hematoma formation.

Suspect an anastomotic aneurysm if your patient develops an aneurysm at an anastomosis site. The doctor will repair the aneurysm surgically.

Thoracic/abdominal aortic aneurysms—*continued*

hemorrhage, or rupture; bowel or spinal cord ischemia; anastomosis aneurysm; or sexual dysfunction.

Distal embolization (also called "trash foot") may also develop if luminal plaques dislodge during or just after surgery and travel to distal vessels. (Keep in mind that an aneurysm contains intraluminal thrombi and plaque fragments from atherosclerosis.)

Evaluation

Base your evaluation on the expected outcomes listed on your nursing care plan. To determine whether your patient's improved, ask yourself the following questions:
• Does the patient have adequate tissue perfusion and blood pressure?
• Can he maintain urine output of at least 30 ml/hour?
• Does he appear alert, awake, and oriented?
• Can he move his legs and distinguish pain and temperature sensations in them?
• Does he have adequate pedal pulses?
• Do his legs feel warm and have normal color?
• Have his bowel sounds returned; has he passed stools?

The answers to these questions will help you evaluate your patient's status and the effectiveness of his care. Keep in mind that these questions stem from the sample care plan on page 117. Your questions may differ.

Other aortic disorders

Aortic dissection

This disorder results from a sudden aortic intimal tear. Arterial pressure then forces blood into the aortic wall, destroying the media and stripping the intima from the adventitia. This creates a false lumen that gradually extends down the aorta or toward the heart. If the condition's not treated, the lumen will eventually rupture.

Acute aortic dissection—potentially fatal—occurs two to three times more frequently than ruptured abdominal aortic aneurysm. An aortic dissection can be ascending (proximal) or descending (distal). (*Note:* You may know this disorder as *dissecting hematoma* or *dissecting aneurysm.* However, many experts now prefer the simpler term, *aortic dissection.*)

Aortic dissection may begin with intimal rupture and secondary dissection into the media. In some cases, it begins with hemorrhage within a diseased media, leading to subjacent intimal disruption (allowing the dissection to extend through the intimal tear). Occasionally, extensive dissection develops with no apparent intimal tear. Hypertension may contribute to dissection regardless of the specific disease process.

The patient's signs and symptoms depend on the dissection's path through the aorta. Dissection can compromise circulation in any major artery arising from the aorta. Dissection that extends into the aortic root can disrupt aortic valve support, causing aortic incompetence. The dissecting column may eventually rupture through the adventitia at any aortic site (most commonly at the left pleural cavity or the pericardial space).

Aortic Disorders

Aortic dissection: DeBakey's classification

Type I. This dissection, the most common and lethal type, starts just above the aortic valve and may reach the aortic bifurcation.

Type II. Remaining within the ascending aorta, this dissection appears most frequently with Marfan's syndrome.

Type III. This type includes two formations. The first, Type III a, starts just beyond the left subclavian artery and remains within the thoracic aorta. The second, Type III b, which has the same origin site, may extend to the aortic bifurcation.

Dissections can also be classified by their location in relation to the aortic valve. Thus, types I and II are proximal; type III, distal.

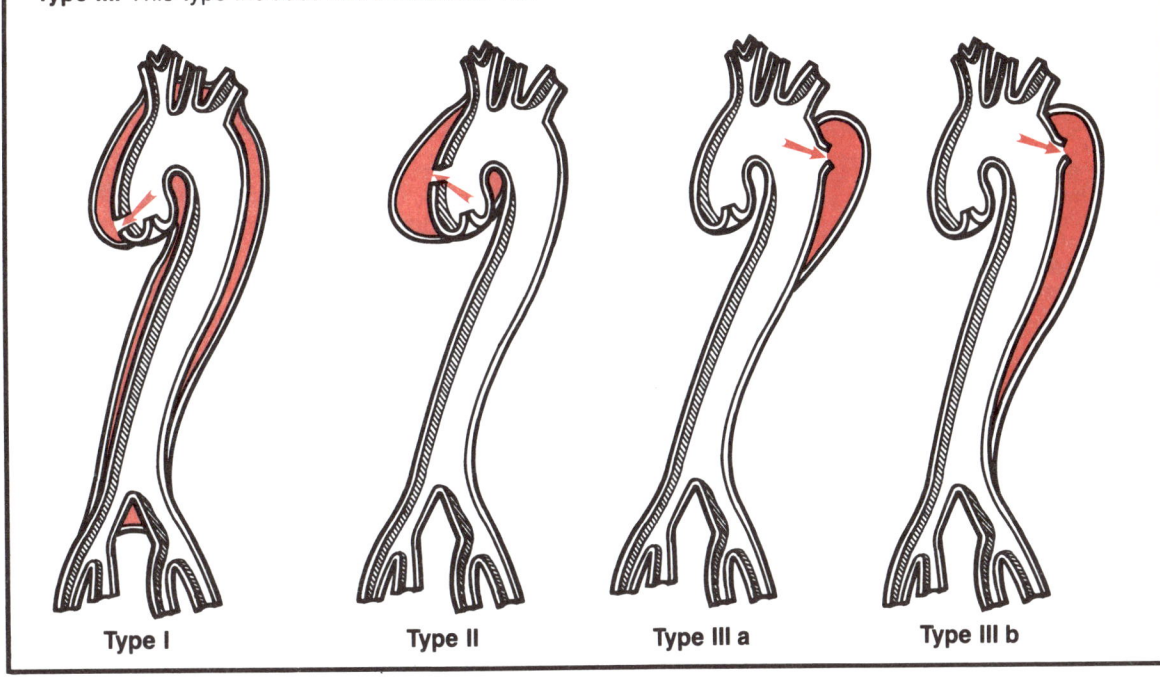

Type I   Type II   Type III a   Type III b

Most aortic dissections start in the ascending aorta within several centimeters of the aortic valve or in the descending thoracic aorta, usually at the ligamentum arteriosum just beyond the left subclavian artery's origin (see *Aortic dissection: DeBakey's classification* for details on dissection locations).

Assessment. Aortic dissection most commonly causes severe pain that the patient may describe as nearly unbearable at its onset. In an attempt to gain relief, he may writhe in agony or pace restlessly.

Suspect aortic dissection if the patient describes the pain as ripping or tearing, especially if it migrates along the path an aortic dissection takes as it extends through the aorta. The pain's location may indicate the dissection's origin. Proximal dissection commonly causes pain that's greatest in the anterior thorax. When pain's most severe interscapularly, suspect a distal origin. With both proximal and distal dissection, the patient may feel pain simultaneously in the anterior and posterior chest. Nearly all patients with distal dissection report back pain. A dissection involving the ascending aorta or arch usually produces throat, neck, tooth, or jaw pain.

A drenching sweat, apprehension, nausea, vomiting, and dizziness frequently occur as pain begins. Other common findings include neurologic deficits, signs and symptoms of congestive heart failure and aortic regurgitation, and pulse abnormalities, such as absence, deficit, and diminution (most common with proximal dissection). The patient may appear to be in shock, despite elevated blood pressure.

Continued on page 122

Aortic Disorders

Aortic dissection: Treatment indications

Expect the doctor to order medical therapy for:
• uncomplicated descending (distal) aortic dissection
• uncomplicated ascending (proximal) dissection with an unknown origin site
• uncomplicated chronic dissection (stable aortic dissection that occurred 2 weeks or more before diagnosis).

Expect the doctor to perform surgery for:
• ascending aortic dissection with a known origin site
• descending aortic dissection that's ruptured or appears likely to rupture (saccular aneurysm), that's compromised vital organs, or that's caused unmanageable pain or blood pressure abnormalities.

Other aortic disorders—*continued*

The doctor may diagnose aortic dissection from the physical examination alone. To help confirm the diagnosis, he'll usually order any of the following studies:
• chest X-ray, which may reveal abnormal aortic widening and aortic knob calcification
• aortography (aortic angiography), which can identify the tear site and assess the dissection's extent
• CT scan or ultrasound with echocardiography, which help define the dissection.

Intervention. Aortic dissection calls for immediate intervention. Although doctors use varying measures, most agree that the patient should be stabilized and given antihypertensive therapy before and during aortography. During this time, prepare the patient for surgery if ordered. Once aortography confirms the dissection, the doctor chooses therapy.

He'll probably order medical therapy and close monitoring for a patient with uncomplicated descending dissection. Surgery's usually too risky for this patient, who's typically elderly and has a history of advanced atherosclerosis or cardiopulmonary disease. (However, aneurysmal rupture requires immediate surgery.)

Medical therapy's goals include:
• reducing the patient's systolic blood pressure to 120 mm Hg (or to the lowest level that maintains vital organ perfusion). The doctor may order sodium nitroprusside (Nipride) or trimethaphan (Arfonad). As ordered, administer Nipride along with a beta-adrenergic blocker, such as propranolol (Inderal).
• diminishing left ventricular ejection velocity (a major stress on the aortic wall contributing to aortic dissection). Expect to administer a drug such as propranolol or reserpine (Serpasil).
• eliminating pain. Administer drugs as ordered or implement comfort measures.

For a patient with ascending dissection, expect the doctor to perform immediate surgery to prevent pulse loss, aortic regurgitation, neurologic compromise, and cardiac tamponade. He'll excise the intimal tear and destroy the false lumen entry by suturing together the aorta's edges proximally and distally. To reestablish aortic continuity, he'll insert a prosthetic sleeve graft between the aorta's edges or join the edges directly.

Aortic arteritis syndromes

Aortic arteritis (also called aortic arterial inflammation) can result from:
• bacterial infection, most commonly by *Staphylococcus aureus* and *Salmonella*
• a syphilitic aortic lesion
• a nonspecific or autoimmune disorder.

Bacterial aortic arteritis. In this disorder, organisms travel through the bloodstream, entering the arterial wall through an injury site. However, organisms sometimes invade the arterial wall directly from other infected tissues or enter through the vasa vasorum. Common entry points include an aortic aneurysm or an intraaortic

123 Peripheral Vascular Disease

Aortic Disorders

Aortic trauma

Blunt aortic trauma. This most commonly stems from a sudden, high-speed deceleration injury. As the body jolts to a stop, its abrupt deceleration produces tremendous shearing forces that act at points where a highly mobile aortic region joins a fixed segment. Occasionally, a pressure or blast injury may rupture the aorta—probably from dramatically increased intraaortic pressure created by aortic blood compression and intensified by cardiac systolic force. Aortic rupture instantly kills about 80% of its victims.

Assessment. You may have trouble assessing for blunt aortic trauma because of the patient's other injuries. However, if the aorta's ruptured, the patient may complain of back and chest pain similar to that caused by an aortic dissection. Patients with a ruptured aorta have increased arterial pressure and pulse amplitude in the arms, decreased pressure and pulse amplitude in the legs, and superior mediastinal widening.

Intervention. The doctor will resect the torn aortic segment and interpose a prosthetic graft into the aorta's two ends.

Distal embolization complicates blunt aortic trauma. Embolization usually occurs in a patient with preexisting aortic disease involving intraluminal thrombi. Sufficient force applied to such diseased aortic sections can cause a thrombus to break loose and embolize distally (for example, a jackhammer resting against the abdomen could provide enough force).

Penetrating aortic trauma. This can result from puncture or laceration, particularly by a gunshot or stab wound. Many victims experience massive hemorrhage leading to rapidly fatal exsanguination.

Assessment. Signs and symptoms depend on the perforation's site and severity. Perforation within the pericardial sac may cause cardiac tamponade. Perforation elsewhere may result in massive hemorrhage with hematoma-induced compression of surrounding structures. Check for signs and symptoms of cardiac tamponade and massive hemorrhage.

Intervention. Expect the doctor to perform immediate surgery.

balloon pump (IABP) insertion trauma site. A patient with infective aortic valve endocarditis also risks bacterial arteritis if valvular organisms invade the adjacent aortic wall.

Assessment. Suspect aortic arteritis in any patient with a history of aortic surgery and a persistent, unexplained fever. Periodic unexplained fever also suggests aortic arteritis. Fever results from episodic bacterial emboli seeding from the infected aorta, which triggers the immune system.

Because direct aortic culturing proves impractical, the doctor must rule out other disorders to diagnose aortic infection. During the patient's febrile episodes, take blood cultures, as ordered, to identify the organism.

In a patient with no history of aortic surgery, diagnosis usually proves harder to confirm. However, suspect arteritis if your patient has any of the following history findings:
- endocarditis
- aortic manipulation (as with IABP insertion)
- adjacent organ infection (such as a liver or kidney infection).

Abdominal ultrasound or CT scans help identify the involved area. A gallium scan helps detect any abscesses.

Intervention. Bacterial aortic arteritis treatment centers on aggressive antibiotic therapy. In a patient with concomitant aortic aneurysm, the doctor will also perform surgery.

Takayasu's arteritis. Probably an autoimmune disorder, Takayasu's arteritis causes vasa vasorum destruction and fibrosis and degeneration of the artery wall's elastic medial layer. The wall's inner (intimal) and outer (adventitial) layers thicken and gradually destroy the vessel lumen, impairing blood flow to the arms and legs. The disease usually affects the thoracic and abdominal aorta—especially the aortic arch—and renal arteries.

Assessment. Expect significant pulse deficits in the patient's arms and legs and possible hypertension, renal failure, and heart failure. Some patients also have a reversed aortic coarctation causing absent or diminished upper body pulses and barely detectable blood pressure in the arms.

Intervention. Treatment focuses on corticosteroid therapy to slow disease progression. The doctor may also order an anticoagulant and/or an antiplatelet drug to treat signs and symptoms and prevent embolic complications. Surgery—endarterectomy, bypass, or graft placement—may also be necessary.

Giant cell arteritis. A disease of unknown origin, this arteritis form usually strikes women over age 50. Although it commonly involves medium-sized arteries, it sometimes affects the aorta and its major branches. The medial arterial layer typically develops granulomatous inflammation and infiltrate, leading to lumen obstruction.

Assessment. The patient will probably report severe headache, marked malaise, and fever. With aortic or major aortic branch involvement, expect signs and symptoms resembling those caused by Takayasu's arteritis. The patient will also have an abnormally high sedimentation rate. If possible, the doctor will confirm the diagnosis with an arterial biopsy.

Continued on page 124

Aortic Disorders

Mural thrombus development

Initial arterial dilation
Dilation increases an artery's radius while decreasing its thickness. As a result, arterial tension mounts, enlarging the aneurysm.

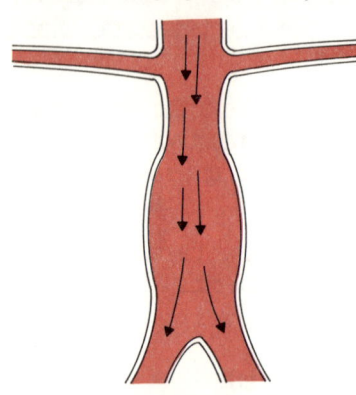

Progressive arterial dilation
With progressive dilation, blood flow velocity near the arterial wall decreases, resulting in turbulence. This leads to arterial wall vibration and weakness.

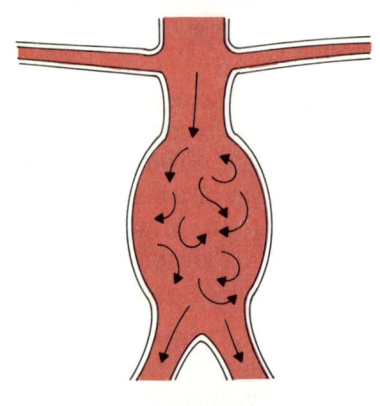

Mural thrombus formation
Turbulence and arterial wall lining abnormalities promote formation of a mural thrombus—platelets, blood cells, and cellular debris interlaced with fibrin.

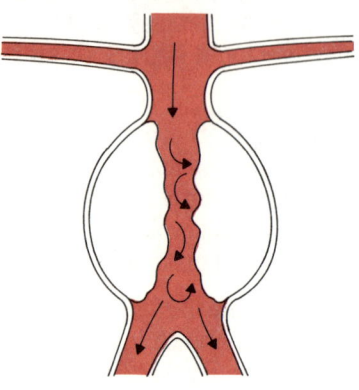

Other aortic disorders—continued

Intervention. High-dose steroid therapy usually reverses the disease and prevents its progression.

Aortic embolism

An aortic embolus may originate from the heart or from diseased vessel sections, such as an aortic aneurysm (mural thrombus). When it occurs at the aortic bifurcation (most common), it's called a saddle embolus.

The following conditions may predispose a patient to aortic embolism:
- known aortic disease
- episodic or sustained hypertension
- abdominal surgery
- altered coagulation
- direct aortic manipulation, which can cause distal embolization.

Twisting, bouncing, heavy lifting, or other activities causing aortic trauma may also make emboli more likely. Occasionally, plaques or thrombi dislodge along the aortic wall for no obvious reason.

Assessment. The patient with a saddle embolus may complain of sudden, severe, bilateral pain that extends downward from the midthigh but may also involve the buttocks, lumbosacrum, and perineum. The patient's legs suddenly become cold, numb, and mottled (or pale). Distal pulses become unpalpable, and paralysis and/or paresthesia may develop.

If ischemia persists, muscle cells may necrotize, releasing muscle breakdown products into the bloodstream. This can lead to shock, hypotension, hyperkalemia, myoglobinuria, and acute tubular necrosis. Sepsis may also occur. If impaired perfusion persists for several hours or more, the patient will probably die.

Angiography confirms aortic embolism. However, the doctor may diagnose the disorder from the patient's history and physical findings and begin treatment at once. A Fogarty balloon-tipped catheter inserted transfemorally can sometimes remove a saddle embolus. If this procedure fails, the patient will require direct aortoiliac incision and removal.

Intervention. If the disorder's diagnosed soon after its onset, thrombolytic agents such as streptokinase may prove useful. A new thrombolytic agent used at some medical centers—recombinant human tissue plasminogen activator—has a more thrombospecific effect than streptokinase and avoids widespread coagulatory disturbances. The doctor may perform surgery if drug therapy fails. Postoperatively, the patient may need long-term anticoagulant therapy.

Vascular Problems

Peripheral Vascular Disease

Peripheral Arterial Disorders: Chronic Occlusion and Other Problems

Patricia L. Baum wrote this chapter. A Peripheral Vascular Nurse Consultant, Ms. Baum lectures nationally on peripheral vascular disorders. Formerly a Peripheral Vascular Nurse Specialist at the University of Massachusetts Medical Center, Worcester, she earned her BSN from St. John's College, Cleveland.

Because all arteries except the pulmonary artery carry oxygenated and nutrient-rich blood to body cells, an arterial disorder can cause tissue damage or even death. In this chapter, we'll review peripheral arterial disorders—particulary chronic disorders of the legs, the most commonly affected areas. For information on coronary artery disorders, see the NURSEREVIEW section on "Cardiac Problems"; for information on cerebrovascular disorders, see the NURSEREVIEW section on "Neurologic Problems."

To help give the best care possible to a patient with a peripheral arterial problem, first review arterial structure and function by reading the next few pages.

An artery has three layers:
* tunica adventitia—the fibrous outer layer
* tunica media—the muscular middle layer
* tunica intima—the thin inner layer.

An artery receives its blood supply from the vasa vasorum and from blood flowing through the vessel lumen. Nerves innervating an artery originate from the autonomic nervous system.

Continued on page 127

Inside an artery

As shown below, an artery has three layers. Arterial and venous capillaries link the artery to a vein.

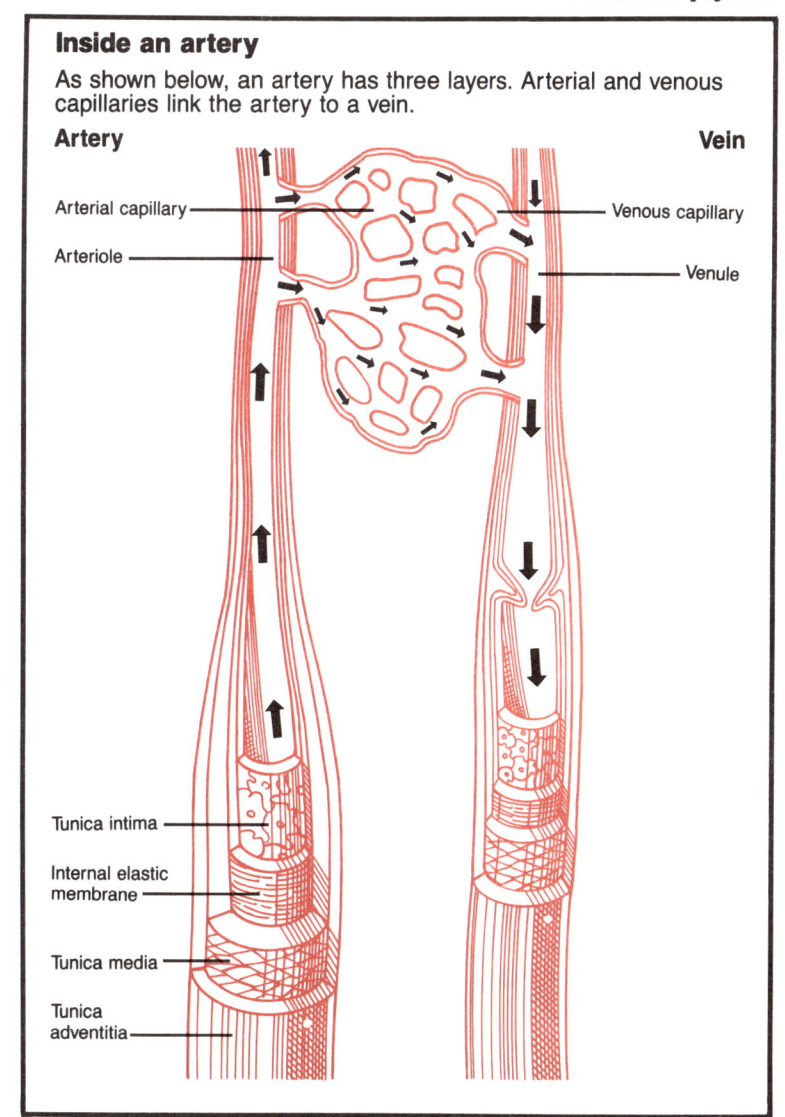

Artery — Vein

- Arterial capillary
- Arteriole
- Venous capillary
- Venule
- Tunica intima
- Internal elastic membrane
- Tunica media
- Tunica adventitia

Vascular Problems

Peripheral Vascular Disease

Peripheral Arterial Disorders

Tracing the arterial tree

The arterial system originates from the ascending aorta. This artery forms three main branches:
- the innominate artery (brachiocephalic), which splits into the right common carotid and the right subclavian arteries
- the left common carotid artery
- the left subclavian artery.

The common carotid arteries fork into the external and internal carotid arteries. The external branch supplies the face and neck with blood. The internal branch, which supplies the brain, further splits into the anterior and middle cerebral arteries, which join at the circle of Willis.

As they branch, the right and left subclavian arteries form the vertebral arteries, which then merge to become the basilar artery supplying the brain stem and cerebellum. The basilar artery ends as the posterior cerebral artery, which also supplies the circle of Willis.

Both subclavian arteries flow laterally beneath the clavicles; each then becomes the axillary artery at the first rib level. The axillary artery extends as the arm's brachial artery. Separating just distal to the elbow, the brachial artery becomes the radial and ulnar arteries. Where these arteries join in the hand, they form superficial and deep palmar arches. The arm's terminal arteries—the digital arteries—supply each finger.

The descending thoracic aorta originates under the left subclavian artery. It enters the diaphragm just left of midline, reappearing as the abdominal aorta. This vessel produces several major visceral branches.

The first branch, the celiac axis, quickly splits into the splenic, left gastric, and hepatic arteries. These vessels supply the liver, duodenum, gallbladder, pancreas, and stomach. Just beyond the celiac axis, the superior mesenteric artery carries blood to the small bowel (except the proximal duodenum), cecum, and ascending and transverse colons. The right and left renal arteries supply the kidneys. The inferior mesenteric artery supplies the descending and sigmoid colons and the rectum. At its bifurcation, the aorta spills into the common iliac arteries at the third or fourth lumbar vertebral level. One iliac vessel extends to each leg.

The internal iliac artery, a common iliac artery offshoot, supplies the pelvic organs. The external iliac artery, a common iliac artery extension, leaves the pelvic cavity as the common femoral artery.

As it forks, the common femoral artery forms the deep and superficial femoral arteries. The deep femoral artery supplies thigh muscles; the superficial femoral artery passes through these muscles, reappearing as the popliteal artery. This vessel provides blood to skin and muscle near the knee joint. After giving rise to the genicular artery, a major collateral circulatory source to the calf, the popliteal splits into three vessels supplying the lower leg and foot: the anterior tibial artery, which becomes the dorsalis pedis artery at the foot; the posterior tibial artery, which courses under the calf muscles, then travels behind the medial malleolus; and the peroneal artery, which supplies the heel and the lower leg.

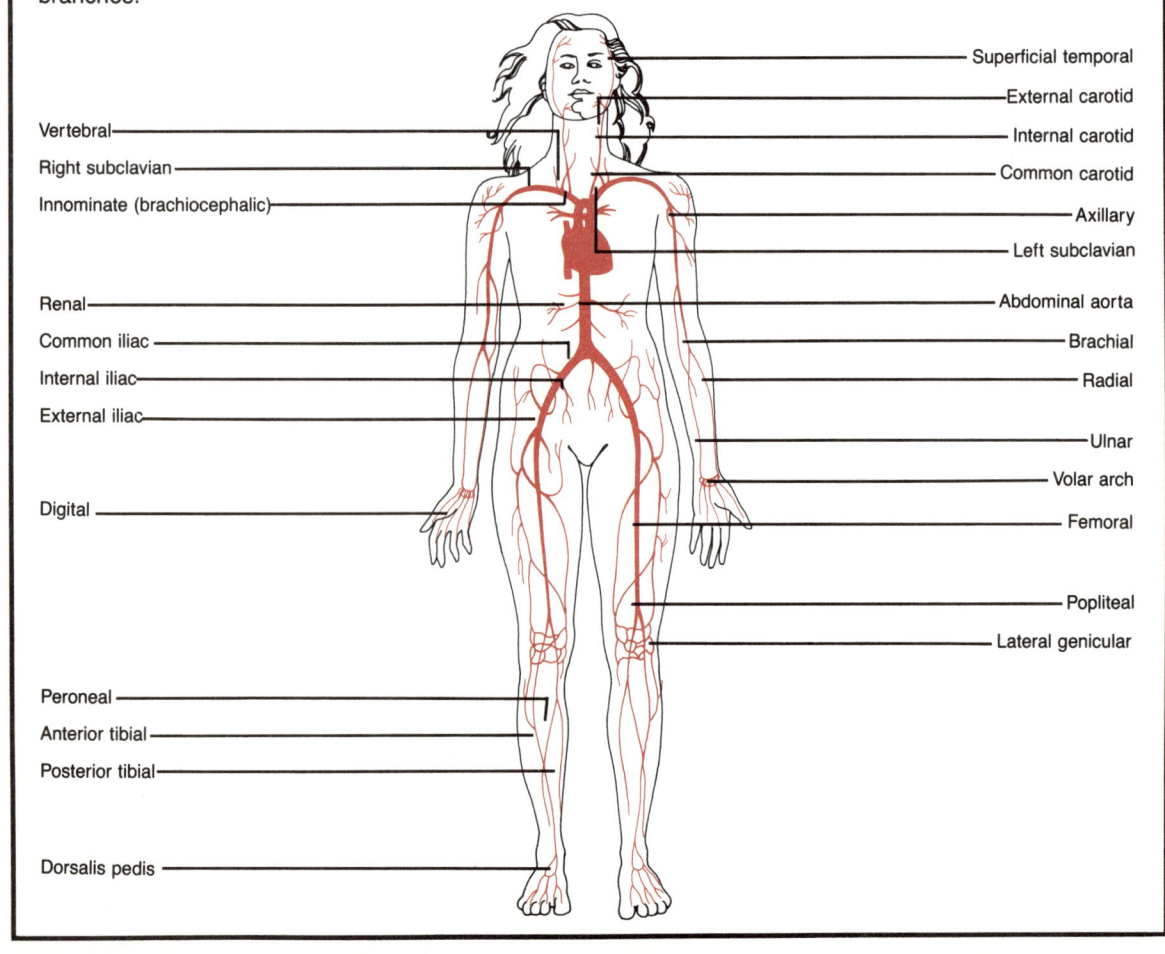

127 Peripheral Vascular Disease

Peripheral Arterial Disorders

Continued

The aorta, the body's largest artery, acts as a transport vessel. It branches first into large arteries, then into smaller arteries, and finally into arterioles. Arterioles have thin walls with an endothelial lining and a single smooth-muscle cell layer encircling them. Because they constrict and dilate according to cellular metabolic needs, they're known as resistance vessels.

Capillaries arise from arterioles. Where the capillary leaves the arteriole, it's surrounded by spiraling smooth-muscle fiber called the precapillary sphincter, which controls blood flow to the tissues. Capillaries exchange nutrients and waste products between the tissues and blood; their single endothelial cell layer promotes rapid exchange. Blood flows out of the capillaries, entering first venules, then veins. (For more information on venules and veins, see Chapter 9.) In some body areas, channels called arteriovenous anastomoses provide direct communication between venules and arterioles, bypassing the capillary network.

A pressure gradient within the vessels permits blood flow. This gradient results as the contracting left ventricle forces blood into systemic circulation. The amount of blood flow reflects the blood volume leaving the ventricle (cardiac output).

Arterial blood flow may be laminar or turbulent. Laminar flow predominates where all blood particles flow parallel to the vessel wall. Turbulent flow—random particle movement—occurs where arteries branch, narrow, taper, or curve.

Blood flow also depends on resistance (impedance to flow). Blood viscosity, the vessel wall's frictional resistance, and peripheral vascular resistance (determined by arteriolar diameter changes) all affect flow. (To review blood flow through the arterial system, see *Tracing the arterial tree*.)

Chronic peripheral arterial occlusion

This disorder—also known as atherosclerosis obliterans, arterial insufficiency, or, more commonly, peripheral vascular disease—may be acute or chronic and may involve any artery. However, because it usually affects the legs, we'll concentrate on chronic occlusion of the legs. (For information on *acute* peripheral arterial occlusion, see *Acute arterial occlusion*, page 130.)

Atherosclerosis, which usually causes chronic peripheral arterial occlusion, narrows the arterial lumen and may advance to thrombotic occlusion or intimal ulceration. Although researchers haven't pinpointed the exact disease mechanism, they believe endothelial injury and lipid infiltration may play a part. Altered intimal permeability may permit lipids and other reactive particles to enter the endothelium. Lipid plaques called atheromas then form. Increased permeability may stem from local intimal injury (for example, from hemodynamic stress). Intimal injury may also permit platelet aggregation and adhesion. Reactive or reparative thickening caused by smooth-muscle cell proliferation may also contribute to atherosclerosis. (For more information on atherosclerosis, see the NURSEREVIEW section on "Cardiac Problems.")

Continued on page 128

Peripheral Arterial Disorders

How atherosclerosis progresses
A fatty streak develops in a normal artery, leading to atheromatous plaque formation. Eventually, the plaque grows to include hemorrhage and a thrombus, completely occluding the arterial lumen.

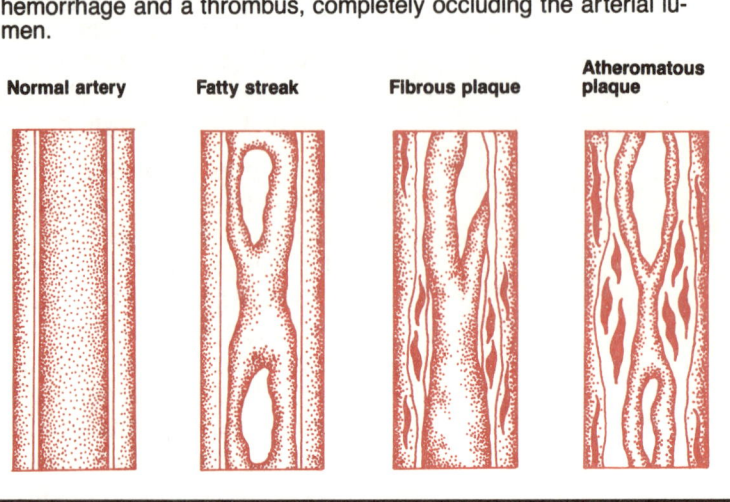

Normal artery   **Fatty streak**   **Fibrous plaque**   **Atheromatous plaque**

Common occlusion sites
Atherosclerotic plaques typically develop at the sites shown in the illustration below.

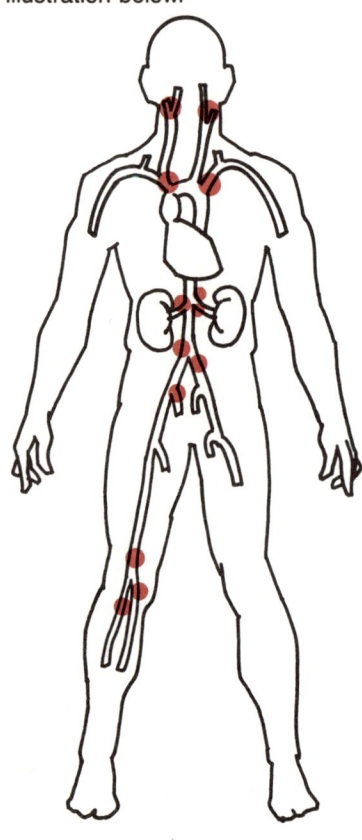

Chronic peripheral arterial occlusion—*continued*

Blood flow through atherosclerotic arteries depends on plaque size, the pressure gradient across the lesion, and arterial resistance. Any collateral circulation affects tissue viability beyond the lesion. Because peripheral arterial occlusion usually becomes chronic, most patients develop collateral circulation in areas beyond the occlusion.

Atherosclerotic lesions usually arise where arteries branch, curve, taper, or narrow. Laminar flow disruption in these areas creates eddies that damage the intima and contribute to plaque formation.

Despite the disease's systemic nature, lesions tend to be localized or segmental, suggesting vessel patency proximal and distal to the lesion. Compromised blood flow to distal tissues causes various effects, depending on the lesion site and severity, metabolic tissue needs, and collateral circulatory adequacy.

Atherosclerosis most commonly occurs in the arterial segment that serves as a transition between the distal superficial femoral and the popliteal arteries. Plaques occur almost as frequently on the common femoral artery's posterior wall and extend into the proximal superficial femoral and deep femoral arteries. Atherosclerosis typically affects the infrarenal abdominal aorta—particularly just beyond the inferior mesenteric artery's origin.

Assessment
The doctor can usually diagnose peripheral arterial occlusion from the patient's history and physical examination.

History. When taking the history, evaluate the patient for potential risk factors by asking him about his diet, health habits, and any diagnosed illnesses.

Risk factors for peripheral arterial occlusion resemble those for coronary artery disease. Uncontrollable risk factors include age and sex. The disease occurs mainly in men aged 50 to 70. Postmeno-

Peripheral Arterial Disorders

Peripheral arterial occlusion assessment: Ruling out other causes

Symptoms of peripheral arterial occlusion can mimic those caused by a neurogenic or musculoskeletal disorder. To rule out these other disorders, ask yourself the following questions as you take the patient's history:
• What symptoms does the patient have? Peripheral arterial occlusion causes muscular weakness, cramping, fatigue, and pain. A neurogenic problem usually causes tingling, numbness, and clumsiness. A musculoskeletal problem results in a constant throbbing ache.
• Did the symptoms arise gradually? Suspect occlusion. Did they arise suddenly? Suspect a neurogenic or musculoskeletal cause, but stay alert for possible *acute* peripheral arterial occlusion.
• When do the symptoms occur? If they occur after exercise (such as walking), suspect occlusion. If standing, sudden movement, or straightening the back precipitates symptoms, suspect a neurogenic problem. If symptoms arise when the patient's resting but don't worsen with exercise, suspect a musculoskeletal problem.
• Where do symptoms occur? Unilateral leg discomfort suggests occlusion. Bilateral lower back discomfort that radiates down the legs may indicate a neurogenic problem. Unilateral or bilateral discomfort confined to joints and surrounding tissue usually signifies a musculoskeletal problem.
• What relieves the patient's symptoms? Occlusion symptoms usually subside after a short rest (about 5 minutes). Neurogenic or musculoskeletal symptoms usually disappear when the patient sits or reclines for an extended period.

While examining the patient, check for palpable pedal pulses, which suggest a neurogenic or musculoskeletal problem. If he has absent pedal pulses, palpable pedal pulses that disappear with exercise, or bruits, suspect occlusion.

pausal women and others with decreased ovarian function have a higher disease incidence than other women.

Controllable risk factors include hyperlipidemia, diabetes mellitus, hypertension, and cigarette smoking. Patients with hyperlipidemia show increased serum levels of cholesterol, low-density lipoprotein (LDL), and very low-density lipoprotein. LDL may also disturb platelet function and promote smooth-muscle cell proliferation and cholesterol synthesis.

Exactly how diabetes mellitus predisposes a person to peripheral arterial occlusion remains unknown. However, some experts suspect that altered glucose and fat metabolism promote atherogenesis.

A patient with sustained hypertension more greatly risks severe atherosclerosis and faster disease progression than a person with normal blood pressure. Damage from persistent hypertension may explain why most plaques occur at arterial branching points, where flow turbulence and blood pressure increase.

Because most patients with peripheral arterial occlusion smoke cigarettes, experts believe that smoking poses a strong atherogenic risk. Smoking may precipitate atherogenesis directly, by an immune mechanism leading to increased endothelial permeability, or indirectly, by causing release of platelet constituents. Smoking also exacerbates preexisting arterial disease.

Smoking affects peripheral arteries in several ways. Nicotine, a vasoconstrictor, reduces skin temperature and arterial blood flow. Smoking increases carboxyhemoglobin levels, which presumably injures the intima and impairs oxygen transport to ischemic tissues. By disrupting platelet function and thus increasing adhesiveness, smoking also makes thrombus formation more likely and sets the stage for plaque formation by reducing oxygen levels and raising carbon dioxide levels. Studies also suggest that smoking causes endothelial damage from hypoxemia and subsequent release of vasoactive amines and bradykinin (a potent vasodilator).

Factors that contribute to peripheral arterial occlusion include stress, obesity, and gout. Stress can trigger hypercholesterolemia, increase platelet levels, reduce clotting time, and exacerbate hypertension through hormonal stimulation. However, the link between stress and atherosclerosis remains somewhat controversial. Obesity, too, plays an unclear role in atherosclerosis development because it typically accompanies hypertension. Increased uric acid levels associated with gout may intensify the atherosclerosis risk by promoting cholesterol deposition, which increases intimal permeability.

Suspect peripheral arterial occlusion if your patient reports intermittent claudication—leg pain, aches, cramps, fatigue, or weakness. Probably caused by inadequate muscle oxygenation, intermittent claudication occurs with exercise and disappears with rest. Question the patient carefully about the pain's nature, location, and duration, and about any precipitating or alleviating factors. Because pain usually develops one or more segments below the occlusion, its location suggests the occlusion site. For example, a patient who complains of calf pain may have superficial femoral artery disease.

Continued on page 130

Peripheral Arterial Disorders

Acute arterial occlusion

Acute arterial occlusion most commonly arises when a clot obstructs a major artery. Such obstruction usually stems from an embolus originating in the heart.

Emboli typically lodge in the arms and legs, where blood vessels narrow or branch. In the arms, emboli usually lodge in the brachial artery but may occlude the subclavian or axillary arteries. Common leg sites include the iliac, femoral, and popliteal arteries. Emboli originating in the heart can cause serious neurologic damage if they enter the cerebral circulation.

Atheromatous debris from proximal arterial lesions may also intermittently obstruct small vessels (usually in the hands or feet). These plaques may also develop in the brachiocephalic vessels and embolize to the cerebral circulation, where they lead to transient cerebral ischemia or infarction.

If thrombosis occurs in a patient with preexisting atherosclerosis and marked arterial narrowing, acute intrinsic arterial occlusion may occur. This complication typically arises in areas with severely stenotic vessels, especially in a patient who also has congestive heart failure, hypovolemia, polycythemia, or trauma. Thrombosis has become the most common cause of acute arterial occlusion.

Acute arterial occlusion may also stem from insertion of a medical device, such as a catheter, or from intraarterial drug abuse or peripheral arterial injection of foreign material.

Extrinsic arterial occlusion can result from direct blunt or penetrating arterial trauma.

In many cases, acute occlusion comes on without warning. Diminished or absent blood flow past the obstruction results in tissue ischemia. Consequently, you can assess acute peripheral occlusion by the five *Ps*:
- *pain*—the most common symptom. This usually has a sudden onset and remains localized to the involved arm or leg.
- *pallor*—caused by vasoconstriction. This usually appears at and beyond the obstruction site.
- *pulselessness*—unpalpable pulses at and beyond the obstruction site.

Continued

Chronic peripheral arterial occlusion—*continued*

Ask the patient how far he can walk before symptoms begin. This helps determine the disease's severity and serves as a guide for future assessment.

The patient may also complain of persistent, severe, burning foot pain that keeps him awake at night (ischemic rest pain). This pain, which usually indicates a more advanced disease state, results from severe nerve and skin tissue ischemia caused by inadequate arterial blood flow.

Ischemic rest pain always develops first in the foot (usually in the toes or heel). It typically occurs at night when the patient's in bed or when he elevates his legs while supine (from decreased blood flow). The pain usually subsides with a dependent leg position (below heart level). The patient may report that he must frequently get up during the night to walk a few steps or must sleep while sitting in a chair.

Be sure to ask the patient if he's taking any medications. Beta-adrenergic blocking agents and ergotamine preparations may bring on or worsen arterial occlusion.

Physical examination. When performing the physical examination, focus on the peripheral arterial system, using inspection, palpation, and auscultation. (Percussion rarely helps assess peripheral arterial disease.)

Inspection may reveal shiny, scaly skin, subcutaneous tissue loss, nail deformities, hairlessness on the affected arm or leg, pallor with limb elevation, and rubor with limb dependency (in a patient with severe ischemia). Also check for arterial (ischemic) ulcers—those with a pale gray or yellowish hue—especially on the ankles.

Pulse and skin palpation can reveal important information. When palpating peripheral pulses, assess their quality and symmetry and check for a thrill (a palpable bruit). Assess the carotid, brachial, radial, ulnar, abdominal aortic, femoral, popliteal, posterior tibial, and dorsalis pedis pulses. (If possible, have the patient lie down for at least 5 minutes before assessing distal pulses.)

Pulse palpation can also give clues to an occlusive lesion's location. Pulses beyond the occlusion usually diminish or disappear. (If you have trouble palpating these pulses, use a Doppler device.) If you suspect peripheral arterial occlusion in a patient with palpable pulses, ask him to exercise the affected limb. Consider peripheral arterial occlusion likely if pulses then disappear.

Palpate the patient's skin with the back of your hand to detect any temperature changes. Coolness may signal arterial occlusion beyond the palpated area. When assessing capillary refill, keep in mind that a delay indicates inadequate circulation to the involved arm or leg. For example, if the patient's toe doesn't rapidly return to normal color after you compress it, suspect arterial occlusion (the delay's usually directly proportional to the degree of arterial insufficiency).

Auscultation may reveal a bruit. A sign of turbulent blood flow, a bruit may suggest arterial occlusion or its cause or may indicate

Vascular Problems

Peripheral Vascular Disease

Peripheral Arterial Disorders

Acute arterial occlusion
Continued

• *paralysis and paresthesia*—from disturbed nerve endings or skeletal muscles (especially sensitive to hypoxia). These symptoms may provide clues to ischemia's extent.

A sixth *P—poikilothermy*—can result in temperature changes below the occlusion level, usually making the skin feel cool.

Diagnosis of acute arterial occlusion usually comes from the patient's history and physical examination. In some cases, the doctor will order diagnostic tests such as arteriography.

Time proves critical in managing the patient with acute arterial occlusion. Without good collateral circulation, he'll suffer muscle necrosis or irreversible arterial changes 4 to 6 hours after occlusion's onset. Treatment aims to revascularize the area and prevent limb loss.

To protect the vascular bed beyond the obstruction, the doctor may order immediate systemic anticoagulation with I.V. heparin or thrombolytic therapy (streptokinase). To enhance microcirculatory blood flow and impede intravascular thrombosis, he may order Dextran infusion.

The patient will probably need surgical revascularization, such as embolectomy. Before surgery, protect the ischemic arm or leg from extreme heat, cold, and pressure.

arterial stenosis (for example, from an aneurysm). Be sure to auscultate the abdominal aorta and any areas over which you've palpated a thrill.

To determine the ankle/brachial index (ABI), auscultate systolic and diastolic arm blood pressure and ankle systolic pressure (for best results, use a Doppler device).

To calculate the ABI, divide ankle systolic pressure (either dorsalis pedis or posterior tibial pressure—usually the higher one) by brachial artery systolic pressure.

$$ABI = \frac{\text{Ankle systolic pressure}}{\text{Brachial systolic pressure}}$$

Normal ABI equals or exceeds 1.0 (100%). The lower the ABI, the more severe the occlusion. Most patients with intermittent claudication have an ABI of 0.45 to 0.75 (45% to 75%). An ABI below 0.25 (25%) means severe ischemia and impending gangrene.

Note: When assessing your patient's arms and legs, be sure to check for motor and sensory deficits.

Diagnostic studies. To confirm peripheral arterial occlusion, evaluate the disease's extent, or assess the patient's response to therapy, the doctor may order the following tests:
• *Doppler ultrasonography*, which typically reveals a relatively low-pitched sound and a monophasic waveform
• *segmental limb pressures*, which help evaluate the occlusion's location and extent
• *pulse volume measurements*, which also help evaluate the occlusion's location and extent
• *exercise testing (treadmill test)*, which may reveal the occlusion's severity. (The doctor probably won't order this test for a patient with severe ischemia.)

Other tests that help evaluate peripheral arterial occlusion include arteriography, standard ultrasonography, computed tomography, digital subtraction arteriography, and radionuclide studies. (See Chapter 6 for more information on assessment.)

Planning
Before determining your nursing care plan, develop the nursing diagnosis by identifying the patient's problem or potential problem, then relating it to its cause. Possible nursing diagnoses for a patient with peripheral arterial occlusion include:
• comfort, alteration in (intermittent claudication); related to arterial occlusion
• tissue perfusion, alteration in; related to arterial occlusion
• knowledge deficit; related to newly diagnosed disease
• activity intolerance; related to intermittent claudication
• sleep pattern disturbances; related to ischemic rest pain
• skin integrity, impairment of; related to tissue ischemia
• noncompliance with therapy; related to inadequate health teaching
• anxiety; related to possible surgery.

The sample nursing care plan on page 132 shows expected outcomes, nursing interventions, and discharge planning for one nursing di-

Continued on page 132

Peripheral Arterial Disorders

Sample nursing care plan: Peripheral arterial occlusion

Nursing diagnosis	Expected outcomes
Comfort, alteration in (intermittent claudication); related to arterial occlusion	The patient will: • experience less leg discomfort. • understand what's caused his discomfort.

Nursing interventions	Discharge planning
• Discuss disease and its process with patient and his family. • Teach patient and his family about medications, if indicated. • Evaluate for medication's effectiveness, if indicated. • Discuss with patient and his family arterial disease risk factors, including ways to modify them to reduce leg discomfort (such as by avoiding stress and cigarette smoking, losing weight, and reducing dietary cholesterol). • Advise patient to sit down and rest when leg discomfort occurs. • Encourage patient to exercise, especially by walking. Advise him to walk to the point of discomfort, rest until the discomfort disappears, then continue walking. Explain how exercise promotes collateral circulation.	• Reinforce discussion of disease and its process with patient and his family. • Teach patient and his family about medications, if indicated. • Discuss risk factor modification as indicated. • Encourage patient to continue exercising. • Advise patient when to seek medical attention, such as when symptoms of acute arterial occlusion occur. • Arrange for follow-up care as indicated.

Chronic peripheral arterial occlusion—continued

agnosis listed on page 131. However, you'll want to individualize each care plan to fit the patient's needs.

Intervention

Peripheral arterial occlusion can cause severe disability or limb loss. Because occlusion usually results from atherosclerosis, the doctor must consider both local occlusive effects and systemic atherosclerotic effects when ordering treatment. Management may be medical or surgical or a combination of both, depending on the patient's signs and symptoms. The doctor will probably order medical therapy for a patient with mild signs and symptoms; surgery for a patient with severe signs and symptoms or a threatened limb.

Medical management includes risk factor reduction, exercise, foot and leg care, medication, and percutaneous transluminal angioplasty (PTA).

To minimize risk factors, the doctor will order therapy to control hypertension, diabetes mellitus, or hyperlipidemia. Also encourage the patient to stop smoking. Explain to him that smoking speeds atherosclerosis and increases the risk of limb loss and blood clots (from blood vessel spasm, which causes effects lasting 20 to 50 minutes after each cigarette). Warn him that pipes, cigars, and chewing tobacco carry the same risk because nicotine's absorbed through oral mucous membranes.

An exercise program helps increase activity tolerance in a patient with intermittent claudication. Encourage him to walk a distance he can tolerate comfortably several times a day and to gradually increase the distance.

Proper foot and leg care can help relieve ischemia and prevent ulcers and gangrene. Encourage your patient to take good care of

---

Chronic peripheral arterial occlusion: Patient instructions

If your patient has chronic peripheral arterial occlusion, advise him to follow these guidelines to relieve symptoms and prevent complications:
• Avoid all tobacco products.
• Avoid extreme heat or cold. If you must go outside in cold weather, dress warmly (taking special care to protect your feet). If your feet become cold, don't apply heat to warm them. Instead, use lukewarm water or another warming agent that's below body temperature.
• Follow this daily foot-care regimen: Wash your feet with mild soap and water. Examine them carefully for cuts, blisters, ulcers, or infections. Lightly powder them with talc if they're sweaty; apply hydrous lanolin ointment if they're dry or scaly. Wear only clean cotton socks.
• Protect your feet from injury by never walking barefooted and by having a doctor trim your toenails and shave any corns or calluses. Always wear shoes that fit properly and that have soft tops and thick soles.
• If you have foot or toe pain at night, sleep with your head elevated and your feet below heart level (for example, by placing 15- to 30-cm blocks under the head of your bed).
• Try to walk 1 to 2 miles each day in 6 to 10 sessions. Stop if leg pain develops.

133 Peripheral Vascular Disease

Peripheral Arterial Disorders

Percutaneous transluminal angioplasty

In percutaneous transluminal angioplasty, the doctor introduces a catheter into the artery, threads a pliable radiopaque guide wire through the catheter, then advances the wire fluoroscopically to the desired location. Next, he advances a dilatation catheter over the wire, positioning a balloon in the lesion's center. Multiple balloon inflations (each taking 30 to 60 seconds) achieve dilatation. After balloon deflation and artery recanalization, the doctor removes the catheter and applies manual pressure to the puncture site for 10 to 15 minutes to stop bleeding.

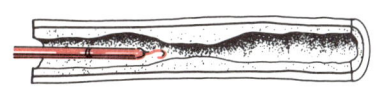

Catheter insertion

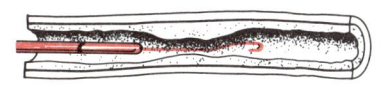

Guide wire advancement

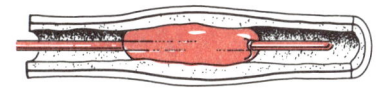

Balloon inflation

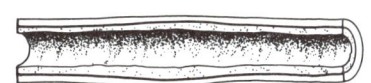

Recanalized artery

his feet, especially if he's diabetic, and to avoid temperature extremes. If he has ischemic rest pain, advise him to keep his feet below heart level to promote blood flow (for example, by placing 15- to 30-cm blocks under the head of his bed). If he has ischemic ulcers, the doctor may order debridement with wet-to-dry dressings. Expect the doctor to order wet-to-wet dressings for a patient who needs granulation promotion.

For a patient with intermittent claudication, the doctor may order pentoxifylline (Trental) to decrease blood viscosity, increase red blood cell flexibility, and improve blood flow through small vessels. He may also order a vasodilator such as isoxsuprine (Vasodilan), tolazoline (Priscoline), or cyclandelate (Cyclospasmol). However, these drugs sometimes prove ineffective and may be contraindicated in severe atherosclerosis. For a patient with ischemic rest pain, the doctor will probably order analgesics.

PTA, a nonsurgical procedure, can sometimes relieve peripheral arterial occlusion. Using fluoroscopy and a special balloon catheter, the doctor dilates the stenosed or occluded artery to a predetermined diameter without overdistending it. This treatment's most effective with a single stenosis site or with multiple focal stenoses of the iliac or femoral arteries. PTA avoids surgical risks. In some cases, the doctor may perform PTA as an adjunct to surgical revascularization.

Prepare the patient for PTA as you would for arteriography. As ordered, administer antiplatelet and anticoagulant drugs (PTA may lead to platelet aggregation and thrombus formation by roughening the intimal surface).

Surgery. The doctor may perform bypass graft surgery, endarterectomy, or embolectomy to revascularize the involved artery. In a few cases, he may perform sympathectomy.

Considered the most effective surgical treatment, bypass graft surgery uses a graft to divert blood flow around the occlusion. The graft may be an autograft or prosthetic material such as expanded Teflon (most commonly, polytetrafluoroethylene [PTFE]) or knitted Dacron. The graft used depends partly on the involved vessel's size. Because autografts prove too small to replace a defective aorta or vena cava, a patient who needs replacement of one of these vessels will receive a prosthetic graft, which has a larger caliber and higher flow. On the other hand, a prosthetic graft may cause thrombosis in small-vessel replacement, so a patient needing such replacement will probably receive an autograft.

The graft may be placed anatomically or extraanatomically. With extraanatomic bypass (EAB), the doctor tunnels the graft subcutaneously. This method's especially useful for a patient who couldn't withstand the trauma of intraabdominal bypass surgery or who has an existing bypass that's become infected or obstructed (see *Classifying bypass grafts,* page 134).

When caring for a bypass graft patient postoperatively, be sure to review his preoperative circulatory assessment (palpable pedal pulses and ABI). Check for adequate perfusion by monitoring vital

Continued on page 134

Peripheral Arterial Disorders

Subclavian steal syndrome

Subclavian steal syndrome develops when blood flows backward in the ipsilateral vertebral artery beyond proximal subclavian (or, more rarely, innominate) artery stenosis or occlusion. Reduced pressure causes blood to flow up the vertebral artery on the unaffected side, into the basilar artery, and down the vertebral artery on the affected side. This blood supplies collateral circulation to the subclavian and its subsidiary branches. Other arteries can then "steal" basilar artery blood supply and possibly compromise the brain stem's blood supply. Atherosclerosis almost always causes proximal subclavian obstruction.

Suspect subclavian steal syndrome in a patient with signs and symptoms of vertebrobasilar arterial insufficiency, at least 30 mm Hg difference between right and left arm brachial systolic pressures, and a bruit at the neck base or in the supraclavicular area on the affected side.

Neurologic signs and symptoms include vertigo, limb paresis, paresthesia, and, less frequently, syncope, bilateral vision disturbances, ataxia, and dysarthria.

Angiography confirms the diagnosis. Treatment may be medical or surgical, depending on the severity of the patient's signs and symptoms. Surgical interventions include vertebral artery ligation on the affected side, aorta-to-subclavian-artery bypass graft, or subclavian endarterectomy.

Classifying bypass grafts

Femoropopliteal bypass graft. Because the segment between the femoral and popliteal arteries most commonly becomes occluded by atherosclerosis, femoropopliteal bypass graft surgery helps treat a patient with disabling intermittent claudication. This procedure can also prevent leg loss. The preferred treatment for leg artery revascularization, this surgery carries a lower postoperative risk than intraabdominal surgery.

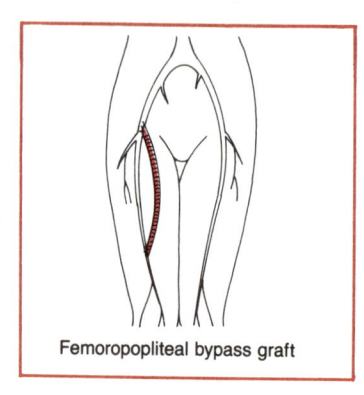

Extraanatomic bypass (EAB) graft. The doctor may perform femorofemoral or axillofemoral graft surgery or he may combine the two (axillobifemoral graft).

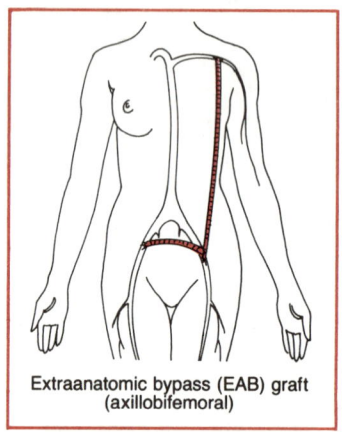

Aortofemoral bypass graft. This procedure helps treat a patient with disabling claudication. It requires major abdominal dissection and aortic manipulation.

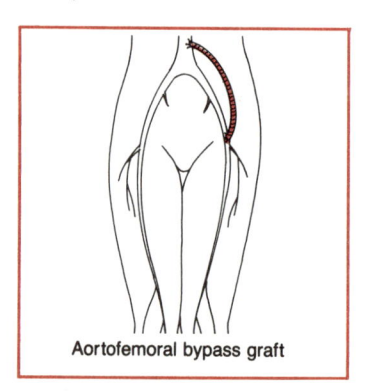

Chronic peripheral arterial occlusion—*continued*

signs; distal pulses; and the affected leg's skin temperature, color, and motor and sensory function every hour for the first 12 hours. Expect edema and erythema from increased blood flow and lymphatic drainage changes. Notify the doctor immediately if the patient has absent or weakening pulses, cold skin, excruciating pain, limited movement, or paresthesia. These findings may signal graft thrombosis. As ordered, administer antibiotics to avoid potential wound infection.

The doctor will probably order strict bed rest for 1 to 3 days, then restricted activity. Encourage your patient to walk, but warn him to avoid acute knee or hip flexion lasting more than 30 to 45 minutes (depending on graft location). Flexion can cause graft kinking or thrombosis. Before discharge, show your patient how to check his graft pulse to help ensure that the graft remains patent. Also make sure he knows when to seek medical care. If the patient has an EAB graft, warn him not to lie on the graft site or wear tight clothing over the graft.

Peripheral Vascular Disease

Peripheral Arterial Disorders

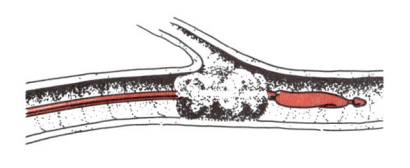

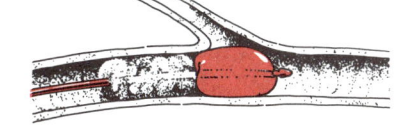

Besides the usual postoperative complications, the patient with a bypass graft risks thrombosis, limb edema, graft site bleeding or infection, hematoma or false aneurysm formation, graft occlusion (1 or 2 days after surgery), and intraoperative embolization. Complications associated with an EAB graft include brachial plexus injury, subclavian and axillary artery injury, arm emboli, and subclavian steal syndrome (see *Subclavian steal syndrome*).

Endarterectomy combined with embolectomy removes the occluding lesion and restores blood flow to the affected area (see *Arterial occlusion removal techniques*). Endarterectomy may also be used in conjunction with bypass graft surgery.

Evaluation

Base your evaluation on the expected outcomes listed on the nursing care plan. To determine the patient's status, ask yourself the following questions:
- Has the patient's leg discomfort decreased?
- Does he understand his disease and its process?
- Does he know how to reduce discomfort by modifying his risk factors?
- Does he understand the benefits of an exercise program?
- Does he know when to seek medical care?

The answers to these questions will help you evaluate your patient's care and determine his future needs. Keep in mind that these questions stem from the care plan on page 132. Your questions may differ.

Other peripheral arterial diseases

Raynaud's syndrome
Raynaud's syndrome—episodic digital ischemia—results from vasospasm. The patient develops pallor, cyanosis, and rubor (usually in the hands or fingers) after exposure to cold temperatures or emotional stress. The disorder affects more women than men.

Raynaud's syndrome may result from deficient basal heat production, which limits cutaneous vessel dilation. Its suggested link to emotional stress may stem from sympathetic nervous system stimulation, which causes release of vasoconstrictive catecholamines and subsequent peripheral vasoconstriction. (*Note:* Until recently, this disorder was called *Raynaud's phenomenon* when it presumably stemmed from connective tissue disease; *Raynaud's disease* when it stemmed from idiopathic vasospasm. However, current terminology favors *Raynaud's syndrome* for either disorder.)

A classic Raynaud's episode occurs after exposure to cold as skin on the patient's fingers or toes turns numb and blanches from severe cutaneous vessel vasoconstriction. Once the patient enters a warm environment, the numb areas usually turn cyanotic as capillaries and venules dilate, blood flow slowly resumes, and extra oxygen moves into the tissues. Finally, the skin turns red from reactive hyperemia as vasoconstriction ends. At this point, the patient may experience pain, throbbing, and burning.

Assessment. Suspect Raynaud's syndrome in a patient with a history of finger or toe pallor or cyanosis brought on by cold temperatures or emotional stress.

Continued on page 136

Arterial occlusion removal techniques

In an *open endarterectomy,* the surgeon cuts the diseased artery lengthwise over the involved segment, then removes the occlusion.

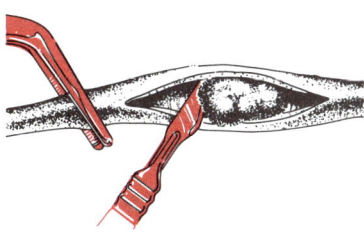

In a *closed endarterectomy,* he inserts an intraarterial stripper to remove the atherosclerotic intima.

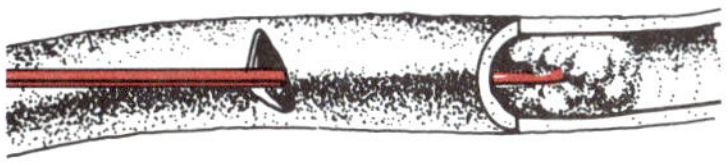

To remove occlusion caused by an embolus, the surgeon may perform *Fogarty balloon catheter embolectomy.* First, he threads a deflated catheter past the embolus, then inflates it. Next, he carefully withdraws the inflated catheter along with the embolus.

Peripheral Arterial Disorders

Other peripheral arterial diseases—*continued*

An ice-water immersion test can verify the diagnosis. In this test, the patient immerses his hand in ice water for 30 seconds after fingertip pulp temperature measurement with a thermistor probe. Then the patient's hand is dried and repeat pulp temperatures are taken every 5 minutes for 45 minutes until the temperature returns to normal. Ordinarily, this takes 10 minutes or less; in a patient with Raynaud's syndrome, it takes much longer. Other diagnostic tests for Raynaud's syndrome include hand arteriography and digital photoplethysmography.

Intervention. Although Raynaud's syndrome can't be cured, the patient can avoid future episodes by taking precautions, for example, avoiding cold temperatures and smoking (which cause vasoconstriction) and avoiding certain drugs, including birth-control pills, beta-adrenergic blockers, and ergotamine preparations. To treat signs and symptoms, the doctor may order a drug such as nifedipine (Adalat), reserpine (Serpasil), phenoxybenzamine (Dibenzyline), or guanethidine (Ismelin) combined with prazosin (Minipress). Biofeedback training may help if the disorder results partly from emotional stress.

Thromboangiitis obliterans

Also known as Buerger's disease, thromboangiitis obliterans involves segmental inflammatory obliteration of small to medium-sized leg and arm arteries and veins. The disease affects the legs more commonly and more severely than the arms and typically occurs in young men who smoke cigarettes. All vessel wall layers become inflamed. Thrombosis also occurs, but without vessel wall necrosis. The disease can cause limb loss.

No one knows what brings on thromboangiitis obliterans, but its high incidence in smokers suggests smoking as a possible cause.

Assessment. The patient usually has a history of intermittent claudication (typically in the foot's arch), ischemic rest pain, and/or diminished or absent arm and leg pulses. These signs and symptoms result from arterial blood supply interruption. When assessing the patient, consider his age, any associated diseases, risk factors, involved sites, and other findings.

Intervention. Urge the patient to avoid tobacco in any form, and warn him that continued tobacco use can lead to disease progression. Explain that if he stops smoking, his circulation might improve—providing no new occlusions arise and he develops collateral anastomotic channels. The doctor may order a vasodilatory drug or perform regional sympathetic ganglionectomy to help increase blood flow.

Thoracic outlet syndrome

In thoracic outlet syndrome, the brachial plexus, subclavian artery, and/or subclavian vein become compressed or irritated as they pass through the thoracic outlet and costoclavicular space (see *Thoracic outlet syndrome*). Causes include congenital fibrous band or cervical rib anomaly, reduced shoulder girdle muscle tone, first thoracic rib abnormality, abnormal clavicle, sagging shoulders, pendulous breasts, poor posture, shoulder muscle hypertrophy, and whiplash injuries (neck hyperextension-flexion).

Peripheral Arterial Disorders

Assessment. Signs and symptoms depend on the involved structure: the brachial plexus (most common), subclavian artery, or subclavian vein. With brachial plexus involvement, expect neurologic signs and symptoms, including pain, weakness, numbness, tingling, paresthesia, or decreased or absent motor or sensory function in the arm, hand, or fingers. Suspect subclavian artery involvement if your patient has decreased or absent arm pulses, numbness, pallor, fatigue, and pain. Arm pain or swelling and reddish blue discoloration suggest subclavian vein involvement. The patient may also have superficial vein distention when he raises his arm.

To ensure accurate assessment, obtain a detailed history and perform a thorough physical examination. The patient will probably describe a gradual, intermittent symptom onset, then progressive worsening. He may also report that arm exertion and elevation intensify his symptoms (arm abduction closes the clavicle and first rib like scissors).

Usually, thoracic outlet syndrome affects all arm nerves without dermatomal preference; however, with preference, it usually affects the ulnar nerve area (C8 to T1) from the axilla to the inner brachium and medial forearm into the last two fingers.

During the physical examination, carefully evaluate the patient's neck, shoulders, arms, and hands. The doctor may order diagnostic studies such as chest and cervical spine X-rays to detect cervical rib or anatomic abnormalities; angiography or photoplethysmography to detect arterial or venous compression; or myelography, electromyography, and nerve conduction velocity studies to check for nervous system involvement.

Intervention. Treatment for thoracic outlet syndrome varies with the disorder's severity. To enlarge the outlet, the doctor may order

Continued on page 138

Thoracic outlet syndrome

The brachial plexus and subclavian artery and vein pass through the thoracic outlet before entering the arm. The clavicle forms the compartment's roof; the first thoracic rib forms its floor. Normally, the thoracic rib joins the first thoracic vertebra (see left illustration). The right illustration shows a cervical rib, a common cause of thoracic outlet syndrome.

Normal thoracic outlet

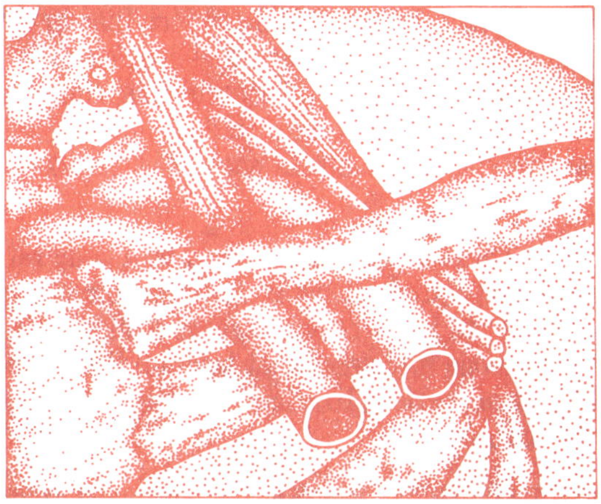

Thoracic outlet compression

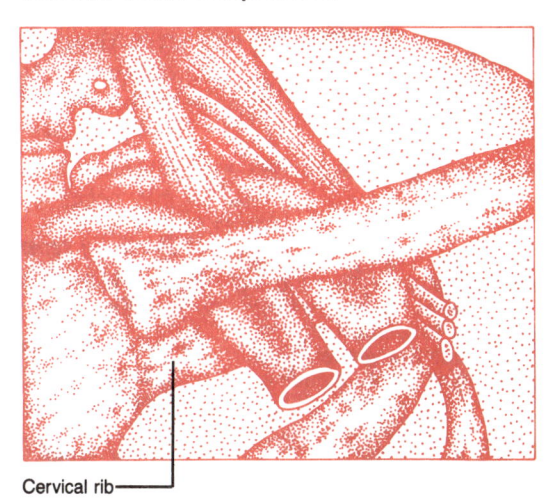

Cervical rib

Peripheral Arterial Disorders

Other peripheral arterial diseases—continued

physical therapy, which helps improve the patient's posture and strengthen his shoulder and suspensory muscles. Or he may order antithrombolytic therapy if the patient's signs and symptoms result from venous thrombosis. Nerve or vessel damage or loss of arm function and strength usually warrants rib resection or arterial surgery. Resection may involve the first thoracic rib or any cervical rib or fibrous bands. Resection widens the compartment, releasing pressure on the brachial plexus and subclavian vessels. The doctor may perform a cervicothoracic sympathectomy along with resection.

After surgery, provide the usual postoperative care and perform frequent neurologic and peripheral circulatory checks. The patient may experience numbness for a few months.

Arterial trauma

The result of blunt or penetrating injury, arterial trauma may result in a completely or partially severed artery or in a nonsevered artery.

Completely severed artery. This commonly stems from a penetrating wound caused by a knife, missile, or surgical instrument. The severed artery's ends usually constrict as the circular muscles contract and pull back into adjacent tissues. These tissues act as a tourniquet to stop bleeding. A clot then develops in the severed artery's ends.

Assessment. To assess for this injury, check the patient's distal pulse first—it usually disappears immediately from wall disruption and lost blood flow in the involved artery. Distal pulse loss may be the earliest—or even the only—sign.

To assess ischemia's severity, consider the trauma site; collateral vessel size, number, and condition; and the demands of tissues supplied by these vessels. However, keep in mind that the patient may lack ischemia signs and symptoms until a distal clot enlarges enough to destroy collateral circulation.

Also keep in mind that the six Ps—pain, pallor, pulselessness, paresthesia, paralysis, and poikilothermy—won't appear for several inches (or at least one major joint) below the severance site.

In some cases, a completely severed artery bleeds excessively or recurrently. For example, the intercostal and common iliac arteries border structures that prohibit retraction or allow little constriction of the severed ends. If the patient has atherosclerosis, the artery can't constrict fully. If he has a clotting disorder, clot plugs may not form or may dissolve spontaneously. In each case, hemorrhage may occur.

Partially severed artery. This can stem from injury by a penetrating object, such as a needle or catheter used in angiographic study or cardiovascular monitoring. In a few cases, it accompanies a closed injury, for example, from bone fragments that lacerate the adjacent arterial wall. In either case, serious bleeding, false aneurysm, and arteriovenous fistulas can result.

Unlike complete severance, partial severance leaves some arterial wall portions undamaged so the vessel can't pull back into surrounding tissues for the tourniquet effect. Consequently, circular

---

Arterial injury mechanisms

Completely severed artery. In this injury, the artery's ends constrict and retract, adjacent tissues become compressed, and a clot plug forms. This injury causes minimal bleeding.

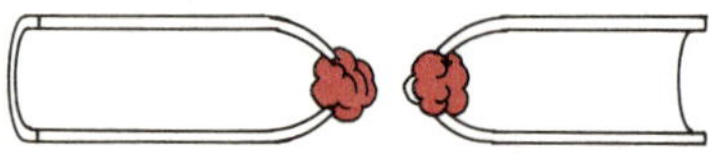

Partially severed artery. This injury results in a gaping wound and massive bleeding that prevent vessel retraction.

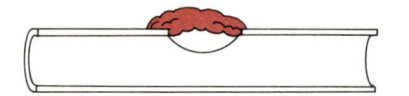

Nonsevered artery. This injury, which disrupts the artery internally, leads to a clot that gradually occludes the vessel. This injury doesn't cause bleeding.

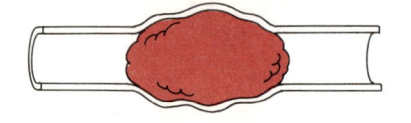

Vascular Problems

Peripheral Vascular Disease

Peripheral Arterial Disorders

Carotid artery occlusive disease

If your patient has a transient ischemic attack, reversible ischemic neurologic deficit, or cerebrovascular accident, don't assume the disorder resulted from a neurologic problem. Carotid artery atherosclerosis may be the cause.

To help prevent these neurologic signs and symptoms, assess any patient with peripheral arterial disease for carotid artery occlusion or stenosis. (For assessment information, see Chapter 6.)

Medical treatment for carotid artery occlusive disease may include the use of anticoagulants, such as warfarin or heparin, and antiplatelet drugs, such as aspirin or sulfinpyrazone. Surgical intervention includes carotid endarterectomy. (For more information on these disorders, see the NURSE-REVIEW section on "Neurologic Problems.")

muscle-coat constriction and retraction of the severed parts cause a gaping wound that bleeds profusely. If blood escapes from the body surface or adjoining cavity, rapid hemorrhaging may occur. More commonly, overlying muscles and skin contain the blood clot temporarily. On careful examination, you may note a pulsating hematoma (from direct communication with the arterial lumen). Its gradually increasing size and pressure can cause life-threatening hemorrhage.

Assessment. Because partial severance rarely narrows the arterial lumen, blood that doesn't escape the injury site still flows distally and may prevent serious ischemia. Undamaged arterial wall portions continue to transmit a pulse wave, so expect normal or only slightly diminished distal pulses.

Unfortunately, a partially severed artery may go unrecognized because the overlying hematoma limits blood's escape from the arterial defect. Consequently, the patient may not seek medical attention until several days after the injury. At this time, he'll probably complain of discomfort in the hematoma area as the mass expands and stretches the overlying tissues. The mass may feel warm and tender and the overlying skin may redden.

Diagnosis usually comes from injury site examination or from angiography.

Nonsevered artery. This injury commonly develops from blunt force or excessive stretch on the arterial wall, such as from high-velocity missile impact near the artery or a needle or catheter wound that pierces the artery but spares most of its outer circumference. The artery's blood flow decreases or disappears, so no serious external bleeding occurs.

Assessment. The injury site may show minimal damage and the region beyond it may look normal at first. However, ischemia and pulse loss develop eventually. An intimal tear, intimal flap, or intramural hematoma may gradually obstruct the arterial lumen.

Intervention (for all trauma types). Depending on the injury's site and type, initial treatment usually involves firm pressure applied directly over the arterial bleeding site. Almost all patients need surgical repair. Time proves critical in treating these injuries; surgery within 4 hours minimizes distal clot formation and helps preserve collateral flow. Every hour of delay intensifies ischemia and reduces the chance for a successful repair.

Vascular Problems

Peripheral Vascular Disease

Peripheral Venous Disorders: Deep-Vein Thrombosis and Other Problems

John and Sharon VanRiper wrote this chapter. John, who received his BSN from Wayne State University, Detroit, is an Intensive Care Nurse in the Cardiac Catheterization Laboratory at the University of Michigan Medical Center, Ann Arbor. Sharon, who received her MS from the University, is Assistant Head Nurse at the Medical Center. She has also earned her CCRN.

Most venous disorders stem from increased venous pressure caused by occlusion (usually from thrombus formation) or valvular incompetency (from injury, inflammation, stretching, or a vein wall defect). Like any vascular problem, a peripheral venous disorder can be acute or chronic and can affect the arms or legs. In this chapter, we'll focus on the legs—the most commonly affected area.

Before reviewing these disorders, however, take the time to read *Vein structure and function.* Then study the next few pages to trace the venous system from head to toe.

Head and neck veins. Major systemic veins that drain capillary networks in the head and neck include the cranial venous sinuses and the internal and external jugular veins.

A series of channels between the dura mater's two layers, the *cranial venous sinuses* drain orbital and cranial cavity structures. *Internal jugular veins* start at the skull's base and travel down the neck beside the common carotid arteries. Each vein joins with the ipsilateral subclavian vein, forming the brachiocephalic (innominate) veins. The internal jugular veins gather blood from the brain, eyes, neck, and superficial facial areas. *External jugular veins* begin on either side of the mandibular angle, draining blood from the skull's exterior, the neck, and deep facial areas. They end in the ipsilateral subclavian vein.

Arm veins. These veins can be superficial or deep; the two types join at many points. Superficial veins, such as the cephalic and basilic veins, contain more valves then deep veins.

Deep arm veins run parallel to the arteries; the same sheath usually encloses both. Most deep veins run in pairs known as venae comitantes (companion veins), separated by the parallel artery. These veins—the *radial, ulnar, brachial, axillary,* and *subclavian*—collect blood from deep arm structures. The arm's venous system ends with the subclavian vein, which extends to the clavicle's sternal end and joins with the internal jugular vein to create the *brachiocephalic vein.*

Thoracic veins. These vessels, which empty into the *superior vena cava,* include the brachiocephalic veins and the azygos vein system. The internal jugular and subclavian veins on either side join to form the brachiocephalic (innominate) veins. Thoracic veins, in turn, combine to form the superior vena cava. Major brachiocephalic branches (besides the internal jugular and subclavian veins) include the *vertebral, internal thoracic,* and *inferior thyroid veins.*

The azygos vein system includes the *azygos, hemiazygos,* and *accessory hemiazygos veins.* These veins gather blood from various thoracic structures and link the superior and inferior vena caval systems. If the inferior vena cava's obstructed, azygos veins return blood from the lower body through collateral channels with the common iliac, renal, and lumbar veins.

Leg veins. Superficial leg veins include the great and small saphenous veins and their many branches. The *great saphenous vein,* the body's longest, starts at the medial end of the foot's dorsal venous arch and empties into the femoral vein in the groin. The

Peripheral Vascular Disease

Peripheral Venous Disorders

Vein structure and function

Veins return blood to the heart from the capillary beds, help regulate vascular capacity, and serve as part of the peripheral pump mechanism (described later). Along with capillaries, veins also help regulate body temperature.

Systemic veins contain approximately two thirds of the body's blood volume (mostly in the deep veins). Blood flows from the capillaries into the venules—the smallest veins—then into progressively larger veins until reaching the heart.

Like arteries, veins have walls containing three layers—tunica intima, tunica media, and tunica adventitia. A vein's tunica media has only a thin smooth-muscle layer and sparse elastic fibers. This makes it thinner than an artery wall and accounts for the comparatively low blood pressure within it.

However, because veins can stretch considerably, they can actively constrict to maintain venous blood pressure and move blood from the periphery to the heart. Like collapsible tubes, veins can undergo venous volume changes with little venous pressure change. Venous system pressure peaks in venules (approximately 15 to 20 mm Hg) and falls lowest in the superior vena cava (approximately 0 to 6 mm Hg).

Many veins have valves that help prevent blood backflow. Each valve consists of a pocketlike endothelial fold reinforced by connective tissue; usually, two folds face each other on the vein wall. Valves attach to the vein wall in a way that permits free blood flow to the heart. However, any backflow makes the pockets expand and fill with blood. This temporarily blocks the vein and stops blood's return to the capillaries.

Arm and leg veins contain the most valves—particularly the legs, where veins must move blood against gravity. Other veins have only one or two valves; a few (such as the vena cava) have none.

Blood and nerve supply. Vein walls contain a network of tiny blood vessels—the vasa vasorum—that nourishes vein cells. Veins also receive nourishment by diffusion from the bloodstream. A vein's nerve distribution resembles an artery's (however, veins contain fewer nerves).

Each arm and leg contains three structurally and functionally distinct groups of veins.
- *Superficial (subcutaneous) veins.* These have relatively thick, muscular walls that nonetheless provide little support. Major superficial vein trunks run in tunnels formed by superficial fascia condensation and lined by areolar tissue. Each arm or leg contains two main superficial vein systems that freely communicate with each other and with deep veins. Each superficial system ends as it penetrates the deep fascia and enters a major deep vein.
- *Deep (intermuscular or intramuscular) veins.* These thin veins have little muscle and receive support from surrounding tissues. Intermuscular veins run parallel to arteries, forming a plexus below elbow or knee level and a single deep major vein at the limb's root.
- *Perforating (communicating) veins.* Also thin, these veins run through the deep fascia to link the superficial and deep vein systems. Their one-way valves typically prevent blood reflux from the deep to the superficial systems.

The venous system also contains the musculovenous pump mechanism, which propels blood to the heart when leg muscles (for example, in the calf) contract around the intramuscular and surrounding veins. The pump's major reservoirs include the soleus and gastrocnemius sinusoids.

The musculovenous pump also helps the heart circulate blood during exercise. This relieves leg vein congestion, increases central blood volume, decreases peripheral edema, and promotes blood flow through active muscles.

Other mechanisms that help venous blood return to the heart include venous valves, nervous stimulation, and respiratory inspiration.

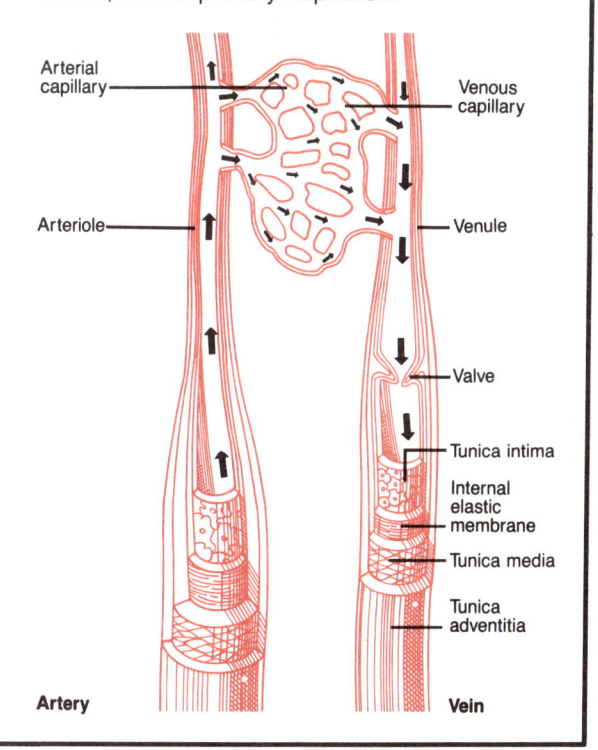

---

small saphenous vein, which runs up the back of the leg, empties into the popliteal vein behind the knee.

Deep leg veins travel parallel to the arteries and collect blood from structures along their path. Many run in pairs, as in the arm. *Posterior tibial veins*, behind the medial malleolus, receive the peroneal veins and other branches as they pass upward. They join with the anterior tibial veins just below the knee. The *anterior tibial veins* form upward extensions of the *dorsalis pedis vein*. They combine

Continued on page 142

Peripheral Venous Disorders

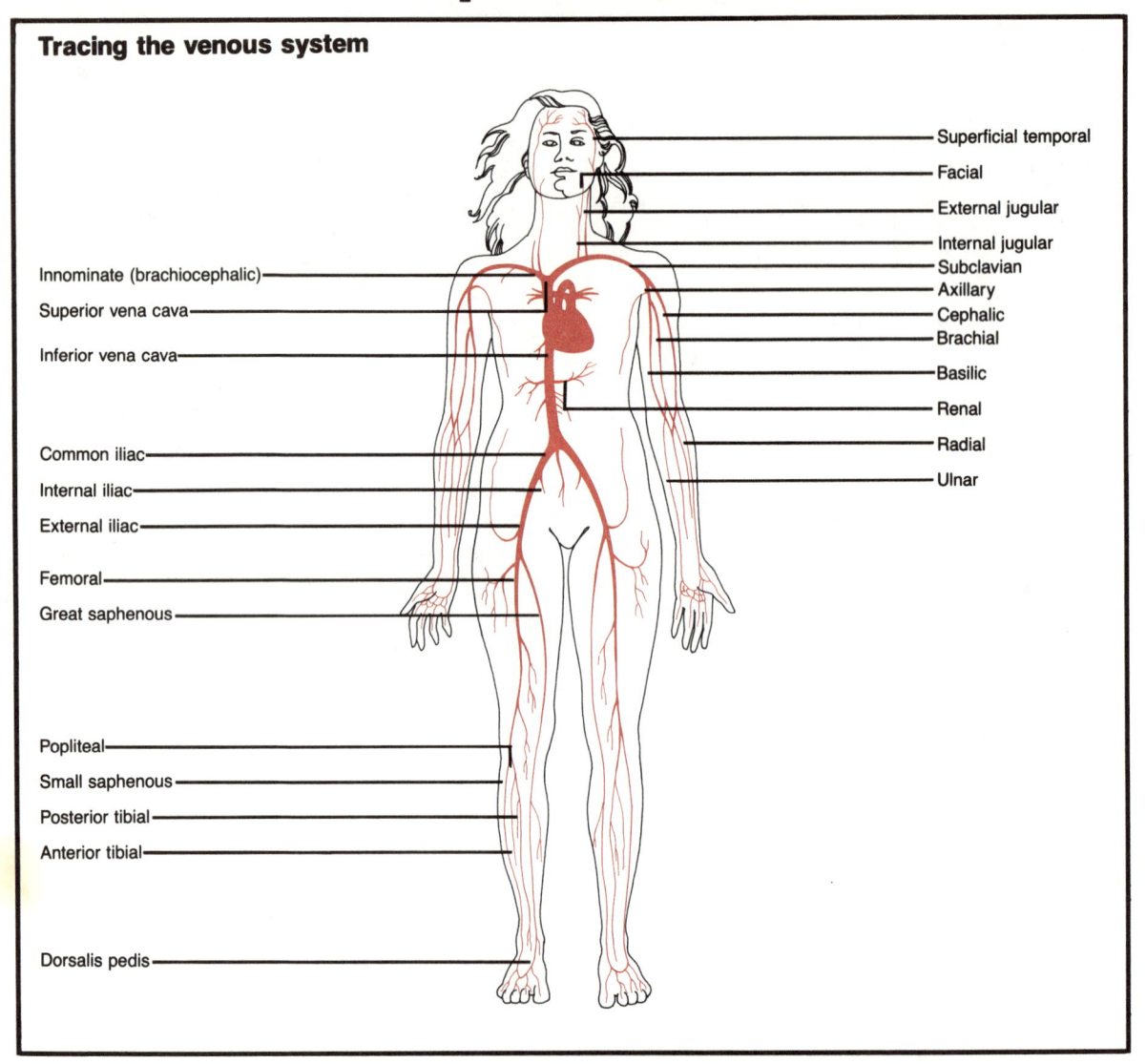

Tracing the venous system

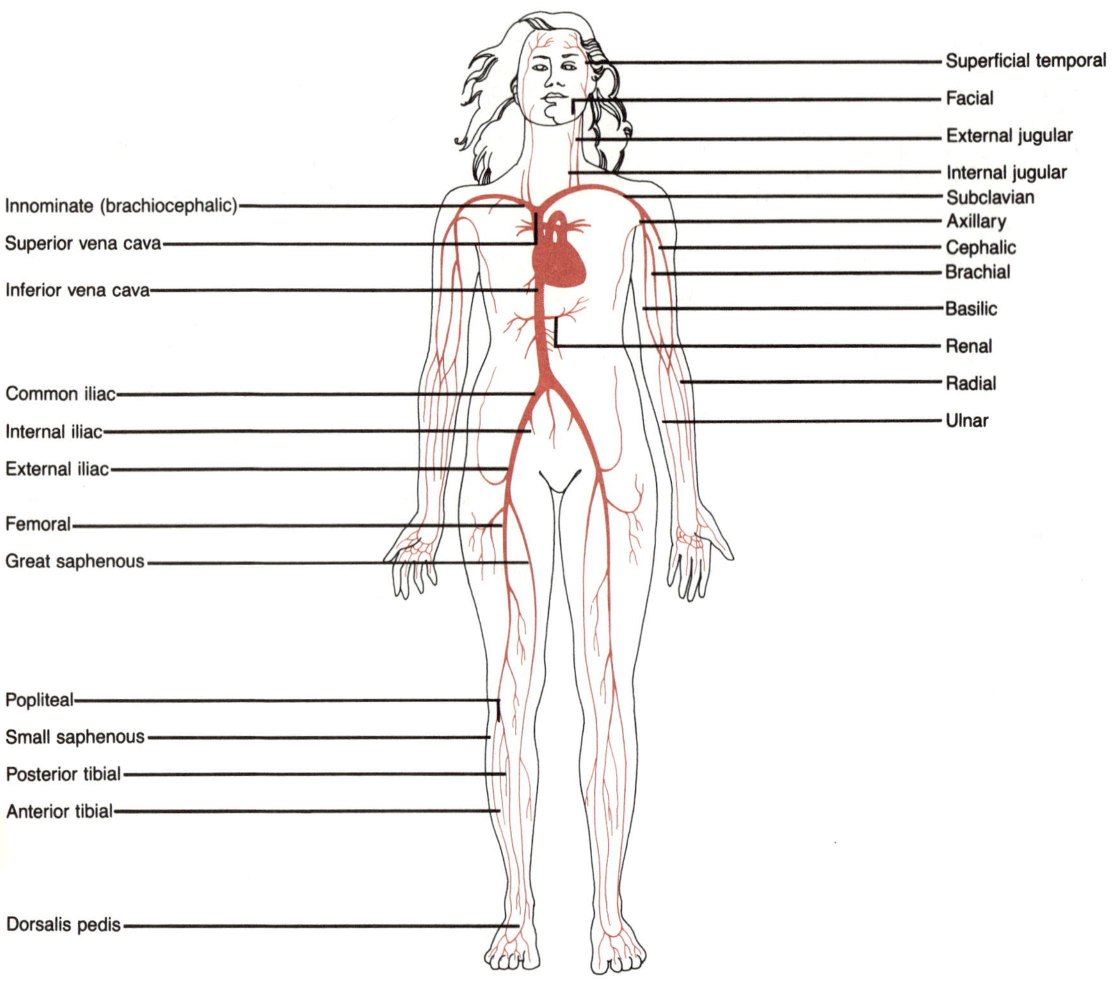
Superficial temporal
Facial
External jugular
Internal jugular
Subclavian
Axillary
Cephalic
Brachial
Basilic
Renal
Radial
Ulnar
Innominate (brachiocephalic)
Superior vena cava
Inferior vena cava
Common iliac
Internal iliac
External iliac
Femoral
Great saphenous
Popliteal
Small saphenous
Posterior tibial
Anterior tibial
Dorsalis pedis

Continued

with the posterior tibial veins to create the popliteal vein. Collecting blood from muscular and articular branches and the small saphenous vein, the *popliteal vein* becomes the femoral vein just above the knee. The *femoral vein* courses under the inguinal ligament in the groin, continuing as the external iliac vein.

Pelvic veins. These parallel the pelvic arteries, draining the general areas that these arteries feed. The *external iliac veins* directly continue the right and left femoral veins. The *internal iliac (hypogastric) veins* drain blood from the pelvic wall, pelvic viscera, buttocks, external genitalia, and the medial thigh aspect. Each joins with the ipsilateral external iliac vein. The internal iliac and external iliac veins combine to form the *common iliac veins,* which, in turn, link as the inferior vena cava at the fifth lumbar vertebral level.

Abdominal veins. The body's largest vein, the *inferior vena cava,* forms from the two common iliac veins. It ascends in front of the vertebral column to the aorta's right, eventually entering the right atrium. Blood from the common iliac veins, *spermatic vein* (in men), *ovarian veins* (in women), *renal veins, suprarenal vein, inferior phrenic veins,* and *hepatic veins* empty into the inferior vena cava.

Peripheral Vascular Disease

Peripheral Venous Disorders

Reviewing common terms

Clot: a semisolid mass, for example, lymph or blood.

Embolus: a plug, such as a clot, carried by the blood from one vessel and forced into a smaller one, thus impeding blood flow.

Phlebitis: vein inflammation, marked by vein-wall infiltration and thrombus formation.

Phlebothrombosis: a clot within a vein that doesn't cause vein inflammation.

Thrombophlebitis: vein inflammation associated with a thrombus.

Thrombosis: thrombus presence, formation, or development.

Thrombus: collection of blood factors—mainly platelets, fibrin, and entrapped cellular elements; typically results in vascular obstruction. (*Note:* Some experts differentiate thrombus formation from simple coagulation, or clot formation.)

Superficial venous thrombophlebitis

Although usually a fairly mild, self-limiting disorder, superficial venous thrombophlebitis can recur or persist. Always accompanied by inflammation, the disorder typically stems from a component of Virchow's triad—venous injury, venous stasis, or hypercoagulability. Superficial vein thrombi rarely become emboli because they adhere firmly to the vein wall. However, in a few cases, they enter pulmonary vessels, causing pulmonary embolism.

The patient complains of local tenderness or pain along the vein's path. The vein typically feels hard or cordlike; inflammation may cause redness, warmth, and edema. Doppler ultrasonography usually confirms absent blood flow through the vein.

The doctor will treat the condition according to its cause and extent and the patient's signs and symptoms. Expect the doctor to order symptomatic pain relief, local heat, compression bandaging, and continued ambulation. For acute, large-vein thrombosis, the doctor may express the thrombus through a small venotomy and apply a compression bandage to speed recovery (this permanently destroys the vein).

Veins collecting blood from the spleen, stomach, intestines, pancreas, and gallbladder make up the *portal vein system.* The portal vein arises where the superior mesenteric and splenic veins meet. At the liver, the portal vein splits into right and left branches, which follow the corresponding hepatic artery branches throughout the organ. These vessels nourish microscopic sinusoids separating liver cell plates. Hepatic artery and portal vein blood mix within the sinusoids and reach the hepatic veins, which drain into the inferior vena cava.

Deep-vein thrombosis

A thrombus that lodges in a vein can cause venous occlusion. Such a thrombus typically lodges in a deep vein, resulting in deep-vein thrombosis (DVT). This disorder can lead to severe venous obstruction and injury, depending on thrombus size and collateral circulatory adequacy. (For details on thrombus formation, see *Venous thrombus formation,* page 144.)

A thrombus usually begins in one of the calf's veins, where it remains or lyses spontaneously. However, it may enter a leg or thigh vein (as with iliofemoral thrombosis) or the lungs, where it becomes a potentially lethal pulmonary embolism.

DVT can lead to venous valve malformation (resulting from damage by thrombus recanalization, as in varicose veins and leg ulcers) and continuing venous obstruction, in which the thrombus grows instead of lyses (as in edematous leg swelling). Extremely extensive thrombi can lead to phlegmasia cerulea dolens—massive, tight leg edema; severe leg pain; and cyanotic skin mottling that may advance to cutaneous gangrene.

DVT most commonly occurs in hospital patients, especially postoperative and heart disease patients. However, it can arise without warning in an otherwise healthy young adult. Researchers have linked DVT to Virchow's triad: venous stasis, venous wall injury, and hypercoagulability.

Venous stasis can develop from leg inactivity. Lacking an intrinsic force to propel blood, veins depend almost totally on voluntary muscle stimulation and competent one-way valves. Inactive voluntary muscles or incompetent valves, such as from prolonged bed rest, can cause venous stasis. Other conditions that promote venous stasis include congestive heart failure, obesity, pregnancy, and abdominal cancer.

Venous wall injury, especially to the intimal layer, alters the epithelial lining, impairing the fibrinolytic activity that inhibits thrombus formation. As platelets aggregate at the injury site, some get trapped by fibrin, red blood cells, and granular leukocytes, setting the stage for thrombus formation.

Venous wall injury can occur from trauma, such as a fracture, dislocation, muscle injury, or venipuncture. Chemical agents (for example, X-ray contrast media), some antibiotic solutions, and irritation from an indwelling I.V. catheter may also lead to injury.

Hypercoagulability results when blood coagulates faster than normal, causing thrombin and other clotting factors to multiply. Con-

Continued on page 144

Peripheral Venous Disorders

Venous thrombus formation

A venous thrombus begins to form when platelets adhere to the endothelium and then to each other. This platelet aggregate then becomes coated with a fibrin mesh, inducing further platelet aggregation. Eventually, a macroscopic white thrombus forms, usually in a deep vein. This thrombus commonly obstructs the lumen, stopping blood flow between vein branches. The stagnant blood then clots, forming a mesh of red blood cells, platelets, and fibrin called a red thrombus. Usually forming at a bifurcation, a red thrombus may retract and undergo lysis. With complete occlusion, blood backflow occurs unless sufficient collateral circulation develops.

What happens next depends on two opposing processes. The thrombus dissolves in a few days (in most cases) from the normal fibrinolytic action of the thrombus, vein wall, and plasma. During this phase, large thrombus portions may break off and, as emboli, lodge in the pulmonary arterial tree. Meanwhile, a much slower process also takes place—inflammation in and around the vein wall, then fibroblastic thrombus organization. A thrombus that doesn't embolize may completely dissolve, leaving vein structure almost unimpaired (as with active fibrinolysis and a small thrombus and attachment area). In some cases, however, the thrombus may convert into fibrous tissue (as with weak fibrinolysis and a large thrombus and attachment area). An organized thrombus tends to recanalize over several weeks, usually by numerous small channels.

Venous valves play a key role in venous thrombus formation. The initial platelet aggregate tends to develop in a valve pocket (presumably from eddy currents); if the thrombus organizes and recanalizes, it incorporates and then obliterates valve cusps.

Venous thrombosis usually stems from venous stasis, venous injury, and hypercoagulability (Virchow's triad).

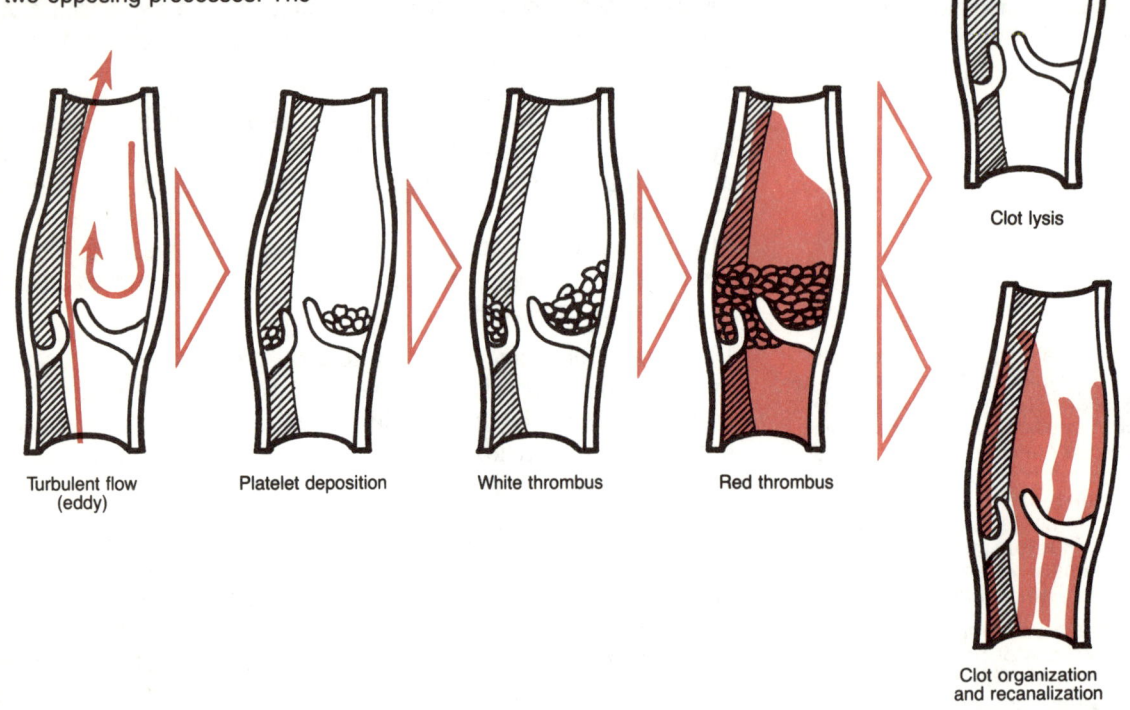

Turbulent flow (eddy) → Platelet deposition → White thrombus → Red thrombus

Clot lysis

Clot organization and recanalization

Deep-vein thrombosis—continued

ditions promoting hypercoagulability include anemia, cancer, polycythemia vera, liver disease, disseminated intravascular coagulation, trauma, and oral contraceptive use.

Assessment
Signs and symptoms of DVT vary, depending on thrombus size and extent, the amount of obstruction, the affected vein's location, collateral circulatory adequacy, and any preexisting medical problems. Typically, the patient complains of deep leg pain of sudden onset that diminishes when he elevates his leg. He may also report leg warmth and swelling. Or he may lack symptoms. When obtaining the patient's history, also determine if he has any conditions suggesting venous stasis, venous injury, or hypercoagulability.

Peripheral Vascular Disease

Peripheral Venous Disorders

Physical examination. Inspection may reveal leg swelling and superficial vein engorgement. Palpation may reveal muscle tenderness and warmth overlying the affected vein. With thrombophlebitis, the patient may have pain when he contracts his gastrocnemius muscle (Homans' sign), as when flexing his foot upward forcefully. (*Note:* Although Homans' sign suggests DVT, it's generally considered unreliable unless accompanied by other findings.)

Diagnostic tests. To identify, localize, and confirm DVT, the doctor may order impedance plethysmography, Doppler ultrasonography, and standard or radionuclide venography.

Impedance plethysmography. This noninvasive study, which can be done at bedside, accurately diagnoses DVT above the knee. The doctor inflates a pneumatic cuff around the patient's thigh to a pressure above baseline venous pressure but below arterial pressure. Electrodes attached to the calf measure electrical resistance (or impedance) resulting from venous volume changes. Normally, venous calf volume rises markedly as blood gets trapped below the cuff. However, if blood's already trapped in the calf, as in DVT, venous volume won't increase as much. In about 45 seconds, calf veins normally fill completely with blood and venous volume reaches a plateau, called the venous capacitance (VC). The cuff pressure's

Continued on page 146

Reviewing edema's causes

A lymphatic or peripheral venous disorder can cause edema—increased interstitial fluid. To understand how, review how fluid exchange takes place through the capillary bed.

Diffusing across the capillary membrane, fluids preserve equilibrium between the vascular and interstitial spaces. Blood pressure (hydrostatic pressure) within the capillary bed—particularly at the arteriolar end—pushes fluid into interstitial spaces. Proteins' weak osmotic action within the tissues (called interstitial colloid osmotic pressure) promotes this movement; hydrostatic tissue pressure hinders it.

As blood flows toward the capillary bed's venous end, hydrostatic pressure falls. Plasma colloid osmotic pressure draws fluid back into the vascular tree. Net fluid flow—formerly directed outward on the capillary bed's arteriolar side—reverses and turns inward on the venous side. Also crucial to this equilibrium, lymphatic capillaries remove excess fluid, including protein, from the interstitial space.

Edema can be general (systemic) or local. Study the information below to review edema's causes and associated signs and symptoms.

Hypoalbuminemia
Mechanism:
Reduced plasma colloid osmotic pressure that permits excessive fluid flow into the interstitial space. Cirrhosis, nephrotic syndrome, and severe malnutrition can lead to hypoalbuminemia.

Distribution:
May initially appear in loose subcutaneous eyelid tissue—particularly after the patient lies down at night—but may also start in the feet and legs. With cirrhosis, ascites may appear first.

Excessive renal retention of salt and water
Mechanism:
Kidneys retain excess salt and water, which enter the interstitial space in small portions. Use of drugs such as corticosteroids, estrogens, and certain antihypertensives can cause salt and water retention.

Distribution:
Usually starts in dependent areas, possibly becoming systemic

Venous stasis (secondary to venous obstruction or insufficiency)
Mechanism:
Thrombophlebitis that obstructs venous drainage; venous valve incompetence (as in varicose veins) or damage (from thrombophlebitis); tumor or fibrosis that compresses veins from the outside (less common). In each case, veins and capillaries have increased hydrostatic pressure, causing excessive fluid loss into the tissues.

Distribution:
Limited to obstruction area (commonly one leg; in some cases, both legs or one arm)

Lymphatic stasis (lymphedema)
Mechanism:
Congenitally abnormal lymph channels; tumor or fibrosis that obstructs lymph channels; inflammation

Distribution:
Local; commonly involves one or both legs

Orthostatic edema
Mechanism:
Prolonged sitting or standing, with inadequate muscle activity to promote venous flow. Because the heart can't accept all venous blood, venous and capillary hydrostatic pressure rise, which causes congestion and fluid loss into tissues.

Distribution:
Initially appears in dependent body areas with maximal hydrostatic pressure (for example, the feet and legs or, in a bedridden patient, the back)

Increased capillary permeability
Mechanism:
Increased capillary permeability that leads to protein leakage into interstitial spaces; this also draws out excessive fluid by increasing colloid osmotic pressure. Causes include burns, snakebite, and allergy.

Distribution:
Usually local, depending on cause; possibly systemic

Peripheral Venous Disorders

Impedance plethysmography

Using temporary venous obstruction created by a pneumatic cuff on the thigh, impedance plethysmography detects venous volume changes in calf veins.

Comparing these typical impedance plethysmography tracings shows how deep-vein thrombosis (DVT) markedly reduces venous outflow. The top tracing shows how venous volume normally rises and then falls as the cuff's removed. The bottom tracing shows how DVT causes venous volume to remain about the same with or without cuff inflation.

Normal tracing

Tracing showing DVT

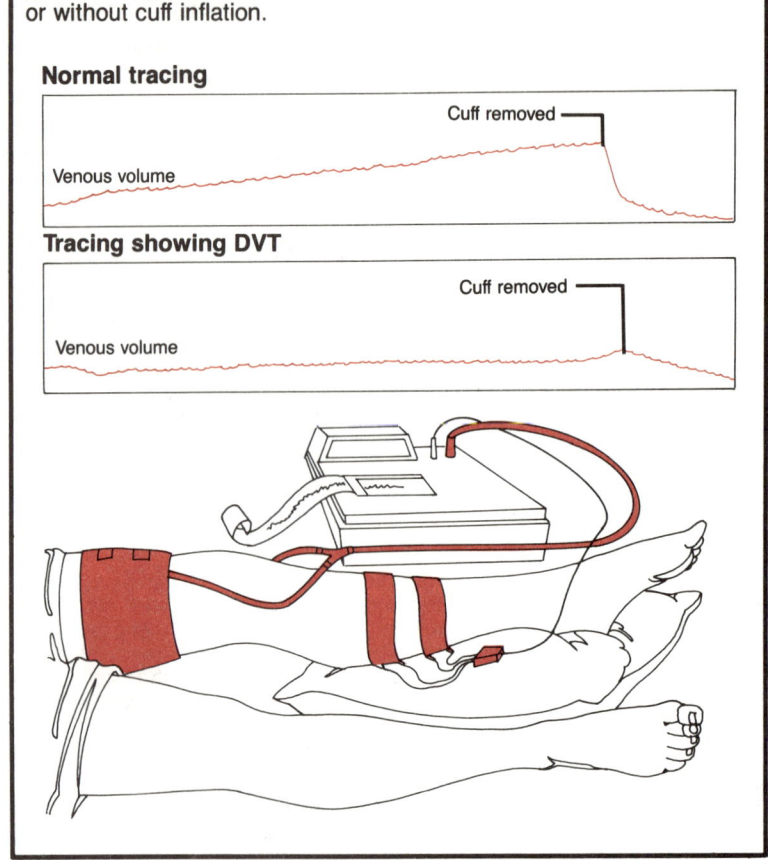

Deep-vein thrombosis—*continued*

then released to allow measurement of volume change (called maximum venous outflow [MVO]). Normally, pressure rapidly returns to baseline from venous runoff. DVT blocks runoff, causing a slower return to baseline; venous volume remains about the same. From cuff inflation and deflation responses recorded on graph paper, the doctor can plot VC against MVO to identify any deep-vein obstruction.

Impedance plethysmography results call for careful evaluation. A false-positive result can stem from pain, low cardiac output, use of vasoconstricting drugs, increased venous tone caused by apprehension, increased venous pressure secondary to congestive heart failure, or external venous compression from a tumor or an abscess. A false-negative result may stem from a longstanding venous thrombus with adequate collateral circulation; superficial phlebitis; or an occluded distal popliteal, tibial, or peroneal vein. However, when combined with Doppler ultrasonography, impedance plethysmography has a 95% accuracy rate.

Doppler ultrasonography. A noninvasive test, Doppler ultrasonography reliably detects thrombi above the knee by assessing such veins as

147 Peripheral Vascular Disease

Peripheral Venous Disorders

the common femoral, superficial femoral, popliteal, and posterior tibial. The technician positions the Doppler probe over the vessel, which he has distally occluded by applying pressure. When he releases the pressure, the probe detects sudden blood flow if the vessel's normal. Unaugmented flow indicates obstruction.

During the test, the patient may be told to hold his breath or perform Valsalva's maneuver. Normally, blood flow through the femoral and popliteal veins decreases during inspiration (the descending diaphragm increases intraabdominal pressure, which briefly slows venous blood's return from the legs). During expiration, the diaphragm rises, intraabdominal pressure drops, and venous blood flows faster. However, as the patient holds his breath or performs Valsalva's maneuver, venous blood flow and the accompanying rushing sound stop. The patient then exhales forcefully, creating the rushing sound as blood flow resumes. If the patient has DVT, the Doppler probe won't detect the rushing sound.

Standard venography. This test uses an I.V. contrast medium and serial angiographic pictures to detect filling defects in the affected veins. Venography visualizes the entire venous system; radiolucent areas indicate thrombi, and blank areas show absent venous filling caused by occlusion.

Although this test definitively diagnoses DVT, it can lead to allergic reaction (from the contrast medium), tissue damage at the injection site, and phlebitis.

Radionuclide venography. These studies record blood's path as it flows through veins. In the technetium 99m isotope test, the doctor injects the radioisotope simultaneously into the veins of each foot. Scintiphotographs taken as the radioisotope enters deep veins record blood flow, revealing DVT directly as a cold spot lacking radioactivity and indirectly by showing collateral channels around an obstructed vein. Residual hot spots and delayed isotope ascent or disappearance also indicate DVT.

This test permits rapid screening for major leg vein thrombosis. Used in conjunction with perfusion lung scanning, it helps detect possible thrombi sources in a patient with suspected pulmonary embolism. Because the test doesn't cause pain, the patient can undergo repeated studies, allowing the doctor to follow the obstruction's course and identify any recurrent thrombi.

By providing excellent views of major intraabdominal veins, this test also helps document caval patency after insertion of an inferior vena cava filter. Used for a patient with suspected subclavian vein thrombosis or superior vena cava syndrome, it permits quick visualization of major arm veins.

Relatively simple, this technique's faster than standard venography and poses little danger of chemical phlebitis or venous thrombosis. However, it's expensive, it must take place in a nuclear medicine laboratory, and it lacks sufficient resolution for visualizing individual calf veins.

In the ^{125}I fibrinogen test, the patient receives an I.V. injection of human fibrinogen labeled with iodine-125 isotope after iodide thy-

Continued on page 148

Superior vena cava syndrome

Caused by obstructed upper-body venous drainage, superior vena cava syndrome results in inadequate drainage. Most patients with this syndrome have an underlying cancerous tumor involving the mediastinum (most commonly upper-right lobe bronchogenic carcinoma).

Signs and symptoms include elevated venous pressure; face, arm, and head edema; dilated chest-wall collateral veins; cyanosis; and neck vein distention. Increased pressure on the esophagus or bronchus may cause dysphagia or dyspnea. The patient may also complain of headache, visual disturbances, and an altered level of consciousness.

The doctor will diagnose superior vena cava syndrome from the patient's history, physical examination, and X-ray findings.

Treatment involves chemotherapy, radiation, or surgery to destroy the tumor. The doctor may try a bypass graft to reroute venous drainage, but this procedure's usually ineffective.

Peripheral Venous Disorders

Deep-vein thrombosis—*continued*

roid blockade. The radioactive fibrinogen concentrates where fibrin forms, indicating a thrombus site. Using a portable scintillation detector probe, the technician scans various major leg vein sites for radioactivity. The first radiation count's usually taken 24 hours after injection; counts are then repeated at selected intervals.

The doctor may order this test to screen a high-risk patient for active DVT or, less commonly, to evaluate a patient with suspected active DVT. The most sensitive test for active arm and leg thrombi (especially isolated calf vein thrombi), this test also helps detect early thrombi that other noninvasive diagnostic tests may miss. And it helps evaluate suspected recurrent venous thrombosis, identify the course of venous disease, and assess for therapeutic or prophylactic effectiveness.

The test's drawbacks include its expense, length (it requires 24 to 48 hours for a definitive diagnosis), and possible hepatitis transmission (from human fibrinogen). Additionally, it can't detect older thrombi that don't incorporate fibrinogen and may miss proximal iliofemoral thrombosis because of the high background activity associated with proximal thigh and pelvic muscle mass. Arthritis, operative wounds, burns, hematoma, trauma, and inflammation can cause false-positive results.

Planning
Before determining your nursing care plan, develop the nursing diagnosis by identifying the patient's problem or potential problem, then relating it to its cause. Possible nursing diagnoses for a patient with DVT include the following:
* skin integrity, impairment of (potential); related to venous stasis
* comfort, alteration in (leg pain); related to venous occlusion
* gas exchange, impaired (potential); related to pulmonary embolism
* anxiety; related to unexpected hospitalization
* knowledge deficit; related to newly diagnosed disease
* noncompliance; related to inadequate health teaching
* injury, potential for (bleeding); related to anticoagulant therapy
* activity intolerance; related to leg pain or swelling.

The sample nursing care plan shows expected outcomes, nursing interventions, and discharge planning for one nursing diagnosis listed above. However, you'll want to individualize each care plan to fit your patient's needs.

Intervention
After the doctor diagnoses DVT, he'll order treatment to prevent further thrombus formation, reduce the embolism risk, and promote systemic fibrinolysis. Treatment usually starts with anticoagulant or thrombolytic therapy. Commonly used anticoagulants include heparin and warfarin. Heparin—the preferred drug—interferes with coagulation by readily combining with antithrombin. This substance helps prevent thrombin from converting fibrinogen into fibrin—a blood clot's basic structure. Although heparin won't break down an existing clot, it can limit clot size and prevent new clot formation. It's usually administered by continuous I.V. infusion.

Peripheral Vascular Disease

Peripheral Venous Disorders

Sample nursing care plan: Deep-vein thrombosis

Nursing diagnosis	Expected outcomes
Skin integrity, impairment of (potential); related to venous stasis	The patient will: • maintain good skin integrity, with no signs of ulcer development or skin breakdown. • demonstrate methods of reducing venous stasis.

Nursing interventions	Discharge planning
• Assess patient's arms and legs for swelling, inflammation, pain, and discoloration at least once each shift. • Check circulation and motor and sensory function at least once each shift. • Protect skin from injury by guarding exposed areas, avoiding placing I.V. catheters in legs, and applying lotion. • Encourage early ambulation. • Discuss with patient methods that help reduce venous stasis: elevating legs during bed rest; wearing elastic support stockings (except when he sleeps or elevates his legs); avoiding cigarette smoking; and practicing deep-breathing exercises to promote venous return. • Discuss appropriate exercises, such as dorsiflexing patient's feet or moving them in a walking motion against the bed's footboard; or, if he must stand for prolonged periods, exercising legs by shifting weight from one leg to another. • If patient can't exercise, perform passive range-of-motion exercises. • Encourage good nutrition and fluid intake.	• Reinforce instructions and discuss how to modify them for home use. • Advise patient when to seek medical care, such as if he experiences sudden pain, swelling, tenderness, or superficial vein dilation. • Arrange for follow-up care. • Instruct patient about discharge medication, if indicated.

Warfarin, also ineffective against an existing clot, prevents vitamin K from synthesizing certain clotting factors. Therefore, it takes effect only after active clotting factor depletion. For this reason, the doctor will probably order heparin before and for a short time after warfarin therapy begins. Warfarin therapy may last several months.

Commonly used thrombolytic drugs include streptokinase and urokinase, which break down clots by dissolving fibrin. Streptokinase, the favored drug, combines with a plasminogen complex to help convert plasminogen to plasmin—an enzyme that lyses clots. However, by producing lysis, circulating plasmin can trigger uncontrollable bleeding. Therefore, the doctor usually orders streptokinase only for a patient at risk for pulmonary embolism.

Urokinase differs slightly from streptokinase in its mechanism of action, but it has the same effect. However, it's more expensive. (*Note:* Expect the doctor to order anticoagulant therapy after thrombolytic therapy ends.)

Because anticoagulant and thrombolytic drugs can cause excessive bleeding, stay alert for blood oozing from I.V. sites. Also assess the patient for neurologic deficits (which may indicate a cerebrovascular accident) and monitor laboratory coagulation test results.

To alleviate leg pain and swelling, the doctor may order bed rest. Elevate the patient's legs, apply local heat, and administer analgesics as ordered. Enforce bed rest as ordered until severe leg

Continued on page 150

Peripheral Venous Disorders

Deep-vein thrombosis—continued

swelling and tenderness subside. Bed rest minimizes leg pain and edema and permits the thrombus to organize and adhere to the vessel wall, which usually takes 1 to 3 days. When the patient resumes activity, make sure he wears an elastic support stocking to minimize pain and swelling.

The doctor will perform surgery only if the patient has severe complications, such as pulmonary embolism. Surgery may entail inferior vena caval ligation or interruption, or umbrella filter placement in the inferior vena cava to trap emboli and prevent them from reaching pulmonary vessels. (For more on pulmonary embolism, see the NURSEREVIEW section on "Respiratory Problems.") Another complication, phlegmasia cerulea dolens, may require thrombectomy with a Fogarty balloon catheter.

The patient at high risk for developing DVT may need preventive measures to manage venous stasis, venous injury, and hypercoagulability. To minimize venous stasis, the doctor may order early ambulation (for a hospitalized patient). Use of support stockings or elastic hose, leg elevation, avoidance of prolonged standing, and active or passive range-of-motion exercises also promote venous blood flow. Also encourage the patient to exercise his legs (using plantar flexion) against a footboard for 5 minutes each hour. This promotes venous flow and may aid fibrinolytic activity, which lyses small clots. To minimize venous injury, advise the patient to avoid injuring leg veins whenever possible.

To reduce hypercoagulability, the doctor may order a prophylactic anticoagulant (such as heparin), low-molecular-weight dextran, an antiplatelet drug (such as aspirin or dipyridamole), or dihydroergotamine mesylate/heparin sodium (Embolex). (See *Embolex: A weapon against deep-vein thrombosis.*)

Evaluation

Base your evaluation on the expected outcomes listed on your nursing care plan. To determine if your patient's improved, you might ask yourself the following questions:
• Do you note leg ulcers, skin discoloration, or cellulitis?
• Does the patient understand his disease and treatment plan?
• Can he demonstrate or explain methods to reduce venous stasis? Does he comply with these methods?
• Does he have adequate nutrition and fluid intake?

The answers to these questions will help you evaluate your patient's status and the effectiveness of his care. Keep in mind that these questions stem from the sample care plan on page 149. Your questions may differ.

Other venous disorders

Varicose veins

Dilated, tortuous surface veins engorged with blood, varicose veins result from intraluminal valvular incompetence. Varicose veins may be primary or secondary. Primary varicose veins, which tend to run in families, affect more women than men and usually occur in both legs. They typically have a gradual onset and progressively

---

Embolex: A weapon against deep-vein thrombosis

The doctor may order Embolex—heparin sodium combined with dihydroergotamine mesylate—to prevent postoperative deep-vein thrombosis and pulmonary embolism after major surgery.

Heparin accelerates formation of an antithrombin III–thrombin complex. It inactivates thrombin and prevents fibrinogen's conversion to fibrin. Dihydroergotamine speeds venous return and therefore inhibits venostasis.

When administering Embolex, keep the following important points in mind.
• Don't administer the drug to a patient with uncontrollable active bleeding.
• Periodically monitor platelet counts, hematocrit, and occult blood in stool tests. Notify the doctor if signs of bleeding occur.
• Before administering Embolex, check the patient's history for lidocaine allergy (Embolex contains lidocaine).
• Administer Embolex by deep subcutaneous injection into an anterior abdominal wall fold above the iliac crest. To avoid hematoma at the injection site, don't administer the drug I.M.
• Stay alert for adverse reactions, such as bleeding, nausea, vomiting, mild local pain and itching, and finger and toe numbness and tingling.

Peripheral Venous Disorders

Incompetent venous valve
The top illustration, below, shows normal venous valves in open and closed positions. The bottom illustration shows an incompetent valve, as in a varicose vein.

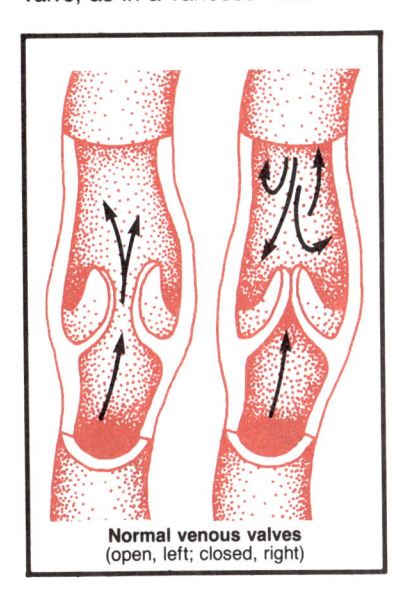

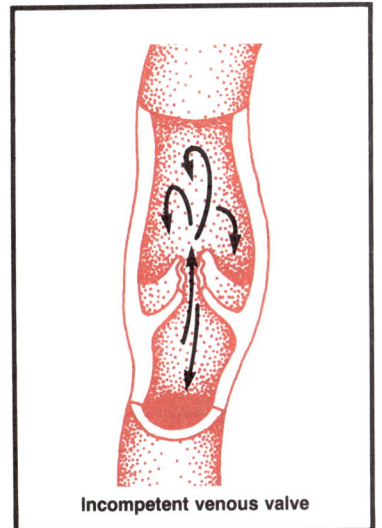

Normal venous valves
(open, left; closed, right)

Incompetent venous valve

worsen. Causes of primary varicose veins include pregnancy and tight clothing. In pregnancy, the expanding uterus (which increases pressure on the inferior vena cava) and increased vascular volume (especially in the pelvis) may impede blood's return to the heart from leg veins. Increased pressure also stresses vein wall integrity, making the vein stretch and grow tortuous. Clothing that restricts blood flow below the waist (such as girdles, skirts or trousers with tight waistbands, and elastic-topped socks or stockings) can also lead to primary varicose veins.

Secondary varicose veins result from venous disorders that cause valvular incompetence, such as venous thrombosis, thrombophlebitis, trauma, and occlusion. These varicose veins, which develop gradually, usually occur in only one leg.

Varicose veins tend to arise in middle to late adulthood. In both types, the initial injury or venous occlusion leads to improper valve closure, resulting in venous blood backflow. As pressure builds, valves become incompetent, causing still more backflow. With progressive blood pooling comes the characteristic leg vein dilation and disturbed tissue oxygen/nutrient exchange. Longstanding or severe varicose veins may produce venous insufficiency that leads to venous stasis ulcers.

Assessment. The patient will probably report dull leg aches accompanied by vague sensations of pressure, fatigue, and heaviness. These symptoms result from increased blood volume and edema in regions with dilated veins. Increased hydrostatic pressure and chronic venous stasis may cause nocturnal calf muscle cramps. The patient may also complain of vein distention in the inner, upper thighs and itching or burning skin over the affected veins. A woman with varicose veins typically has leg heaviness, fatigue, and swelling a few days before menstruation. Fluid retention and the premenstrual rise in circulating estrogens (which may decrease venous tone) probably account for these symptoms.

Keep in mind that the patient's symptoms don't necessarily reflect varicose vein size or severity. A small cluster of dilated veins may cause severe discomfort, whereas swollen, cordlike veins may cause no symptoms.

Ask the patient what seems to bring on his discomfort and what relieves it. He'll probably experience maximum discomfort from prolonged sitting or standing; symptoms may also peak in the evening and in warm weather. His legs may feel best after a night's sleep (unless he suffers muscle cramps) or when he elevates them. He may also report that exercise relieves his symptoms—a sign that calf muscle activity promotes venous blood flow.

During the physical examination, you may note dilated, purplish, ropelike veins within the great or small saphenous system, particularly in the calves. With secondary varicose veins, expect signs and symptoms of venous injury, such as leg edema, ulcers, and discoloration. (For information on two varicose vein assessment tests—the manual compression test and Trendelenburg's test—see *Assessing venous valve competence,* page 152.)

Continued on page 152

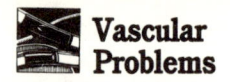

Peripheral Venous Disorders

Assessing venous valve competence

If your patient has varicose veins, consider using one of the tests described below to assess venous valve competence.

Manual compression test. Palpate the dilated vein with the fingertips of one hand. Firmly compress the vein with the other hand at a point at least 8" (20 cm) higher. Feel for an impulse transmitted to your lower hand. With competent saphenous valves, you won't detect any impulse. A palpable impulse indicates incompetent valves in a vein segment between your hands.

Trendelenburg's test (retrograde filling test). First, mark the distended veins with a pen while the patient stands. Then have him lie on the examining table and elevate his legs for about a minute to drain the veins. Next, have him stand while you measure venous filling time. Competent valves take at least 30 seconds to fill. If the veins fill in less than 30 seconds, have the patient lie on the table again and raise his leg for 1 minute. Then apply a tourniquet around his upper thigh. Next, have him stand. If leg veins fill in less than 30 seconds, suspect incompetent perforating and deep-vein valves (functioning valves block retrograde flow).

Now remove the tourniquet. If the veins again fill in less than 30 seconds, suspect incompetent superficial vein valves that allow backward blood flow.

To pinpoint incompetent valve location, repeat this procedure by applying the tourniquet just above the knee and then around the upper calf.

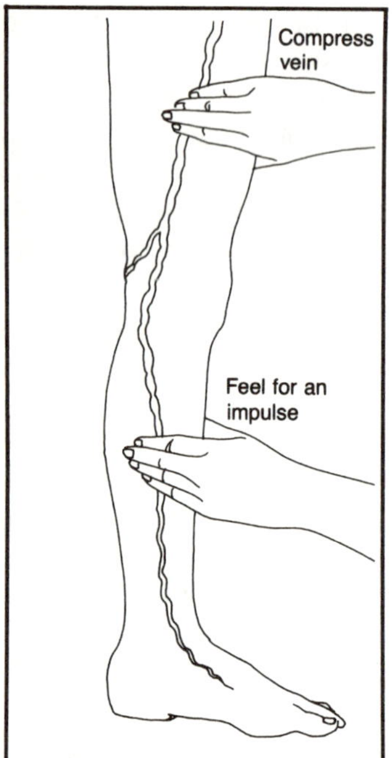

Manual compression test

Compress vein
Feel for an impulse

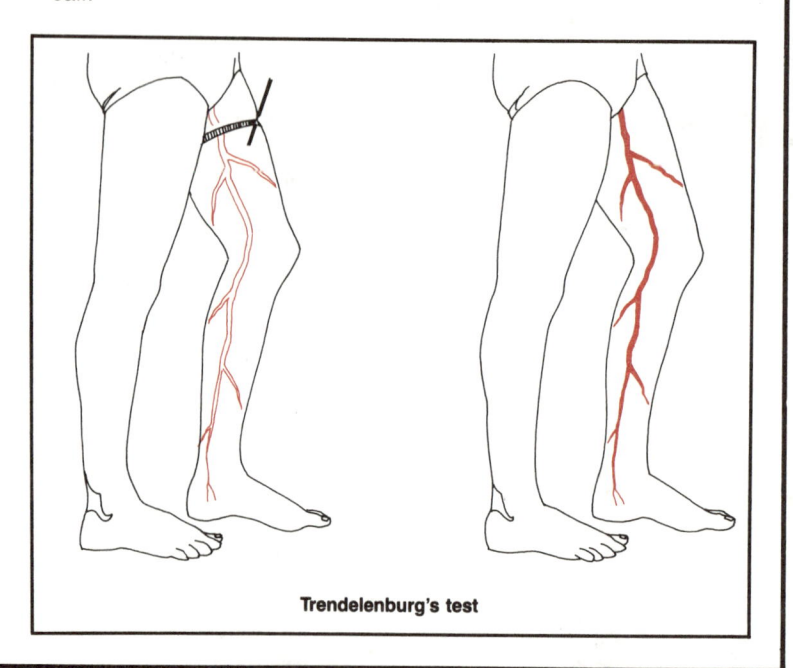

Trendelenburg's test

Other venous disorders—continued

Diagnostic studies that help assess varicose veins include lower-limb venography, plethysmography, and Doppler ultrasonography. In lower-limb venography, which evaluates deep-vein patency or adequacy (especially of the iliac vein and vena caval portions), the patient reclines at a 45-degree angle while a tight tourniquet's applied just above his ankle. After a contrast medium's injected into his foot, he exercises the leg by rising on his toes several times. Serial X-rays taken during this activity reveal venous blood's rate and path up the leg. (Some doctors also place a tourniquet on the upper leg.) After dye injection, the tourniquet's quickly released and the leg's elevated for X-ray imaging.

Intervention. Treatment for varicose veins depends on the disorder's severity. The doctor will try to slow the disorder's progression and reduce blood pooling and venous pressure to prevent complications.

For a patient who has small, relatively asymptomatic varicose veins with competent valves, the doctor may recommend measures to

Peripheral Vascular Disease

Peripheral Venous Disorders

Lymphatic system and lymphedema

The lymphatic system, which acts as a filtering mechanism, has three main elements: lymphatic capillaries, collecting lymphatic vessels, and lymph nodes.

Lymphatic capillaries absorb lymph from various tissues and organs, maintaining fluid balance within the interstitial space.

Collecting lymphatic vessels act mainly as channels for lymph. Running parallel to blood vessels, collecting lymphatics carry lymph to regional lymph nodes, the thoracic duct, and, ultimately, the systemic circulation. Each collecting lymphatic has intimal, medial, and adventitial layers, with smooth muscle and medial elastic fibers in direct proportion to its size. These vessels also contain many valves, which prevent lymph backflow.

Lymph nodes, interspersed throughout collecting lymphatic vessels, filter lymph before its return to the bloodstream. They also produce lymphocytes.

Smooth-muscle contraction in collecting lymphatic vessel walls maintains lymph flow. Skeletal muscle contraction, peristaltic smooth-muscle movement in visceral walls, and arterial pulsations aid this flow by squeezing, compressing, or massaging neighboring lymphatic vessels to force lymph toward veins.

Respiratory movements also promote lymph movement. Inspiration lowers thoracic cavity pressure. The resulting suction makes lymph flow upward from the thoracic duct's abdominal segment.

Lymphedema. This disorder can be primary (caused by a process basic to lymphatic development) or secondary (caused by a pathologic change, such as a tumor, infection, inflammation, or trauma, that obstructs the lymphatic channels).

Whatever the cause, lymph begins to collect in the tissues, creating edema, inflammation, and further lymph stasis as lymph vessels can't remove excess fluid.

Lymphedema's usually unilateral, nonpitting, chronic, and painless. The involved arm or leg may double or triple in circumference and become discolored.

The doctor usually diagnoses lymphedema from the physical examination. He may order lymphangiography to confirm the diagnosis.

Expect the doctor to treat lymphedema with palliative measures that help maintain healthy skin and reduce edema. To maintain healthy skin, try to prevent or control skin infections. To help reduce edema, have the patient elevate the affected arm or leg and restrict his dietary sodium and/or water intake. The doctor may also order a diuretic and external compression, which promote lymph drainage into the venous circulation. To achieve compression, the patient may use custom-made, formfitting, elastic support hose or sleeves; massage; or an intermittent compression pump, which helps prevent fluid accumulation in the tissue and promotes lymph drainage.

Most patients with lymphedema don't require surgery. However, if the doctor does perform surgery, he'll probably use a procedure that excises lymphedematous tissues or that promotes lymph drainage.

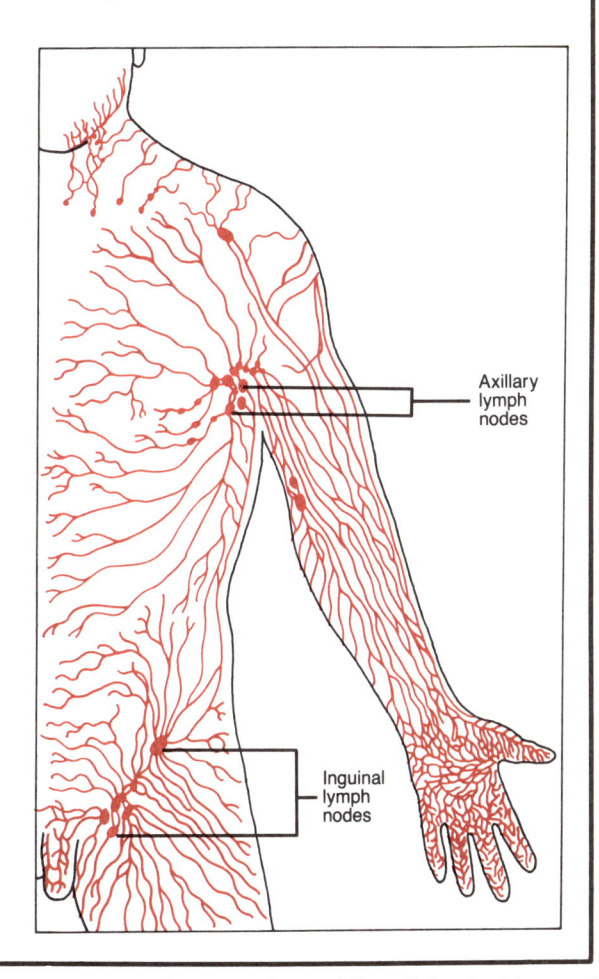

lower hydrostatic pressure, for example, avoiding tight clothing and prolonged standing, exercising frequently (particularly by walking), elevating the legs, and wearing elastic stockings. For a patient with moderate symptoms, he may suggest support hose or mild compression stockings (such as antiembolism stockings), which help compress dilated veins and force blood into more competent veins. A patient with severe symptoms may need custom-fitted, surgical-weight stockings with graduated pressure (highest at the ankle, lowest at the top). Compression stockings drain the veins and help move blood to the heart. Except during sleep and leg elevation (when veins drain naturally), the patient should wear the stockings

Continued on page 154

Vascular Problems

154 Peripheral Vascular Disease

Peripheral Venous Disorders

Comparing arterial and venous ulcers

Arterial ulcers

Location:
Between toes or on toe tips, over phalangeal heads, on heels, above lateral malleolus; in a diabetic patient, over metatarsal heads and on foot's side or sole.

Disease process:
May occur when a blocked or constricted artery causes distal ischemia. As ischemia worsens, capillary perfusion falls, metabolic exchange diminishes, and the skin becomes increasingly fragile and trauma-prone.

Signs and symptoms:
Clearly defined ulcer edges; a deep, pale base; necrosis; no healthy granulation tissue; possibly gangrene. Patient may also have pallor with leg elevation, rubor with leg dependency, cellulitis, and signs of ischemia (such as thin, shiny, dry skin; thickened nails; and absent hair growth). Patient usually reports severe pain.

Precipitating factors:
Chronic peripheral arterial occlusion, atherosclerosis, diabetes mellitus, and cigarette smoking.

Intervention:
To correct the underlying problem—arterial occlusion—the doctor usually surgically revascularizes the artery to restore circulation. If surgery's ineffective, the doctor may amputate the limb. To help debride necrotic areas, use sterile wet-to-dry saline solution dressing changes. Once the area's clean, use a wet-to-wet dressing to promote granulation. The patient may require bed rest to ensure adequate oxygen and nutrients for healing. If infection occurs from ischemia, apply topical antibiotics as ordered. If the patient needs leg immobilization, expect the doctor to use a short-leg fiberglass cast with a cut-in window for dressing changes.

Continued

Other venous disorders—*continued*

at all times. However, warn him that, although the stockings help ease symptoms, they won't cure the disorder.

The doctor may use sclerotherapy for a patient who's a poor surgical risk and who has mild to moderate primary varicose veins that don't respond to other measures. (Sclerotherapy's value in treating large dilated veins, including the great saphenous vein, remains controversial.) In this technique, the doctor injects a sclerosing agent such as sodium tetradecyl sulfate or morrhuate sodium into the dilated vein's lumen. This causes instant phlebitis that destroys the lumen and shunts blood to more competent veins. After destruction of the targeted vein's lumen, the leg's immediately compressed with an elastic bandage or stocking, which the patient must wear for at least 6 hours and possibly as long as 6 weeks. (He must enlist another person to renew the pressure every 6 to 8 hours.) After sclerotherapy, he may have pain and tenderness at the injection site for weeks and permanent pigment stains on the surrounding skin (from an inflammatory reaction to the sclerosing chemical).

The doctor may consider surgical intervention—vein ligation and stripping—for a patient with primary varicose veins causing persistent, severe, or worsening symptoms or superficial thrombophlebitis.

If the doctor chooses surgery, warn the patient that surgery won't prevent varicose veins from recurring and that the procedure may cause scarring. Surgery usually requires only a brief hospital stay. Beforehand, the doctor may mark varicose veins with an indelible pen as the patient stands. This allows quick assessment of their extent and location.

As ordered, encourage the patient to ambulate on the first postoperative day. Also advise him to wear compression bandages or elastic stockings for the next few weeks, as indicated, to decrease edema, prevent bleeding, and help maintain venous return from the lower legs.

Varicose vein ligation and stripping

The doctor inserts a flexible intraluminal vein stripper and threads it upward through the small saphenous vein. He then gathers the small saphenous vein onto the intraluminal vein stripper and removes it.

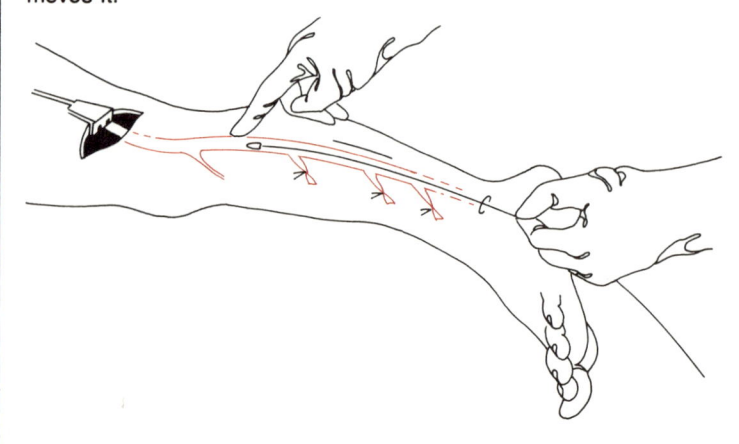

Peripheral Vascular Disease

Comparing arterial and venous ulcers
Continued

Venous ulcers

Location:
Ankle, mostly in pretibial and anteromedial supramalleolar areas

Disease process:
Valvular incompetence first causes blood backflow into superficial veins, resulting in venous hypertension. As pressure rises, red blood cells (RBCs) leak through capillaries into surrounding tissues. RBC breakdown products infiltrate subcutaneous tissues and calf skin, making these areas grow edematous, fragile, and, possibly, ulcerated.

Signs and symptoms:
Superficial ulcer with uneven edges and ruddy granulation tissue. Possible stasis dermatitis and firm (brawny) edema, reddish brown skin discoloration, and dilated, tortuous superficial veins. Patient may report mild pain.

Precipitating factors:
History of deep-vein thrombophlebitis or postphlebitic syndrome, incompetent valves in deep perforating veins, and chronic venous insufficiency.

Intervention:
The doctor will try to correct venous stasis and promote ulcer healing. To correct venous stasis, apply compression bandages and enforce bed rest with leg elevation above heart level. To promote healing, apply porous dressings and change them frequently. The doctor may order medications such as dextranomer (Debrisan) to absorb exudate. For an ulcer needing chemical debridement, use an enzyme product such as fibrinolysin (Elase), as ordered. For infection or cellulitis, administer an appropriate systemic antibiotic as ordered—not a topical ointment. If your patient's ambulatory, the doctor may order Unna's boot—moist gauze impregnated with zinc oxide that hardens when applied in layers. Recurrent venous ulcers may warrant surgery.

Peripheral Venous Disorders

Postphlebitic syndrome

Also called chronic venous insufficiency or chronic venous occlusion, postphlebitic syndrome usually results from damage by thrombophlebitis (especially in deep veins). Longstanding primary varicose veins may also cause this syndrome.

Thrombophlebitis impairs deep-vein valves, typically making them incompetent. Because the musculovenous pump then can't reduce ambulatory venous pressures, the patient has chronic venous hypertension in the lower leg when he stands. Communicating veins transmit these elevated pressures from deep to superficial veins. Venous outflow obstruction usually diminishes with time because deep veins commonly recanalize within 3 to 6 months. Valvular incompetence causes a minimal venous pressure reduction with exercise.

Assessment. Besides a history of thrombophlebitis or longstanding varicose veins, the patient with postphlebitic syndrome usually has leg edema, stasis dermatitis (especially dark ankle pigmentation called hemosiderosis) and, occasionally, skin ulcers—typically on the medial ankle at the lowest perforating vein.

Intervention. To treat postphlebitic signs and symptoms, the doctor may recommend custom-fitted elastic support hose and leg elevation, which help reduce leg edema. Encourage good skin care to help control or prevent dermatitis and ulcers. If ulcers develop, expect the doctor to order measures described in *Comparing arterial and venous ulcers.*

A patient with venous ulcers that recur despite therapy may require surgery. In the Linton procedure, the doctor strips the saphenous veins and ligates incompetent communicating veins. Significant venous occlusion may warrant a vein bypass or crossover graft.

Note: To help prevent postphlebitic syndrome, make sure any patient with thrombophlebitis receives good follow-up care. Encourage him to wear support hose as indicated, to exercise regularly, and to notify the doctor if he experiences leg pain.

Arteriovenous fistula

An abnormal anastomosis between an artery and a vein, an arteriovenous fistula can be *congenital* (most common in the arms and legs) or *acquired* (usually the result of trauma, such as a stab or missile wound). The iatrogenic access fistula, surgically created to institute renal dialysis, has become the most common acquired arteriovenous fistula.

To understand how an arteriovenous fistula disturbs hemodynamics, consider what happens with a *large* fistula: blood readily flows through the abnormal opening (the path of least resistance). As blood shunts from an artery to a vein, cardiac output and heart rate increase, diastolic pressure drops from low peripheral resistance, and blood and plasma volume rise to compensate for increased venous blood volume. A large fistula places a chronic burden on the heart that can eventually cause congestive heart failure.

A fistula can cause local as well as systemic changes. Aneurysmal dilatation generally appears in the artery or vein at the fistula site.

Continued on page 156

Vascular Problems

Arteriovenous fistula: Assessment findings

An arteriovenous fistula causes such systemic changes as increased pulse rate, cardiac output, heart size, and blood volume; and decreased diastolic arterial pressure and peripheral resistance.

It may also cause local changes, including a thrill, a continuous murmur, increased arterial collateral channels, aneurysm formation, and decreased pulse rate with occlusion.

A large fistula produces the most marked circulatory changes; a small fistula causes few or no changes. Late signs of a large fistula include congestive heart failure and pulmonary edema. Left untreated, a large fistula can cause death.

The illustration below shows local changes caused by an arteriovenous fistula. (A small fistula may produce only slight changes.)

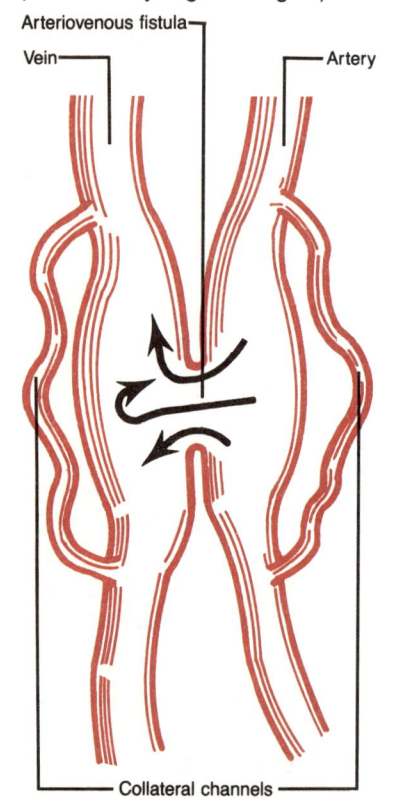

156 Peripheral Vascular Disease

Peripheral Venous Disorders

Other venous disorders—*continued*

Because the fistula markedly reduces distal arterial pressure, extensive collateral circulation develops from arterial branches arising above the fistula to those communicating below.

Assessment. Common signs of an arteriovenous fistula include a pulsating mass, a continuous murmur (palpated as a thrill), edema and phlebitis, cyanosis, erythema, or hemangiomas. With a congenital fistula, the patient may have large varicose veins in and around the fistula. With massive collateral circulation, skin temperature increases. You may also note marked blood pressure changes beyond the fistula site. An arm or leg fistula may result in a lengthened limb. To identify the fistula's location, the doctor may order arteriography.

Intervention. Expect the doctor to surgically close or excise a congenital fistula, usually through direct repair of both artery and vein. In some cases, he'll inject an autologous blood clot or Gelfoam directly into an extensive, diffuse congenital fistula to shrink it.

Self-Test

1. Intermittent claudication may be relieved by:
   a. a dependent foot position   **b.** leg elevation   **c.** exercise   **d.** rest

2. Your patient complains of severe, tearing intrascapular back pain. You suspect:
   a. proximal aortic dissection   **b.** distal aortic dissection
   c. aortic arch rupture   **d.** abdominal aortic aneurysm rupture

3. Intermittent claudication probably stems from:
   a. an inadequate blood supply   **b.** inadequate muscle oxygenation
   c. a dependent leg position   **d.** an elevated leg position

4. The doctor may treat intermittent claudication medically with:
   a. pentoxifylline (Trental)   **b.** PTFE grafts   **c.** analgesics
   d. phenoxybenzamine (Dibenzyline)

5. Virchow's triad consists of all the following components except:
   a. hypercoagulability   **b.** hypocoagulability   **c.** venous wall injury   **d.** venous stasis

Answers (page number shows where answer appears in text)
1. **d** (page 100)   2. **b** (page 121)   3. **b** (page 129)   4. **a** (page 133)   5. **b** (page 143)

Selected References

Books

Bates, Barbara. *A Guide to Physical Examination,* 3rd ed. Philadelphia: J.B. Lippincott Co., 1983.

Braunwald, Eugene, ed. *Heart Disease: A Textbook of Cardiovascular Medicine,* 2 vols., 2nd ed. Philadelphia: W.B. Saunders Co., 1984.

Brunner, Lillian S., and Suddarth, Doris S., eds. *Textbook of Medical-Surgical Nursing,* 5th ed. Philadelphia: J.B. Lippincott Co., 1984.

Carolan, Jacqueline M., ed. *Shock: A Nursing Guide.* Oradell, N.J.: Medical Economics Books, 1984.

Dale, W.A. *Management of Vascular Surgical Problems.* New York: McGraw-Hill Book Co., 1985.

Guyton, Arthur C. *Textbook of Medical Physiology,* 6th ed. Philadelphia: W.B. Saunders Co., 1981.

Guzzetta, Cathie E., and Dossey, Barbara M. *Cardiovascular Disease Nursing: Bodymind Tapestry.* St. Louis: C.V. Mosby Co., 1984.

Hallett, John, et al. *Manual of Patient Care in Vascular Surgery.* Boston: Little, Brown & Co., 1982.

Hurst, J. Willis, ed. *The Heart, Arteries and Veins.* New York: McGraw-Hill Book Co., 1982.

Kotchen, T.A., ed. *Clinical Approaches to High Blood Pressure in the Young.* Littleton, Mass.: John Wright PSG, 1983.

Malasanos, Lois. *Health Assessment,* 2nd ed. St. Louis: C.V. Mosby Co., 1981.

National Heart, Lung, and Blood Institute. National High Blood Pressure Education Program. *1984 Report of the Joint National Committee on Detection, Evaluation and Treatment of High Blood Pressure.* Bethesda, Md.: National Institutes of Health, 1984.

Perry, Anne G. *Shock: Comprehensive Nursing Management.* St. Louis: C.V. Mosby Co., 1982.

Rutherford, Robert B., ed. *Vascular Surgery,* 2nd ed. Philadelphia: W.B. Saunders Co., 1984.

Sabiston, David C., Jr., ed. *Textbook of Surgery: The Biological Basis of Modern Surgical Practice,* 2 vols. Philadelphia: W.B. Saunders Co., 1977.

Scheinman, Melvin M., ed. *Cardiac Emergencies.* Philadelphia: W.B. Saunders Co., 1984.

Shoemaker, William C. *The Society of Critical Care Medicine: Textbook of Critical Care.* Philadelphia: W.B. Saunders Co., 1984.

Underhill, Sandra L., et al., eds. *Cardiac Nursing.* Philadelphia: J.B. Lippincott Co., 1982.

Periodicals

Bastarche, Marie, et al. "Assessing Peripheral Vascular Disease: Noninvasive Testing," *American Journal of Nursing* 83(11):1552-56, November 1983.

Baum, Patricia. "Heed the Early Warning Signs of Peripheral Vascular Disease," *Nursing85* 5(3):50-58, March 1985.

Doyle, Jeanne. "All Leg Ulcers Are Not Alike: Managing and Preventing Arterial and Venous Ulcers," *Nursing83* 13(1):58-63, January 1983.

Fries, E. "Should Hypertension Be Treated?" *New England Journal of Medicine* 307(5):306, July 29, 1982.

Kaplan, N.M. "Therapy for Mild Hypertension: Toward a More Balanced View," *Journal of the American Medical Association* 249(3):365-67, January 21, 1983.

Lucke, W.C., and Thomas, H. "Anaphylaxis: Pathophysiology, Clinical Presentations and Treatment," *Journal of Emergency Medicine* 1:83-95, 1983.

Peterson, F.Y. "Assessing Peripheral Vascular Disease at the Bedside," *American Journal of Nursing* 83(11):1549-51, November 1983.

Prough, D.S., et al. "Recent Advances in Critical Care Pharmacology, Part III: Treatment of Shock," *Hospital Formulary* 20(1):40-48, January 1985.

Rice, V. "Shock Management, Part I: Fluid Volume Replacement," *Critical Care Nurse* 4(6):69-82, November/December 1984.

Rice, V. "Shock Management, Part II: Pharmacologic Intervention," *Critical Care Nurse* 5(1):42-57, 1985.

Sheffer, A.L. "Anaphylaxis," *Journal of Allergy and Clinical Immunology* 75:227-33, 1985.

Zimmerman, T.A., and Ruplinger, J. "Thoracoabdominal Aortic Aneurysms: Treatment and Nursing Interventions," *Critical Care Nurse* 3(6):54-63, November/December 1983.

Index

A
Abdominal aortic aneurysm. *See* Thoracic/abdominal aortic aneurysms.
Acid-base balance, in hypovolemic shock, 35-37
Acidosis, in shock, 3, 6
Adrenergic blockers, 89t
Adult respiratory distress syndrome (ARDS), as complication of hypovolemic shock, 42
Afterload, 43
Aldosterone, role of, in pressure regulation, 75
Ambulatory continuous automatic blood pressure monitor, 85
Anaphylactic shock, 55-63
    allergens and, 55
    assessment, 58-60, 58i
    care plan, 60
    causes, 59
    chemical mediators in, 57
    intervention, 61-63
    nursing diagnoses, 60
    pathophysiology, 56, 56i
    skin changes in, 9
    two-phase response in, 56, 57i
Anaphylactoid reaction, 55
    causes, 59
Anaphylaxis. *See* Anaphylactic shock.
Anastomotic aneurysm, 120
Aneurysmectomy, 118i
Aneurysms. *See also specific types.*
    acquired vs. congenital, 115
    pathophysiology, 113
    sites, 113
Angina, in hypovolemic shock, 27
Angiography, 111-112
Angiotensin I/II, role of, in pressure regulation, 75
Antihypertensives, 88t
Anti-LPS (antiendotoxin) serum, 71
Anxiety, as sign in hypovolemic shock, 26
Aorta, anatomy and physiology of, 114i, 127
Aortic aneurysm. *See* Thoracic/abdominal aortic aneurysms.
Aortic arterial inflammation, 122-124
Aortic arteritis syndromes, 122-124
Aortic disorders, 113-124
Aortic dissection, 120-122
    assessment, 121-122
    DeBakey's classification of, 121i
    intervention, 122
    pathophysiology, 120-121
    signs, 121
Aortic embolism, 124
Aortic trauma, 123
Arterial bleeding, 27
Arterial blood flow, 127
Arterial blood gas analysis, 12, 13, 14t
    in cardiogenic shock, 47
    in hypovolemic shock, 27
Arterial occlusion, peripheral. *See* Peripheral arterial occlusion.
Arterial oxygen content, 20-21
Arterial trauma, 138-139, 138i
Arteries, anatomy and physiology of, 125, 125i, 126i, 127
Arteriography, 111
Arterioles, 127
Arteriovenous fistula, 155-156
Arteriovenous oxygen difference, 20
    in cardiogenic shock, 48
Artificial blood, 37
Atherosclerosis
    as cause of chronic peripheral arterial occlusion, 127-128
    progression of, 128i
Autonomic hyperreflexia, 66
Autotransfusion, 35

B
Bacterial aortic arteritis, 122-123
Balloon tamponade, 119i
Baroreceptors, 74-75
Basophil, 55
Behavior modification, in hypertensive therapy, 86-87
Beta blockers, 87, 89-90
Bigeminal pulse, 103t
Blood chemistry findings, 13t
    in hypovolemic shock, 28
Blood clotting, altered, in shock, 6
Blood groups, 32t
Blood pressure. *See also* Hemodynamic monitoring *and* Hypertension.
    accurate measurement of, 80, 81i, 82
    alternate measurement methods, 7
    in cardiogenic shock, 46
    classification of, 73t
    monitors, automatic, 84
    pediatric, 93i
    in pregnancy, 92i
    regulating mechanism, 73-76
    in shock, 9, 11t
Blood products, 32t
    administration of, 40-41
Blood volume
    in pregnancy, 92i
    as pressure-regulating mechanism, 73
Body fluid(s)
    distinguishing types of, 22i
    loss, causes of, 22
Bruit, 105
Buerger's disease, 136
Bypass grafts, 133-135, 134i

C
Capillaries, 127
Capillary fluid shift, as compensatory mechanism, 76
Capillary refill, in shock, 9
Captopril, 88t
Cardiac failure, in shock, 6
Cardiac index, 20, 43
    in cardiogenic shock, 44
Cardiac output, 19-20, 43
    distribution, normal, 6t
    in shock, 3, 5-6, 9
Cardiogenic shock, 43-54
    assessment, 45-48
    care plan, 49
    classification, 50
    complications, 45
    hemodynamic parameters in, 20, 47-48
    intervention, 50-54
    nursing diagnoses, 49-50
    pathophysiology, 44-45
    PCWP in, 19, 48
    predisposing conditions, 43
    warning signs, 48
Carotid artery stenosis, 106i, 139
    OPG tracings in, 109i
Carotid audiofrequency analysis, 109
Carotid phonoangiography, 109
Cell
    in shock, 3, 5
    structure and function of, 4i
Central nervous system (CNS) ischemic response, as compensatory mechanism in hypovolemic shock, 24
Central venous pressure (CVP) monitoring, 16-17, 17i
Cerebral ischemia, in shock, 6
Chemical compensation, in shock, 3, 5
Chemical mediators, in anaphylactic shock, 57
Chemoreceptors, 75
Chest X-ray, in hypovolemic shock, 28
Clot formation, as local response to hemorrhage, 25i
Coarctation of the aorta, as cause of hypertension, 78t
Colloids, 33, 34t, 35
Compensatory mechanisms, in hypovolemic shock, 23-24
Compression stockings, 153-154
Continuous automatic blood pressure monitor, 84-85
Contractility, 43
Corticosteroids, 38, 62
Cross matching, 32t
Crystalloids, 33, 34t, 35
Cyanosis, in shock, 9, 27

D
DeBakey's classification of aortic dissection, 121i
Decompensatory responses, in hypovolemic shock, 24-25
Deep-vein thrombosis, 143-150
    assessment, 144-148
    care plan, 149
    intervention, 148-150
    nursing diagnoses, 148
    Virchow's triad and, 143-144
Dehydration, as causative factor in hypovolemic shock, 26
Dextran, as volume expander, 34t
Diagnostic studies
    in anaphylactic shock, 59-60
    in cardiogenic shock, 47-48
    in deep-vein thrombosis, 145-148
    in hypertension, 84
    in hypovolemic shock, 27-28
    in peripheral vascular disease, 107-112
    in septic shock, 69-70
Digitalis, 38, 53, 71
Digital subtraction angiography (DSA), 112
Dissecting aneurysm, 115i. *See also* Aortic dissection.
Dissecting hematoma. *See* Aortic dissection.
Disseminated intravascular coagulation (DIC), as complication of hypovolemic shock, 42
Distributive shock, 55-72
Diuretics, 52, 88-89t, 89-90
Dobutamine, 38, 51-52, 71
Doppler ultrasonography, 107, 108i, 146-147
Duplex scan, 107

i refers to an illustration; t to a table

Index

E
Edema, 101-102, 102t
    causes, 145
Efficiency of tissue oxygen extraction (ETOE), 28
Embolex, 150
Embolism, aortic, 124
Endarterectomy, closed vs. open, 135i
Epinephrine, 38, 61, 62
    as hormonal regulator, 75
Episodic digital ischemia, 135-136
Exercise, in hypertensive therapy, 86
Exercise (treadmill) test, 110-111
External counterpulsation device, 53
Extracellular fluid, 20i

F
False aneurysm, 115i
Fluid loss
    causes, 22
    replacement guidelines, 52
Fogarty balloon catheter embolectomy, 135i
Funduscopic examination, in grading hypertensive retinopathy, 82, 83i
Fusiform aneurysm, 115i

G
Giant cell arteritis, 123-124
Glucocorticoids, 38
Guanethidine, 136

H
Heart sounds, in cardiogenic shock, 46-47
Hematocrit values, in hypovolemic shock, 27
Hematologic test findings, 14t
    in hypovolemic shock, 27
Hemodynamic monitoring
    invasive, 15-21
        in cardiogenic shock, 47-48
        central venous, 16-17, 17i
        in hypovolemic shock, 28
        intraarterial, 15-16, 15i
        intracardiac, 17-19, 18i
    noninvasive, 16
Hemoglobin values, in hypovolemic shock, 27
Hemorrhage
    classification of, 24t
    local responses to, 25i
    pressure points to control, 30i
Hetastarch, as volume expander, 34t
Histamine, 57
Hormonal reactions, in shock, 5, 10, 24
Hypercoagulability, 143-144
Hyperdynamic vs. hypodynamic septic shock, 68, 69t
Hypertension, 73-97
    assessment, 79-80, 82-84
    care plan, 85
    in children, 93i
    complications, 94-97
    criteria for, 73, 73t
    follow-up criteria, 82t
    intervention, 85-91, 93-94
    isolated systolic, 94
    malignant, 95

Hypertension—(cont'd)
    patient compliance with therapy for, 90-91, 93-94
    pregnancy-induced, 92i
    pressure-regulating mechanisms and, 73-76
    primary, 77
    risk factors, 76-77
    secondary, 77, 78t
    signs, 79
    vascular injury in, 77i
Hypertensive crisis, 95-97
Hypertensive encephalopathy, 95-97
Hypotension, as sign in hypovolemic shock, 26
Hypothermia, in shock, 9
Hypovolemic shock, 22-42
    assessment, 25-28
    care plan, 29
    compensatory mechanisms in, 23-24
    complications, 40-42
    decompensatory responses in, 24-25
    dehydration as causative factor in, 26
    diagnostic studies in, 27-28
    fluid loss in, 22, 26
    hemodynamic parameters in, 20
    intervention, 30-31, 33, 35-40
    nursing diagnoses, 29
    patient positioning in, 33
    PCWP in, 19
    progression of, 22-25
    signs, 26-27
    skin changes in, 9

I
Ice-water immersion test, 136
Impedance plethysmography, 108, 145-146, 146i
Infected (mycotic) aneurysm, 120
Inotropic agents, in hypovolemic shock, 37
Intermittent claudication, 100
Intraaortic balloon pump, 53, 53i
Intraarterial pressure monitoring, 15-16, 15i
Intracellular fluid, 22i
Intradermal testing, 59
Iodine-125–fibrinogen uptake test, 112, 147-148
Ischemic rest pain, 100-101
Ischemic ulcers, 103-104
Isolated systolic hypertension, 94

K
Kartchner-McRae test, 109

L
Laboratory studies, in shock, 12-14, 13t, 14t
Lactic acid test, serum, 13-14
Left ventricular stroke work, 20
Leg swelling, chronic, differentiating causes of, 101, 102t
Leg ulcers, as complication of peripheral vascular disease, 103-104, 104t
Level of consciousness, in shock, 11t, 12
Lipedema, 102
Lymphatic system, 153i
Lymphedema, 101, 153i

M
Malignant hypertension, 95
Manual compression test, for venous valve competence, 152i
Mast cell, 55
MAST suit, 36i
Mean arterial pressure (MAP), 16
    vascular resistance and, 74i
Mural thrombus, development of, 124i

N
Neurogenic shock, 63-66
    assessment, 64-65
    care plan, 65
    complications, 66
    hemodynamic parameters in, 20
    intervention, 65-66
    nursing diagnoses, 65
    pathophysiology, 63
    PCWP in, 19
    predisposing conditions, 63
Neurotrophic ulcers, 104
Nitroglycerin, 37-38, 52, 71, 96, 97
Nitroprusside, 37, 38, 52, 71
Norepinephrine, 38, 51, 62, 71
    as hormonal regulator, 75

O
Obstructive shock, 72
Ocular pneumoplethysmography (OPG), 109-110, 109i
Oliguria, in hypovolemic shock, 27, 38-39
OPG-Gee Test, 109-110
Orthostatic vital signs, in hypovolemic shock, 28

P
Packed red blood cells, 32t
Pain, in peripheral vascular disease, 100-101
Patch test, 60
Patient compliance, with hypertension treatment, 90-91, 93-94
Patient evaluation
    for hypertension, 79-80, 82-84
    for peripheral vascular disease, 98-112
    for shock, 3-21
Patient positioning, in hypovolemic shock, 33
Pediatric blood pressure, 93i
Pentoxifylline, 133
Percutaneous transluminal angioplasty (PTA), 133, 133i
Periorbital ultrasound examination, 108i
Peripheral arterial disorders, 125-139. See also specific disorders.
    assessment findings in, 107
    signs, 105
Peripheral arterial occlusion
    acute, 99, 130-131
    chronic, 127-135
        assessment, 128-131
        atherosclerosis as cause of, 127-128
        care plan, 132
        contributing factors, 129
        intervention, 132-135

i refers to an illustration; t to a table

Index

Peripheral arterial occlusion—*(cont'd)*
    pain in, 100-101
    patient guidelines in, 132
    risk factors, 128-129
    signs, 129-130
    sites, 128i
Peripheral pulse changes, 102
Peripheral vascular disease, 98-156
    diagnostic studies for, 107-112
    patient evaluation, 98-112
    symptoms, 100-104
Peripheral venous disorders, 140-156
    assessment findings in, 107
    signs, 105
Photoelectric plethysmography, 108
Plasma, 32t
Plasma protein fraction, as volume expander, 34t
Platelet aggregation, as local response to hemorrhage, 25i
Platelets, 32t
Plethysmography, 107-110
Postphlebitic syndrome, 155
Potassium intake, increased, blood pressure reduction and, 86
Pregnancy-induced hypertension, 92i
Preload, 43
Pressure points, to control bleeding, 30i
Prostaglandins, role of, in pressure regulation, 75
Pulmonary artery pressures (PAP), 17-18, 18i
Pulmonary capillary wedge pressure (PCWP), 18-19
Pulsating hematoma, 115i
Pulse
    changes
        in hypovolemic shock, 26
        peripheral, 102
        in shock, 9-10, 11t
        characteristics, 103t
Pulse points, palpation of, 105-106i
Pulse volume measurements, 110, 111i
Pulsus alternans, 103t
Pulsus bisferiens, 103t
Pulsus paradoxus, 103t

R

Radionuclide angiography, 112
Radionuclide phlebography, 112
Radionuclide studies, 112
Raynaud's phenomenon. *See* Raynaud's syndrome.
Raynaud's syndrome, 135-136
Renal failure, as complication of hypovolemic shock, 42
Renin-angiotensin-aldosterone feedback system, 75, 76i
    in pregnancy, 92i
Renin, role of, in pressure regulation, 75
Renovascular hypertension, as cause of secondary hypertension, 78t
Respirations
    in cardiogenic shock, 47
    in shock, 11t, 12
Retrograde filling test, 152i
Rh typing, 32t
Right ventricular pressures, 17

S

Saccular aneurysm, 115i
Saccular dilation, 119
Sclerotherapy, for varicose veins, 154

Scratch test, 59-60
Segmental limb pressure (SLP), 110, 110i
Septic shock, 66-72
    assessment, 69-70
    care plan, 70
    causative organisms, 67-68
    complications, 71
    hemodynamic parameters in, 20
    hyperdynamic vs. hypodynamic, 68, 69t
    intervention, 70-71
    nursing diagnoses, 70
    pathophysiology, 67-68
    PCWP in, 19
    prevention, 70
    risk factors, 66-67
    skin changes in, 9
    temperature in, 9
    ulcers in, 12
    urine output in, 11
Shock, 3-72
    cardiogenic, 43-54
    cell in, 3, 5
    distributive, 55-72
    hypovolemic, 22-42
    pathophysiologic dynamics of, 3-6
    patient evaluation, 3-21
    risk factors, 7
    signs, 8-9, 10-12
    stages of, 4-6, 11t
Smoking
    as cause of thromboangiitis obliterans (Buerger's disease), 136
    as risk factor in peripheral arterial occlusion, 129, 132
Spinal shock, 63, 64-65
Starling's curve, 46i
Stasis ulcers, 104
Stepped-care approach, in hypertensive therapy, 87, 89-90
Straingauge plethysmography, 108
Streptokinase, 149
Stroke index, 20
Stroke volume, 20, 43
Subclavian steal syndrome, 134
Superior vena cava syndrome, 147
Sympathetic response, as compensatory mechanism in hypovolemic shock, 23
Sympathomimetic drugs, 51-52
Systemic vascular resistance, 20

T

Tachycardia
    in hypovolemic shock, 26
    in shock, 9
Tachypnea
    in hypovolemic shock, 26
    in shock, 11t, 12
Takayasu's arteritis, 123
Thermodilution technique, in cardiac output determination, 19-20
Third space shifting, 7, 22
Thirst, extreme, in hypovolemic shock, 27
Thoracic/abdominal aortic aneurysms
    assessment, 116-117
    care plan, 117
    complications, 119-120
    diagnostic studies for, 116-117
    intervention, 118-119, 118i
    nursing diagnoses, 117
    signs, 116

Thoracic outlet syndrome, 136-138, 137i
Thromboangiitis obliterans, 136
Thrombophlebitis, superficial venous, 143
Thrombus scintigraphy, 112
Tilt test, for hypovolemic shock, 28
Toxemia of pregnancy. *See* Pregnancy-induced hypertension.
Toxic shock syndrome, 68
Transfusion reactions, 40-42
Traumatic aneurysm, 119
Trendelenburg's test, 152i
True aneurysm, 115i
    traumatic, 119

U

Ulcers, arterial vs. venous, 154-155
Urine output, decreased, in shock, 10-11, 11t, 47
Urine test findings, 14t
    in hypovolemic shock, 28
Urokinase, 149
Use testing, 60

V

Varicose veins, 150-154
    assessment, 151-152, 152i
    intervention, 152-154
    pain in, 101
    pathophysiology, 151
    primary vs. secondary, 150-151
Vascular injury, in hypertension, 77i
Vascular resistance, as pressure-regulating mechanism, 74, 74i
Vascular stress-relaxation, as pressure regulator, 76
Vascular system, 98i
Vasodilators, 37-38, 52-53, 88t
Vasopressors, 71
Vein ligation and stripping, 154, 154i
Vein structure and function, 141i
Venography, 111-112, 147
Venous bleeding, 27
Venous capacitance, 145
Venous disease, pain in, 101
Venous oxygen content, 20-21
Venous return, compromised, in shock, 3, 6, 9
Venous stasis, 143
Venous system, 140-143, 142i
Venous thrombosis, 101
Venous thrombus, formation of, 144i
Venous valve, incompetent, 151i
    assessment of, 152i
Venous wall injury, 143
Ventricular assist device, 53, 54i
Ventricular function curve, 46i
Vessel spasm, as local response to hemorrhage, 25i
Virchow's triad, 143-144
Volume displacement plethysmography, 107
Volume expanders, 33, 34t, 35, 50-51

W

Water-hammer pulse, 103t
Weight reduction therapy, in hypertension, 85-86
White blood cell count, in hypovolemic shock, 28

i refers to an illustration; t to a table